HEALING THE NATION

HEALING THE NATION

Prisoners of War, Medicine and Nationalism in Turkey, 1914–1939

✦ ✦ ✦

YÜCEL YANIKDAĞ

EDINBURGH
University Press

© Yücel Yanıkdağ, 2013, 2014

First published in hardback in 2013

This paperback edition 2014

Edinburgh University Press Ltd
The Tun – Holyrood Road
12(2f) Jackson's Entry
Edinburgh EH8 8PJ
www.euppublishing.com

Typeset in JaghbUni Regular by
Servis Filmsetting Ltd, Stockport, Cheshire

A CIP record for this book is available from the British Library

ISBN 978 0 7486 9589 8 (paperback)
ISBN 978 0 7486 6579 2 (webready PDF)
ISBN 978 0 7486 6580 8 (epub)

The right of Yücel Yanıkdağ to be identifiedasauthorofthisworkhasbeenasserted in accordance with the Copyright, Designs and Patents Act 1988, and the Copyright and Related Rights Regulations 2003 (SI No. 2498).

Published with the support of the Edinburgh University Scholarly Publishing Initiatives Fund.

Copyright acknowledgements

Part of the below article has been reprinted by permission of the publisher (Taylor & Francis Ltd, http://www.tandf.co.uk/journals):
Yücel Yanıkdağ, 'Educating the Peasants: The Ottoman Army and the Enlisted Men in Uniform', *Middle Eastern Studies* 40 (2004), pp. 92–108.

CONTENTS

Acknowledgements	vii
Author's note on usage	ix
List of maps and figures	x
List of tables	xi
INTRODUCTION	1
1. THE OTTOMAN GREAT WAR AND CAPTIVITY IN RUSSIA AND EGYPT	14
2. IMAGINING COMMUNITY AND IDENTITY IN RUSSIA AND EGYPT: A COMPARISON	46
3. SAVIOUR SONS OF THE NATION: INSIDE THE PRISONERS' MINDS	77
4. PRISONERS AS DISEASE CARRIERS: CASES OF PELLAGRA AND TRACHOMA	119
5. WAR NEUROSES AND PRISONERS OF WAR: WARTIME NERVOUS BREAKDOWN AND THE POLITICS OF MEDICAL INTERPRETATION	171
6. DEGENERATIONIST PATHWAY TO EUGENICS: NEUROPSYCHIATRY, SOCIAL PATHOLOGY AND ANXIETIES OVER NATIONAL HEALTH	208

EPILOGUE: THE SEARCH FOR A USEABLE PAST:
PRISONERS OF WAR, THE
OTTOMAN GREAT WAR AND TURKISH NATIONALISM   249

Bibliography   274
Index   295

ACKNOWLEDGEMENTS

I am happy to be finally able to acknowledge and thank all of the people and institutions who have helped me with this project, beyond and before.

Carter V. Findley and Jane Hathaway have been involved in this lengthy undertaking since its earliest days. I thank them for training and helping me when I was at the Ohio State University, and their continued support, inspiration and motivation since then.

Most recently, I have benefited from the financial support of the US Department of Education's Fulbright-Hays Faculty Fellowship and the University of Richmond (Faculty Research Committee). These and other grants and fellowships allowed me to travel to a number of archives and libraries in Turkey and in the UK: the Ottoman Archives of the Turkish Prime Ministry in Istanbul; the Archives of the Turkish General Staff (ATASE), Ankara; the Public Record Office and Imperial War Museum in London; Atatürk Kitaplığı; Beyazıt Kütüphanesi; Erzurum Atatürk Üniversitesi Kütüphanesi; Milli Kütüphane; İslam Araştırmaları Merkezi (İSAM) Library; IRCICA Library; Boğaziçi University Library. ILL of the University of Richmond's Boatwright Library tirelessly helped me locate numerous books and articles. I also thank my colleagues in the Department of History at the University of Richmond, especially David Brandenberger, who helped me with the cover image. Kim Klinker, director of the University of Richmond's Spatial Analysis Lab, and her students kindly produced the maps for the book.

Mustafa Aksakal, Mehmet Beşikçi, Walid Hamarneh, Erol Köroğlu, Hakan Özoğlu and Sanem Güvenç Salgırlı read individual chapters or more and offered useful detailed criticism. Alan Briceland and Jennifer Fronc read the manuscript at its final stage and offered invaluable criticism and much-needed editorial assistance. Many others offered useful assistance by helping me obtain research material, or offered constructive criticism or encouragement throughout this project: Cemil Aydın, Carl Boyd, John Curry, Boğaç Ergene, Sue Gartner, Nuray Grove, M. Şükrü Hanioğlu, John Herman, Hasan Kayalı, Vangelis Kechriotis, A. Fikret Kirişçioğlu and Martha Rollins. In Istanbul, friends and family helped me obtain books, articles and images while I was in the US, and graciously put up with and hosted me when I was there. My brothers Fatih, Yavuz and Selim and my niece Sümeyye were kind enough to put up with my long-distance requests to photocopy research material located in Istanbul. M. Kudret Kirişçioğlu helped me locate books and assisted with the more than occasional illegible words or passages in Ottoman. I also thank the History Department and the Atatürk Institute for Modern Turkish History at Boğaziçi University for inviting me to share the result of my research at their beautiful campus.

Several people are not with us any longer to see the final product which their help, encouragement and prodding finally brought to fruition: Craig Cameron, David G. Gartner, Patrick Rollins and my father Kadir Yanıkdağ. They are all deeply missed. Craig and Patrick were instrumental as I completed my undergraduate and master's degrees. David G. Gartner made that education possible with his financial support and continued encouragement.

Finally, I am painfully aware that this endeavour has at times been a less than joyous experience for my family – both immediate and extended. I thank my mother Mihri and my aunt Emine for their encouragement. Above all, I am most grateful to my wife Sheryl for her loving support and encouragement. She tolerated my long absences while I was away or even 'at home'. She read over and provided invaluable feedback on the manuscript many times at various stages.

AUTHOR'S NOTE ON USAGE

Scholars and students of Turkish history know that the name Mehmet is sometimes spelt as Mehmed. One of the psychiatrists the reader will encounter in this book wrote his name as both Fahreddin and Fahrettin. The rendering of Ottoman and Turkish names reflects modern Turkish usage, except in cases of direct quotations. Until the summer of 1934, citizens of Turkey did not have last names. At that point, a law was passed requiring the citizens to adopt surnames. For example, Mazhar Osman, another psychiatrist encountered in this book, took on the last name of Uzman or 'specialist'. However, anything he published before 1934/1935 carries only the name Mazhar Osman. In order to avoid confusion in the notes and bibliography, surnames have been placed in brackets.

Similarly, for Ottoman dates, whether expressed in lunar Hijri or the solar Rumi calendars, Gregorian equivalents have been included.

MAPS AND FIGURES

MAPS

1	Select prison camp locations in Egypt	xii
2	Select prison camp locations in Russia	xiii

FIGURES

1.1	Prisoner activities in Egypt	32
1.2	Alexandria – Sidi Bishr [Camp] football team, 1919	33
1.3	Captured Turkish cavalry patrol	35
1.4	Prisoner Lieutenant Mehmet Hüseyinoğlu	36
3.1	Prison camp diploma	92
3.2	Prisoner imagining reception by the 'War Rich'	97
4.1	Pellagra map: 'endemicity return'	125
4.2	Pellagra victim, post mortem	129
4.3	Pellagra victim: skin marks on hands and face	129
4.4	Prisoner of war camp, Kaukab [Iraq]	130
4.5	Prisoners of war being disinfected	143

TABLES

1.1	Ottoman war casualties in World War I	19
1.2	Ottoman prisoners of war in World War I	20
4.1	Ottoman pellagra hospital admissions and deaths	123
4.2	Morbid conditions present in autopsied POWs	131
4.3	Pre-capture and prison camp diets compared	132
4.4	European and non-European POW rations in Egypt	134
4.5	Further comparison of rations: nutritional values	135
4.6	Study of trachoma patients repatriated in August 1919	146
6.1	Distribution of 1,320 mental degenerates	216

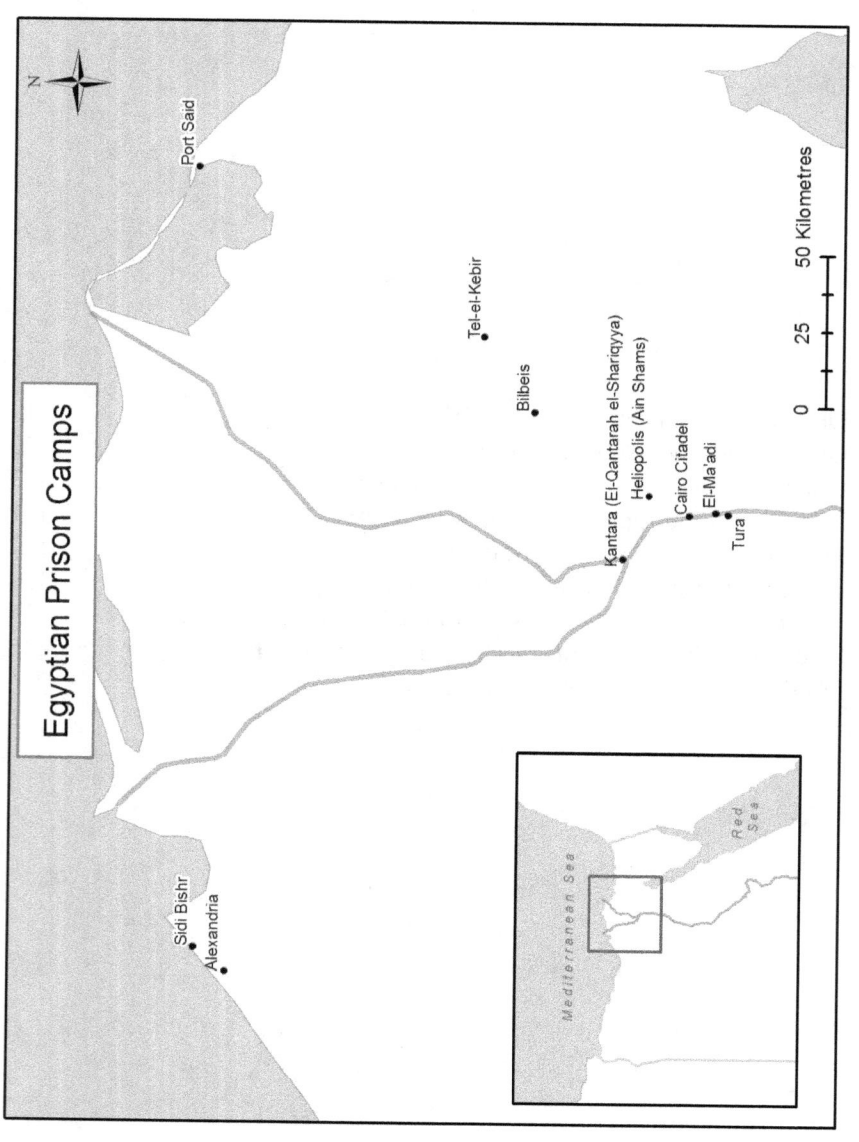

Map 1 Select prison camp locations in Egypt

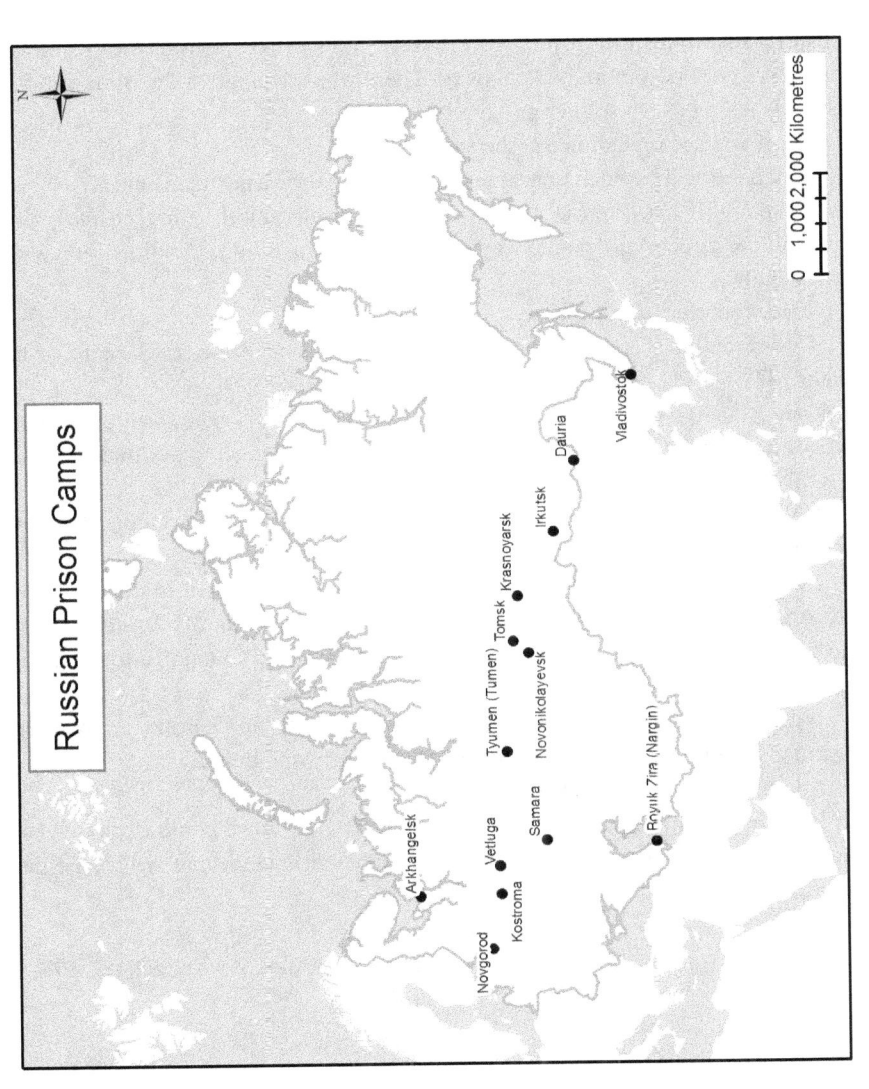

Map 2 Select prison camp locations in Russia

We are now returning only our own selves and our regrets to this Mother (Anatolia-*Anadolu*, 'full of mothers') whose hundreds of thousands of sons we ripped from her bosom and taken away. There was a woman at the train station. She kept asking every soldier passing by:

–'Did you see my Ahmed?' she says.

Which Ahmed? Which one of the hundreds of thousands of Ahmeds?

As she pulls her arm out under her ragged printed-cloth attire (*basma*), she points in the direction opposite way to the train is travelling; the direction away from Istanbul.

–'He went that way', she says.

That direction? To Aden, to Medina, to the Canal Zone, to Sarıkamış, to Baghdad?

Was her Ahmed eaten up by ice, by sand, by water, scurvy sore, or typhus lice? Even if he escaped them all, if you see her Ahmed, you need to ask him too:

–'Did you see my Ahmed?'

No! None of us saw your Ahmed. But your Ahmed saw everything. He saw the hell Allah could not describe even to [Prophet] Muhammad.

Now winds from the West, from the East, from the right, from the left blow into Anatolia whistling together 'rout'. [Mothers and fathers of] Anatolia came and squatted down by railways, paved roads, khans, and fountains, looking for their sons.

Wagons, cars, trucks and all, as if ashamed of it, from Anatolia, are rushing towards Istanbul with curtains pulled down, secretly and quickly.

Anatolia asks of her Ahmed . . .

If we could only tell them how we wasted Ahmed; if we could explain what we won with him to a mother; if we could give some news that will make her proud . . . But we lost Ahmed in a gamble!

Falih Rıfkı Atay, *Zeytindağı*, pp. 108–9

INTRODUCTION

It was almost noon on 25 June 1922, when a ship named *Ümit* (*Hope*) slowly pulled up to the Zeytinburnu port in Istanbul. It was carrying hundreds of Ottoman-Turkish passengers – released prisoners of war – whose long and strange trip had started in a carrier with a Japanese flag from Vladivostok, Russia's major port on the Sea of Japan. The passengers were Ottoman prisoners of war being repatriated after spending years in captivity in Siberia. Everyone was on deck. Those who hailed from the city or had deployed from there were seeing the capital of the Ottoman Empire, or what remained of it, for the first time since their deployment. In 1914, when the Ottomans entered the Great War, Istanbul was bustling with Ottoman soldiers on their way to the scattered fronts where they would be expected to fight for the empire. Now, eight years later, the city to which they returned was under allied occupation, and had been since the end of the war in November 1918. The city was still crowded with soldiers, but this time the soldiers were from the occupation forces.

The newly released prisoners of war on board the *Ümit* expected to be greeted by throngs of citizens, gathered to welcome their repatriation to Turkey. However, the passengers would be disappointed. With the exception of a few locals gathered at the port, the returning soldiers were met by the soldiers of the occupation forces. By late afternoon, the passengers had still not been permitted to disembark the ship. Finally, four officers – two Ottoman and two from the occupation forces – boarded the ship. After a 'general walk around the ship', one of the Ottoman officers turned to the prisoners and announced that those who lived in or had relatives in Istanbul could disembark in Zeytinburnu, provided that they could give a street address.

Among the prisoners on the ship was a certain Lieutenant Halil, who had been captured by Russians on the eastern Anatolian front early in the war. A representative prisoner who wrote a detailed memoir about his captivity and repatriation, Halil did not live in Istanbul, nor could he provide the address of a 'relative', as the authorities demanded. Thus, those who remained on board the *Ümit*, including Halil, were taken to the nearby Selimiye barracks on the Anatolian shore of the city. Hopeful of finding a comfortable bed at the barracks, Halil and his friends experienced more disappointment. After serving their nation and suffering as prisoners of war abroad, they were met with similar conditions at home. The hallways of the barracks were crowded with lice-infested refugees who had fled the war in western Anatolia after the Greeks invaded in mid-1919. Halil and the other former prisoners of war opted to spend the night outside. That night, his compatriots talked, mentioning a coffeehouse in the Beyazıt district frequented by former prisoners of war. The next day, Halil embarked on a shorter journey to the European side of the city to find Eyüp Ağa's coffeehouse. Once there, he quickly assessed the place and observed that 'those who came in were all from our category, repatriated prisoners of war'.[1]

Halil was typical of the repatriated former prisoners who did not get the reception they expected. Mehmet Arif, another lieutenant who had been a prisoner in Russia, escaped in the summer of 1918. Upon arriving in Istanbul in late 1918, he had to prove to the Ministry of War that he had been a prisoner in Russia. While waiting in line at the Ministry, he heard a fellow prisoner begging the officer in charge to speed up the paper work, pleading 'Brother . . . I just arrived after escaping from captivity. My leave is about to end'. The desk officer answered, 'We did not send you a red wax-sealed invitation. You did not have to come back'. Incensed at the disrespectful response, Mehmet Arif noted that the man was merely a clerk officer, who 'did not fight [and instead] spent his life sitting at a desk. And us; were we supposed to be invited with red-sealing wax to our own country?'[2]

Despite the chilly reception at home, Halil and Mehmet Arif were the 'lucky' ones. They had physically survived both war and captivity, and without major psychological breakdowns. Although the trauma of fighting a bloody war and then becoming a prisoner of war likely stayed with Halil and Arif as unforgettable memories for the rest of their lives, these men were not debilitated by their experiences. However, there were thousands of unknown men who had not been as lucky and suffered from physical and mental ailments as a result of captivity.

Dr Mazhar Osman served as a military psychiatrist during the Great War; by 1928, he was a state doctor in charge of the new Bakırköy mental institution in Istanbul. He briefly and passively reflected on the repatriation of the Ottoman prisoners of war, commenting that 'whether returning from Siberia, Egypt or India, among our prisoner-soldiers, after those afflicted with pellagra and blinded with trachoma, [the number of] those who had dementia praecox were horrifyingly high'.³ ('Dementia praecox' is now understood as a variant of schizophrenia.) Dr Mazhar Osman observed that those patients afflicted with dementia praecox looked like 'the living dead' as they returned to their families. As a psychiatrist, though, he did not have much to say about pellagra, a nutritional deficiency that prisoners in camps in Egypt developed. Nor did he discuss in detail the highly contagious eye disease trachoma, which caused blindness of thousands of prisoners.

These were not the only diseases among the former prisoners of war; dysentery, tuberculosis and malaria, among others, afflicted these men. As a result, the former prisoners of war became disease carriers, quickly contaminating the people with whom they came into contact in Anatolia. For example, the eye disease trachoma posed a particular threat to the civilian population. In the later 1920s, the rates of infection forced the Turkish republic to initiate a 'war against trachoma', which took decades to finally put the disease on the retreat.⁴

Unlike the contagious physical diseases, the schizophrenic 'living dead' (and those with other real and presumed mental diseases) constituted a different threat to the new Turkish republic and the nation. Although contemporary medical professionals contended that little could be done for the men suffering from these 'invisible' wounds, they did urge action on the matter because they believed that mental disorders were hereditary. Therefore, doctors advised that more is done to protect future generations from inheriting these diseases and thus undermining the nation's present and future. The construction of mental illness as both invisible (except to the professional medical gaze) and hereditary granted medical professionals great authority in the project of nation-making during the early republican period.

By focusing on the nexus of war, medicine and nationalism, *Healing the Nation: Prisoners of War, Nationalism and Medicine in Turkey, 1914–1939* examines discourses produced by two closely related but distinct groups.⁵ The first is the Ottoman prisoners of war (POWs) held in Russia and in British prison camps in Egypt.⁶ For a variety of reasons, ranging from diplomatic and political to logistical, a majority of Ottoman prisoners were not released or repatriated from captivity in Egypt and Russia until and up to three to four years after the Great War had ended. From their first days in the camps in late 1914 to until their repatriation in the early 1920s, the men in the prison camps engaged in the process of constructing a national identification.

Rather than focusing on the captors' treatment of prisoners, *Healing the Nation* analyses how prisoners understood concepts like nation, culture and tradition, and how they identified with and performed them in their daily lives in prison. In addition, the execrable conditions in the camp, the treatment prisoners endured in them and the people they encountered all played a role in their concerns about the nation they represented. People can reflect critically on their culture if there are others around to which they can compare their own. These encounters produce critical reflexivity toward those differences and heighten the sense of awareness of the meaning of even every day, banal practices. Prisoner of war camps, then, where these Ottomans encountered the cultures and traditions of their captors and those of fellow European prisoners, provided prisoners with both the time for reflection on these concepts, and an unusual 'exile' environment where nationalising became a possibility.[7] Furthermore, the fact that Ottoman prisoners of war were held in camps in Russia and Egypt provides for the examination of these important issues in a comparative light, which allows one to highlight the differences in construction and maintenance of identity resulting from dissimilar experiences of captivity.

The second group on whom this study focuses is the Ottoman-Turkish military neurologists and psychiatrists (hereafter neuro-psychiatrists) who examined and diagnosed prisoners upon repatriation. While these mental specialists were not present in the prison camps, they had actually seen some of these men in 1914, when they conducted initial, cursory examinations of recruits after mobilisation was declared. During and after the war, these neuro-psychiatrists, following the current medical practice in Europe, diagnosed the men who mentally broke down on the front as 'hysterics' and 'malingerers', and those repatriated prisoners as schizophrenics. Rather than being treated as victims of industrialised war, or long years of captivity, these men, especially the 'living dead' prisoners, were perceived by the neuro-psychiatrists as hereditary degenerates or psychopaths, whose experience of war or captivity only served to expose their underlying hereditary condition.[8]

By the end of the nineteenth century in Europe, psychiatry's object of inquiry had already expanded beyond individuals to include populations, nations and even civilisations. In the Ottoman Empire, it took the crucible of the Great War and the physical and demographic destruction that became more visible when the dust finally settled in 1922 for the Ottoman-Turkish neuro-psychiatrists to come to the same view as their European colleagues. For example, during the war, psychiatrists had initially viewed soldiers with mental disorders or trauma as individual degenerates or victims of hereditary failings. But these men soon came to be interpreted as signs of degeneration and threats to the nation – not at the individual level, but at the level of the nation itself. From this new collectivistic and organicist perspective, individual health came to be understood in terms of the needs of the national community. In this way, then, the Great War, with its seemingly endless string of malingerers, deserters, hysterics and schizophrenics, produced the evidence that finally convinced Ottoman neuro-psychiatrists to view individual degenerates as symptoms of a much bigger problem. That problem was the possibility of a national degeneration. By the early 1920s, the neuro-psychiatrists began to view individual degenerates as symptoms of an ailing larger collective, a nation on the verge of biological degeneration. Accordingly, the prisoners are the 'subject' of Chapters 1 to 3 of *Healing the Nation*, but in Chapters 4, 5 and 6 they become 'objects' of discourse and diagnoses in the writings of the neuro-psychiatrists and other doctors.

Healing the Nation takes the Great War as a watershed event to argue that the benchmarks that defined the nation and nationals slowly shifted from 'shared sentiments' to 'biologized' attributes.[9] First, during the war, Turkism, Ottomanism and Islamism coexisted among the prisoners; they were not independent and neatly separable identities. Rather, they converged, overlapped and sometimes clashed. Despite this mosaic of identities, prisoner officers actively policed each others' behaviour in captivity, identifying the absence of 'collective conscience', especially among the 'uncivilized and unhygienic' enlisted men, as pathological and non-national. After 1918, this task fell to the neuro-psychiatrists, who viewed the war's residual psychological and demographic consequences with concern about impending 'national degeneration'. Struggling to address this concern, the neuro-psychiatrists maintained that pre-existing pathological and hereditary conditions, rather than war or captivity, were the causative factors for mental breakdown among the men. Moreover, after the war, they identified one-third of the body politic as suffering from similar forms of degeneration, and as possible contaminators of healthy citizens. Despite the bleak situation, the nation was not 'doomed' to failure or complete degeneration, but capable of being regenerated. They used this argument and their positions as agents of the state, to push for eugenics policies to regenerate the nation in the post-war period.

Healing the Nation examines how the doctors' interpretations of prisoners' health issues led to far-reaching questions about the relationship between the prisoners' physical bodies and mental states, on the one hand, and the body politic and collective mentality of the Turkish republic during the interwar period, on the other. In this way, their diseased or broken bodies and shattered nerves became grounding points of profound social anxieties about the present and future of the nation. Ultimately, *Healing the Nation* demonstrates how wartime and post-war ideas about 'national degeneration' and eugenics among neuro-psychiatrists became instrumental in the creation of a biologisation of national identity without necessarily (ethno)-racialisation during the interwar years. However, this does not mean others did not attempt to racialise national belonging.

Prisoner of war camps provide a unique environment for studying Ottoman and Turkish nationalism. First, captivity brought thousands of Ottomans of differing ethnic, social, economic and educational backgrounds from various parts of the empire together in a foreign (or semi-foreign) land. The experience of war, defeat and captivity, and the 'opportunity' to observe foreigner 'others' prompted those who identified themselves as ethnic Turks to reflect on and articulate the tensions that had always bubbled just below the surface in their multi-ethnic and multi-religious empire. The fact that this empire was now in clear and present danger of survival made all these issues all the more important. Lengthy captivity created conditions and produced mentalities that motivated these Ottoman prisoners to reflect on the problems and develop solutions to the ills of their community, nation and state. Those who engaged in this examination of the empire and the nation were almost exclusively junior officers of the regular army or reserve officers.[10] These men accused their senior officers of not caring enough to participate in such soul-searching.[11] Were it not for the unfortunate experience of captivity, these junior officers likely would not have written down their thoughts and experiences, nor would they have produced camp newspapers and captivity narratives. In this sense, then, their captivity gave them the opportunity to observe and to record on paper a range of voices and opinions about the strengths and deficiencies of the empire, nation, culture and religion.

Thus the prisoners of war produced unique sources that provide an otherwise unavailable glimpse into the lives and minds of those held in camps in Russia and Egypt. The most important of these are the 'prison camp newspapers'. These so-called newspapers were handwritten by the prisoners in the camps under difficult conditions. They range in size from two to twenty pages and in frequency of 'publication'. Contributions from readers were always welcome. For 'distribution', some were copied by hand multiple times, or single copies were passed around from prisoner to prisoner. In the Egyptian camps, some newspapers may have been mimeographed, increasing the number of available copies for the larger number of readers. A few of the newspapers openly stated their aim in the first issue.[12] For instance, *Vaveyla* [*Lament*], in Krasnoyarsk, Siberia, stated that, in addition to serving as a memento of captivity, it 'would be the lamenting organ of the unfortunate prisoners in these remote places'.[13] These newspapers are especially useful as sources because they provide direct access to the thoughts of the prisoners in the editorials and essays they wrote. Although they are individual opinion pieces, they nonetheless represent a collective, rather than individual, commentary.

The second type of sources on which *Healing the Nation* relies, although not as unusual as camp newspapers, have nevertheless been under-utilised. They include the medical books, articles and reports produced by medical professionals, particularly psychiatrists, during the period under study. These medical sources share more with the camp newspapers than is evident at first glance. Neither the camp newspapers nor many of the medical sources were written for 'public' consumption; rather, the former were produced only for those in prison camps and the latter for an audience of doctors who read specialised books and journals. Moreover, these authors did not self-censor – certainly, nowhere near as much as authors of similar sources meant for public consumption. Therefore, these sources provide candid and immediate reflections on the issues with which they are concerned.

This book is as much about nationalism and identity as it is about the prisoners in prison camps and the neuro-psychiatrists who examined them upon their repatriation. Using these unique sources, *Healing the Nation* expands on the scholarship on nationalism by including both ideological and biological factors, and examining how they influenced each other. Medicine, a supposedly 'objective' field of inquiry, shaped the ideological contents of national and cultural identities. Science is not a domain separate from culture or existing outside of history. Consequently, the kinds of scientific questions that emerged in the period under study were motivated by social anxieties about nation, race, gender, sexuality, health and disease.

NATIONALISM

It is necessary to offer a brief conceptual framework of the theories of nationalism that inform this book. First, the book is predicated on the assumption that there is no single 'grand theory' of nationalism that explains much more than the specificity of any particular instance of nationalism. Therefore, we need to examine particular instances of nationalism and identification at particular conjunctures or moments. Theories of Benedict Anderson and Partha Chatterjee are familiar and useful in explaining the origins and development of nationalism, or its anti-colonial form, in 'exilic' environments and in encounters with Westerners – the same kind of situation in which the prisoners found themselves. The prisoners' captivity and environment was a dislocatory event; the neuro-psychiatrists perceived the Great War and its aftermath as a critical juncture when the nation was about to or had entered a state of crisis in the form of a possible national degeneration. For both groups, their experiences brought to the surface the affective and visceral dimensions of identification. *Healing the Nation* accepts the premise that 'nationalism works through people's hearts, nerves, and gut', and 'is an expression of culture through the body'.[14] Readers will recognise the influence of Anderson and Chatterjee in this work, but their theories do not go far enough to explain the affective aspects of identification and nationalism. It is this affective, or emotional, side of nationalism that some scholars argue is what allows the ideology to be sustained by the people. The work of theorist Slavoj Žižek serves to complement the sociological and historical models offered by Anderson and Chatterjee, among others. Žižek's theory of nationalism illuminates the hows and whys of the development and sustaining of identification with nation in the prison camps and in Turkey during the republican years.

While nation and national identity were always on the minds of the self-proclaimed nationalists, they did not think or write about them directly but thought, wrote and acted *with them in mind*. Because of this, they did not write about the nation or nationalism directly. However, they wrote about what threatened, weakened and undermined it, and what could be done to secure it, heal it, masculinise it and strengthen it.[15] Since the existence of 'Others' remains necessary for the definition of the self, nationalism thrives easily in places and during times where and when Others seem more plentiful and always interrupting the fulness and realisation of the nation. That 'threat' to the nation can come from many fronts: the ethnic Other; those who ape foreign behaviour and ideologies; those who lack any ideology (nationalism) or a 'national aim'; the ignorant peasants. Yet, that real or imagined 'threat' can also come from the degenerate or psychopathic Others, who put the nation's future and survival in danger both by their existence and presumed proclivity towards procreation.[16]

Nationalism, according to Žižek, is supported by a fantasy structure that attempts to conceal a constitutive lack that is always present within the ideology. This social fantasy serves national or nationalist ideology by stigmatising an 'Other' – often an ethnic but also domestic Others – as the enemy of, or threatening to, the nation. The fantasy can be expressed in positive terms, stating the nationalist desire, 'if we only had educated peasants and people with a national aim (*gaye*) we would fulfil the nation'. However, it is usually expressed in negative terms, singling out threats and obstacles: 'if only peasants' ignorance and degenerates did not exist, we would fulfil the nation'. Therefore, the presence of the Other threatens the well-being and fulfilment of the nation.[17]

PRISONERS OF WAR, NEURO-PSYCHIATRISTS AND TURKISH NATIONALISM

The nationalism of the Young Turk elites and, later, the leaders of the Independence movement in Anatolia has been the subject of a number of studies.[18] These major works skilfully examine the self-identification and nationalisation of intellectual and political leadership. However, we do not know if those views and identifications were shared by those outside the small, yet influential, ruling minority.

Outside the political and intellectual elite, educated Ottomans served as the link to the common people; this was especially visible in the prison camps. Among the junior officer prisoners, surely some were the sons of pashas or members of the affluent classes. However, of those junior officers who left behind captivity memoirs, most came from relatively humble provincial Anatolian backgrounds – places like Kayseri, Erzurum, Çorum, Tokat, Ürgüp and Niksar.[19] They were literate and could read the works of the intellectuals. At the same time, both on the battlefield and in captivity, they had close and extended contact with enlisted peasant soldiers, whose problems and shortcomings they attempted to diagnose in service to the larger project of nationalism. As such, these men's writings serve to bridge the gap between the political and intellectual elite, whom other scholars have discussed, and the almost completely voiceless peasants. The junior officers did not always understand the peasants, or were not always sympathetic to them, but through direct contact with them, they reported on their encounters and their understanding of peasants' problems. Thus the junior officers' writings permit a closer look at the peasant soldiers. What the junior officers produced is still a representation, but this representation is the result of intimate contact with the peasant soldiers during the experience of war and captivity. Therefore, these representations may be more credible than those produced by the political and intellectual elite, some of whom were ideologically and culturally distinct or cut-off from the majority of the society.[20] In addition, the camp newspapers produced by the prisoner officers occasionally featured or recorded the direct voice of the peasant soldier – even if only fleetingly or after the enlisted men had been educated in prison camp schools.

Just as the officers' voices and concerns serve as a better reflection of society in general than those of the political and intellectual elite because they represent the larger literate segment of Ottoman and early republican society, the worries and concerns of the mental health professionals also allow us to see a different angle of Turkish nationalism in the later 1920s and 1930s. Other scholars have noted that Turkish nationalism took an 'ethno-religious' turn in the later 1920s and early 1930s, breaking away from the cultural nationalism of the earlier period.[21] Neuro-psychiatrists' biologisation of national belonging might have possibly given fodder to those who were interested in achieving this 'ethno-religious' turn. By approaching identification and nationalism from the perspectives of prisoners of war and neuro-psychiatrists, and by using hitherto unexamined sources, *Healing the Nation* reveals a number of levels of internal and external alterities in the construction of the national community. *Healing the Nation* examines two important and neglected sites of nationalism that are significant in their own right, as they reveal the tensions that existed in the larger body politic.

TERMINOLOGY AND SOURCES

Something needs to be said about the diseases, especially mental ones, encountered in this study. From hysteria to neurasthenia, this work treats the disorders as diagnosed by the neuro-psychiatrists as both real and constructed. Therefore, no attempt is made to judge the validity of these diagnoses by today's diagnostic standards. Every attempt is made not to retrospectively diagnose past suffering, even though in some cases the neuro-psychiatrists seem to have done that themselves. In a couple of places this book re-examines the diagnoses of the neuro-psychiatrists – not to question their credibility as men of medicine, but to show how various social and pseudo-scientific ideas came to influence their diagnostic practices.[22]

Furthermore, there was a great deal of confusion and lack of precision in making diagnoses among the neuro-psychiatrists themselves, and they admitted this freely. This was not at all particular to the Ottoman-Turkish men of medicine; the same was true for their European colleagues. As the reader will discover, meanings and interpretations of diseases and pseudo-diseases evolved significantly even within a relatively short period of time. *Healing the Nation* has dealt with such pitfalls and diagnostic confusion accordingly.

STRUCTURE OF THE BOOK

Healing the Nation is structured both thematically and roughly chronologically. Chapter 1 provides a historical background of the Ottoman Great War and comparatively examines the daily experiences of the Ottoman prisoners in Russia and Egypt. The next chapter argues that differences in the way the prisoners experienced captivity in the two disparate locations directly influenced the nature and the process of identification and nationalisation that took place. While Chapter 2 mostly uses the captivity narratives to do this, Chapter 3 heavily relies on those unique prison camp newspapers. Chapter 3 analyses what the prisoners thought were the problems with nation, empire, culture and religion, and what they offered to solve these problems. Chronologically, Chapter 4 starts in the prison camps during the war, but stretches all the way to the later 1930s. It examines two major diseases that killed or blinded thousands of prisoners of war while they were in the camps; the second half of the chapter deals with what the state did to eradicate the eye disease trachoma for which the prisoners were blamed for reintroducing and spreading into Anatolia. Moving from physical to mental disorders, Chapter 5 also starts with war years to study how the neuro-psychiatrists interpreted and diagnosed various mental breakdowns found among both the prisoners and the non-prisoners. Chapter 6, covering the Turkish republican period until 1939, scrutinises the fears of and solutions offered by the neuro-psychiatrists to the problems they believe plagued the veterans, former prisoners and the nation at large. The epilogue considers how individuals and the nationalist state dealt with the problem of remembering and forgetting the traumatic experience of the Great War and captivity. It explores how strategic remembering and forgetting makes and unmakes national histories and how this refashioning of history serves the state in its effort of nation building.

NOTES

1. Halil Ataman, *Esaret Yılları*, pp. 297–8.
2. Mehmet Arif Ölçen, *Vetluga Irmağı*, p. 243. Actual Turkish wording is rather obscene, '*Kırmızı götlü balmumu ile davet etmedik. Gelmeseydiniz*'.
3. Mazhar Osman [Uzman], *Akıl Hastalıkları*, p. 418.
4. Not being contagious, pellagra among the former prisoners either killed them or eventually disappeared as the men began to consume more nutritious food than the camp rations.
5. This book studies Ottoman and Turkish nationalism from 1914 to 1939. Aside from the obvious fact that World War II began in 1939, the year is also important for reasons pertinent to this study. Turkey's declared neutrality in 1939 was seen as a 'eugenic' victory by neuro-psychiatrists. Secondly, the Seventh Turkish National Medical Congress, which was scheduled to meet in October 1938, may have actually met in 1939 due to Mustafa Kemal's illness. One of the most important topics for discussion at this Congress was whether a more thorough eugenics policy should be adopted by the state or not. The 1939 Turkish decision for neutrality in World War II is actually an important marker for the end of this study. As will be clear later in this book, neuro-psychiatrists, having seen the medical and demographic damage caused by World War I, added their voices to others opposed to entering the second war for demographic reasons. The republican state's announcement of its neutrality in late1939, as Europe was engulfed in war once again, was interpreted by the likes of neuro-psychiatrists as a eugenic victory.
6. Although there were Ottoman prisoners in a number of other locations, this work focuses only on these two locations because of the availability of sources.
7. Umut Özkırımlı, Contemporary Debates on Nationalism, p. 81. Özkırımlı's work introduced me to many other nationalism scholars. See Yael Tamir, *Liberal Nationalism*, p. 30. On the subject of exilic environments, see Benedict Anderson, *Imagined Communities*, chapter 4.
8. Ottoman and Turkish doctors used the words *tereddi*, adopted from Arabic, and *dejenere*, a corruption of *dégénéré* to refer to degeneration.
9. The War of Independence is not directly and separately examined in this work mostly because many of the prisoners were still in captivity when that war began, although many others returned in time to join the war effort. Among the neuro-psychiatrists only Nazım Şakir seems to have been fully involved in the War of Independence. The others remained in Istanbul after the end of the Great War even though they clearly supported the nationalist forces.
10. On the reserve officers, see Mehmet Beşikçi, 'İhtiyat Zâbiti'nden 'Yedek Subay'a'.
11. In a society where the overall literacy rate was roughly 5 per cent, the peasant soldiers were illiterate and did not leave behind any written records.

12. Almost exclusively in Egyptian camps, a number of prison camp newspapers existed for the sole purpose of providing news, mostly translations from local or British newspapers. Two such camp newspapers are: *Esaret* (*Captivity*) and *Garnizon* (*Garrison*).
13. 'Mukaddime – Gazetenin mesleği hakkında birkaç söz', *Vaveyla*, 1 (1 Teşrin-i Sani 1331/14 January 1915), p. 1.
14. Gregory Jusdanis, *The Necessary Nation*, p. 31.
15. See Umut Özkırımlı, *Contemporary Debates on Nationalism*, p. 55.
16. In this connection, we should mention Michel Foucault who wrote of anatomo-politics of the human body and biopolitics of the population. The former centred on the 'body's disciplining, the optimization of its capabilities'. The latter, coming later, 'focused on the species of the body, the body imbued with the mechanics of life and serving as the basis of the biological processes'. While anatomo-politics and biopolitics are different from each other at the level of intervention mechanism, they nevertheless support and complete each other. From the nineteenth century on, natality, mortality, hygiene and the prevention of disease, among others, become areas of intervention by the state to 'improve' life. Biology, demography, statistics and epidemiology made it possible to analyse processes of life on the level of populations and to govern both individuals and collectives. From vaccination to hygiene and eugenics, the state was concerned with the body as the site of power as it regulated life. In this work, we encounter both anatomo-politics and biopolitics in the early republican Turkey. M. Foucault, *A History of Sexuality*, vol. I, p. 139.
17. Žižek suggests that 'the element that holds together a given community cannot be reduced to the point of symbolic identification: the bond linking together ... [a community] always implies a shared relationship toward a Thing ... National identification is ... sustained by a relationship toward the Nation qua Thing', or 'Nation as Thing'. This 'Thing' is that unique 'set of properties that make up the specificity of the nation, our particular-universal. The "Thing" is imagined as the producer of our rituals, our ceremonies and practices', which are assumed to possess some unique sensibility. What we fear in the Other is that they might steal our Thing. Imagining of a theft conceals the fact that we never had it in the first place. Žižek augments his theory of nationalism by employing the psychoanalytic concept of 'lack', and experience thereof, as an essential part of the human condition. He argues that a community can never achieve a full or completed identity because of that lack, which produces antagonism within a society. Nationalism, according to Žižek, is supported by a fantasy structure that tries to conceal this constitutive lack by stigmatising or blaming an Other. The presence of the Other always threatens the well-being and fulfilment of the nation. But the nation Thing is never actualised because it cannot be. The paradox is that the 'national Thing' is both threatened by the Other and at the same time utterly inaccessible to him. In this way, the Others – the peasant, the ethnic Other, the 'aimless', the psychopath or the degenerate – both conceal and embody the lack of fulness of a community. Thus, the national Thing has to both cause the subject to try to attain its fulfilment and at the same time be unattainable. The threat from the Other is not really to our identity, but a reminder of our own inner tensions and feelings. These tensions and feelings are projected onto the Others. Alan Finlayson, 'Psychology, Psychoanalysis and Theories of Nationalism', pp. 154–5. Slavoj Žižek, *Tarrying with the Negative*, p. 201; see also his, 'Eastern Europe's Republics of Gilead', pp. 50–62.
18. For an admittedly cursory summary of these, see Chapter 3 of this book.
19. I realise that they had to be comparatively well-off enough to be able to afford education rather than having to work to support their families. Among the prisoners who left

behind memoirs are students or graduates of madrasas, military high schools and even a *Mülkiye* graduate. Although these prisoners mention that while in captivity they met other Ottoman prisoners who had been educated in European universities such as the Sorbonne, none of these seem to have left behind captivity memoirs. It is possible that they wrote in prison camp newspapers, but there is no way to trace this as they did not talk about themselves. One exception to this in both regards is Faik Tonguç, a *Mülkiye* graduate who went to London to 'bolster his education' (*Birinci Dünya Savaş.nda*, p. 15 and inside back cover).

20. Gayatri Spivak makes a distinction between representation and re-presentation. See her, 'Practical Politics of the Open End', pp. 397–404. For subaltern studies and the debate about the agency of the subaltern, see various articles in the journal *Subaltern Studies*; Rosalind O'Hanlon, 'Recovering the Subject: Subaltern Studies and Histories of Resistance in Colonial South Asia', pp. 189–224; Gayatri Chakravorty Spivak, 'Can the Subaltern Speak?', pp. 271–313; Gyan Prakash, 'Subaltern Studies as Postcolonial Criticism', pp. 1475–90; Gyan Prakash, 'Writing Post-Orientalist Histories of the Third World: Perspectives from Indian Historiography', pp. 383–404.
21. For example, Soner Çağaptay, *Islam, Secularism, and Nationalism in Turkey*.
22. See Mark S. Micale and Paul Lerner 'Trauma, Psychiatry and History', p. 24.

CHAPTER

1

THE OTTOMAN GREAT WAR AND CAPTIVITY IN RUSSIA AND EGYPT

Weep oh heart, weep for my state
A curtain of darkness fell over my bright future.
Tuberculosis ruined my youth and existence
Fate wrecked me and made me wretched
At a young age, destiny turned youth's joy into torment
In the end, doctors became my only true friends.

M. Feyyaz Efendi, '*Hatırat*' (unpublished), p. 54[1]

This chapter does two things. The first quarter provides historical background, explaining why the Ottomans entered the Great War, how the war unfolded and how many prisoners were taken by other powers. The remainder of the chapter uses a comparative approach to examine the capture and captivity experiences of Ottoman prisoners in Russia and Egypt. The latter section explores the similarities and differences in the captivity experiences and analyses how they contribute to the project of nationalism. Conclusions reached in that section form the basis of the argument constructed in Chapter 2.

THE OTTOMAN GREAT WAR: HISTORICAL BACKGROUND

In late October of 1914, the Ottoman Empire entered what would soon be known as the Great War on the side of Germany and Austria-Hungary. This new conflict came soon after the disastrous Balkan Wars of 1912–13, in which the Ottomans lost nearly all of their Balkan territories, retaining only parts of Thrace. In the First Balkan War, even the city of Edirne, the former Ottoman capital and only 220 kilometres (135 miles) from Istanbul, was lost to the Bulgarians. The enemy forces made it to within 50 kilometres (30 miles) of Istanbul before an armistice was reached. The Second Balkan War started when the victors quarrelled over the spoils of the first war. Ottomans took advantage of the Bulgarian diversion and retook the city of Edirne in the Second Balkan War.

Overall, the Balkan Wars represented a major defeat for the Ottomans. In his recent work examining the reasons why the Ottomans entered the Great War, Mustafa Aksakal argues that apprehension of dissolution and partition, which drove Ottoman officials to join the war in 1914, derived from the disastrous Balkan Wars of 1912 and 1913. Shared by many beyond the political elite, these apprehensions and insecurities were based on real and perceived threats to the survival of the empire. As individual Ottoman offers of alliance to Entente powers were rebuffed, Ottoman concerns about Entente plans for the Ottoman Empire increased. Consequently, in August 1914, a few Ottoman leaders signed a secret treaty with Germany, marking the beginning of an uneasy relationship between these two allies. Since the treaty was supposedly secret, the Ottoman authorities announced that they would mobilise but remain neutral.[2] As the treaty was signed, Ottoman Minister of War, Enver Pasha, requested that the German battle cruiser *Goeben* to be dispatched to Istanbul. Enver's request was seconded by General Liman von Sanders, the head of the German military mission in the Ottoman Empire. They thought that the *Goeben* would strengthen the Ottoman naval forces against the Russian Black Sea fleet. Soon the *Goeben* arrived, along with the *Breslau*, at the Dardanelles with the British in pursuit. These two ships entered Ottoman naval service, retaining their German crew, but changing their names to *Yavuz* and *Midilli* respectively.

The Russian declaration of war came within three months, soon after 29 October 1914, when an Ottoman squadron of warships – notably the *Yavuz* and the *Midilli* under the command of Admiral Wilhelm Souchon, the German admiral now in Ottoman uniform as part of the German military mission to the Ottoman Empire – sailed into the Black Sea and bombarded several Russian Black Sea ports. Although some of the leadership at the time suggested that Souchon had acted on his own initiative, thereby dragging the Ottoman Empire into war, in reality he had Enver Pasha's written order. The Ottoman leadership, namely the Grand Vizier Said Halim Pasha, had delayed the entry into the war as long as he could by claiming the Ottomans were not yet ready and needed military and financial assistance from the Germans.[3]

Despite nearly three months of mobilisation, the Ottoman Empire, which was not nearly as industrialised as the European powers, entered the war with many shortcomings. A significant amount of recently purchased heavy equipment and weapons had been lost or abandoned during the retreats and surrenders of the Balkan Wars.[4] Therefore, there were shortages of weapons, equipment and ammunition. Upon the signing of the alliance treaty, Germans started to supply the Ottomans with much-needed materials. However, Bulgaria was still neutral at that time and shipping war supplies to the Ottomans by rail through Bulgarian territory depended on its willingness to allow passage. It was only after the Bulgarians finally formed an alliance with the Germans and Ottomans and entered the war on the side of the Central Powers that the Ottomans received significant shipments of weapons and ammunition from Germany.

In addition to the empire's limited industrial capability and shortage of railroads, mobilisation of soldiers was also slow due to changes within the recruitment system. While the military solved the mobilisation problem and, within months, military strength reached over a million men with a combat strength of 820,000, it still encountered logistical problems. In some cases, men who showed up at the recruitment stations could not be fed and were sent home and told to return later. While the number of men mobilised was relatively impressive, there was a significant shortage of officers: only one officer could be assigned to sixty-five men.[5] In order to deal with the shortage of officers, the military command took some shortcuts. Military Academy cadets were immediately assigned to units as brevet lieutenants (*Zabit Vekili*). Senior cadets of the military secondary schools and civilian high school graduates or students were introduced into the military as officer candidates (*Zabit Namzedi*) after brief training.[6] Many of the diaries and memoirs utilised in this study were kept by these *zabit vekilleri* and *namzetleri*.

While probably none of the European belligerents could have predicted that the Great War would become so 'great' and last as long and demand as much as it did, the Ottoman Empire was less prepared for the industrial, economic and logistical demands of such a protracted war than the other belligerents. It did not have nearly enough rail lines and those that existed were incomplete in places; in many places different gauges meant that material being shipped from Istanbul sometimes had to be loaded and unloaded three times before it reached its final destination. Russian control of the Black Sea and British and French blockades ended coastal shipping completely. Of course, this meant that many more men and even more pack animals had to be allocated to sustain the deficient lines of communication.[7] The Entente blockade was also instrumental in starving about 500,000 civilian Ottoman subjects in places like the Syria-Lebanon coastline.[8] According to scholars Mesut Uyar and Edward Erickson, more food and fodder was lost during transfer and storage and to the black markets than was actually consumed by men and military animals.[9] The medical system in place was 'notoriously bad' and 'was instrumental in the loss of 10 to 11 times more men than were lost in combat'. For example, in eastern Anatolia, in the Third Army zone of combat, from late 1915 to late 1918, only 14,000 men were killed in action or because of wounds, but 110,000 men fell prey to epidemics (spotted typhus, dysentery, cholera, etc.), simple diseases and unhealed combat wounds.[10]

The Ottoman Empire was a multi-ethnic, multi-religious empire even to its last days, though with continually shrinking borders and loss of the Balkan provinces, it had become a mostly Muslim empire well before the Great War. Yet, its Muslimness, which stood at 74 per cent in 1906–7, did not mean that it was mostly a Turkish empire. Large numbers of Arabs, Kurds, Circassians and other non-Turkish Muslims represented a significant part of those numbers. Still, more than 20 per cent of the population was non-Muslim.[11] The military also reflected this demographic diversity. We do not have exact numbers, but a report by an Ottoman officer in 1917 gives us some idea of the ethno-religious make up at that time. Hüseyin Hüsnü Emir, reporting on the ethnic composition of infantry divisions, noted 66 per cent as Turkish, 26 per cent as Arab, and 8 per cent as others.[12] Apparently, because this roughly corresponded to the ethno-religious makeup of a group of 7,233 Ottoman prisoners captured by the British in 1917, Hüseyin Hüsnü's estimates have been accepted as an accurate reflection of the Ottoman military's ethnic make-up. In 1917, the British reported the following demographics for the 7,233 prisoners: 64 per cent Turks, 27 per cent Arabs and 9 per cent Greeks, Armenians and Jews.[13] However, the situation is more complicated than that. Two things must be kept in mind. First, Hüseyin Hüsnü probably only reported on infantry divisions, while many more non-Muslims likely served in labour battalions rather than in infantry divisions.[14] Serving in labour battalions is still military service even if Hüseyin Hüsnü was likely more concerned about fighting forces. Second, despite the fact that prisoner of war statistics provided by the British in this case closely corresponded to the estimates of Hüseyin Hüsnü, the 'randomness' of being captured in wartime has to be kept in mind. For instance, at a later date, the British reported significantly different statistics on the Ottoman prisoners of war captured by the Egyptian Expeditionary Forces (EEF). Of the 101,836 total Ottoman prisoners the EEF alone captured 5,703 were officers and 96,133 other ranks. They reported 80.9 per cent of the officers and 77.3 per cent of the men as Turks; Arabs stood at 10.62 per cent of officers and 15.12 per cent of men; Greeks were 1.44 per cent and 2.62 per cent; Jews 0.022 per cent and 0.03 per cent; others 6.85 per cent and 4.6 per cent, respectively.[15] What this means is that we do not really have accurate statistics of the ethno-religious make-up of the Ottoman army in World War I. All we have are some estimates at specific time periods. However, what we know is that whatever the exact ethno-religious makeup, the army was composed of mostly illiterate peasants. Of course, linguistic diversity also created communication problems. Many Arab soldiers, but some of the others as well, did not speak Turkish.

Estimating other statistics in the Ottoman Great War – number of men fielded, casualties and prisoners of war – is also a difficult task, as many of the reported numbers vary significantly from one source to another. Contemporary writers were not very accurate about reporting numbers, but some later writers have also added to the confusion. For example, based on work done at the Military Archives in Ankara, the commonly accepted estimate for the number of soldiers the Ottoman military fielded during the whole length of the war stands at 2,850,000. Edward Erickson, whose important *Ordered to Die* both synthesises the official Turkish military histories and features his own original interpretations, puts the number of mobilised at 2,873,000.[16] This is a difference of 23,000 men; while not an insignificant number, it is still within an acceptable range. What seems to be more exact is the number of men fielded up to July 1915: 1,943,700.[17] So far those numbers correspond and are not a cause of concern. In 1932, Colonel Baki, basing his information on the wartime Ottoman military records being organised into the Military Archive in Ankara, the same one from where the two numbers above were derived, placed the number of men fielded at 3,059,205.[18] This is a difference of 209,205 men, or more than 7 per cent, and certainly represents a significant variation from the other later estimates. While giving us a rough sense of the numbers involved, such a variance also highlights the difficulty of dealing with statistics from this time period; it reminds us that they are merely good estimates.

Similar kinds of problems also plague the statistics relating to Ottoman prisoners of war that this book studies. These men were taken captive in a number of places. Those in Russia were mostly captured on the eastern Anatolian front, after the disastrous Sarıkamış campaign. We do not know exactly how many soldiers died and were captured in Sarıkamış. Out of about 118,000 combat troops on 22 December 1914, only 8,900 remained 'available' after the campaign. Most men did not die in combat, but likely froze to death in the high altitudes due to their inadequate gear.[19] It is likely that some of whom the Ottoman military authorities presumed died were actually taken captive by the Russians. This may partially explain the discrepancy between the significantly lower numbers of prisoners Ottoman officials assumed the Russians took, as opposed to the statistics the Russians reported on captured Ottomans. Smaller number of Ottomans who were captive in Russia also came from another front, a 'foreign' front against the Russians. In 1916, Ottomans had sent the Fifteenth Army Corps, consisting roughly of 33,000 men, to Galicia to help out the Austro-Hungarians.[20] As many as 10,000 Ottomans may have been captured in Galicia by the Russians. Those in British captivity were taken on the Gallipoli, Syria, Palestine, Gaza, Yemen and Mecca-Medina fronts. Ottomans captured in what is now Iraq were usually sent to India or Burma for internment, but large numbers were also interned in Iraq. All of the prisoners were eventually sent

Table 1.1 Ottoman war casualties in World War I[21]

Source[a]	Combat dead	Disease dead	Wounded	POWs	MIA[b]/Lost	Deserters
E. Erickson	243,598	466,759	1,066,903	145,104	61,487	500,000
C. Taşkıran	85,000	240,000	400,000	202,152	n/a	n/a
Colonel Baki	112,473	388,618	n/a	66,391	37,340	n/a
M. Larcher	85,000	240,000	400,000	n/a	n/a	n/a

[a] *Sources:* Edward Erickson, *Ordered to Die*, p. 189; Cemallettin Taşkıran, *Ana Ben Ölmedim*, pp. 47 and 51; Miralay Baki, *Yurt Müdafaası*, p. 132; Maurice Larcher, *La Guerre Turque*, p. 590.
[b] MIA, missing in action.

to Egypt after the war, as part of the British effort to consolidate its places of internment. It was not only those in Russian captivity who were not repatriated until well after the end of the Great War. As of 19 May 1920, the British still held some 32,968 'Turks' in Egypt.[22]

Presumably, scholar Cemalettin Taşkıran, the author of the only other work on the Ottoman-Turkish prisoners of war, based his statistics for Ottoman dead and wounded on Maurice Larcher, the French commandant who wrote in the mid-1920s on the Ottoman participation in the Great War. Upon closer examination, Colonel Baki's statistics seem to more accurately reflect the number of dead, but not the prisoners. Erickson's statistics on the prisoners, taken by some other scholars to represent the total number, actually do not include those Ottomans who returned (on their own) in 1918. Earlier in his work, Erickson gives the 1918 returnees as roughly 9,000, which would bring the total number of prisoners to 154,104.[23] Taşkıran, whose work suffers from citation problems, breaks down the number of Ottoman prisoners according to captors. He notes that the British captured 134,447 Ottomans and the Russians 65,000. France, Romania and Italy captured a total of 2,705 Ottomans, which brings the grand total to 202,152.[24] While his number for other captors are presumably accurate, Taşkıran's statistics for those prisoners in British captivity are notably lower than what the British themselves reported officially in published works.

As mentioned earlier, contemporary sources are not always clear in the numbers they report. For example, within a single official British source, one finds inaccurate terminology: *Statistics of the Military Effort of the British Empire*, a compilation of statistical reports submitted by various wartime units and individuals within them, refers to all Ottomans as 'Turks' on one page, but just a few pages later, separates Greeks, Arabs, Jews and 'Others', from

Table 1.2 Ottoman prisoners of war in World War I

	Ottoman POWs in Russia		Ottoman POWs in British captivity	
	According to Austrian sources[a]	According to Russian sources[b]	According to British sources[c]	According to Austrian sources[a]
Officers	950	n/a	7,751	822
Men	50,000	n/a	142,290	41,700
Total	50,950	64,505	150,041	42,522
Dead	10,000 (20%)	582 (0.09%)	10,738 (7.1%)	4,500 (10.5%)

[a] Hans Weiland and Leopold Kern, *In Feindeshand*, 2d volume, pull-out appendix.
[b] Nicholas Golovine, *The Russian Army*, p. 74.
[c] War Office, *Statistics of the Military Effort*, pp. 630, 634.

'Turks'. The source is still helpful for figuring out rough estimates, but problems do arise. For instance, 'non-Turkish' Ottomans are sometimes thrown into the larger category of 'Others', which included 'men of friendly nationalities such as Poles, Czecho-Slovaks, &c'.[25] In short, when the same work reports that 150,041 'Turks', were 'captured and interned', we can be only partially certain that 'Turks' included all Ottomans. Similarly, one cannot determine clearly whether the total of 150,041 included the 10,738 'Turks' who died in captivity.[26]

Yusuf Akçura, the Ottoman Red Crescent representative in Russia at the end of the war, estimated that there were between 60,000 and 70,000 Ottoman POWs in that country. Accordingly, while Golovin's estimated number of Ottoman dead is clearly too low, his actual number for the captured men might be closer to reality.[27] *Novoe Vremya* newspaper published in Piatigorsk, located in Stavrapol Krai, trans-Caucasian Russia, reported that by 14 February 1915, 49,527 Ottoman (527 officers and 49,000 men) prisoners had passed through the railway station town of Mineralnye Vody of the same district. This was February 1915 and still very early in the war. Presumably, those Ottoman POWs who died after capture in such places as Nargin Island (Böyük Zira) on the Caspian or otherwise on the way to Mineralnye Vody would not have been counted among those who passed through the town. Being conservative and assuming that the Russians captured only 65,000 Ottomans by the end, the total number of men captured by Russia and England comes to just over 214,546. When one includes those prisoners held by the French and Italians, then we arrive at the rough number of 217,251 prisoners. Because of the difficulties outlined above, that number should be regarded as an absolute minimum. Actual numbers might be closer to 250,000.[28]

CAPTIVITY IN RUSSIA AND EGYPT: A COMPARISON

An anonymous folk song from the Çorlu region of Turkey reminds its listeners of the Great War and its prisoners with these words:

> The war has ended. Where are those who were supposed to return home?
> They did not come, the young men; they remain in captivity.
> They have fallen into foreign lands, save them, oh God.
> Some remain in wintry places, some remain in summery places.

This second half of this chapter uses a comparative approach to examine the experiences of Ottoman prisoners in the 'summery places' of Egypt and the 'wintry places' of Russia. This comparative account gives the reader a sense of what the daily lives of the prisoners were like in each locality, in addition to how and why various differences existed. It also lays the foundation for the following chapter, which examines the ramifications of these differences.

Capture, transport and camp life

Ottoman prisoners were captured on the eastern Anatolian 'Russian' front, where the climate was bitter cold during the winter, and on the Syria-Palestine 'British' front, where it was unbearably hot during the summer. Neither was a pleasant situation, but the bitter cold in the mountainous terrain was the greater enemy. Even without the war, surviving 'General Winter', as one prisoner called the numbing cold, would have been a difficult task in itself.[29] To begin with, Ottoman soldiers were improperly clad for the deadly Anatolian winters. Because of ill-planning and a limited industrial mobilisation capacity, Ottomans had to manage with light coats and shoddy, or even missing, footwear. Missing footwear means either that they never really had anything that could withstand the harsh conditions or that what they had simply wore away. Officers regularly reported that their men only had makeshift shoes, fashioned from the hides of animals they had slaughtered for food. Because of the inadequacy of their own uniforms, Ottomans of all ranks regularly appropriated the great coats, boots and clothing of Russians killed in battle.

While plundering Russian clothing provided some warmth and comfort for the Ottoman troops, it also led to a dangerous situation in the event of capture. The captors stripped captives of all items belonging to their own dead, no matter the weather conditions; thus, some men found themselves in extremely dire situations. Witnessing a number of barefooted men marching into captivity in ice and snow, one Ottoman officer observed, 'they were all doomed to die'.[30]

So pathetic were the conditions of the Ottoman soldiers that their plight moved a local Russian woman to tears as she watched them march through town; the woman took off her own shoes and gave them to one of the shoeless soldiers.[31] In other instances, Russian women offered bread to the miserable-looking soldiers or berated the Ottoman officers in charge for their men's condition. Likely, these Russian women were compassionate towards the prisoners because they worried that their husbands or sons might be experiencing similar conditions. If they could not help their sons and husbands, some could certainly offer help to the Ottoman prisoners as surrogates.

The initial shock, and sometimes shame, of captivity pushed some prisoners to resignation, whereas others mentally prepared for life in captivity.[32] Following capture, the prisoners were moved behind the Russian lines to be sent to a staging camp. These were basically temporary camps employed by the Russians. The staging camp served two purposes. First, it served to collect enough prisoners until they could all be loaded on trains to send to permanent camps. Second, although not always openly admitted to, staging camps also served as quarantine camps. The prisoners would be kept there long enough to see if any diseases appeared among them before they were sent to larger camps, where they would be mixed in with others.

Usually intended for transporting animals, overcrowded boxcars (called *teplushki*) served as the main mode of transport to permanent camps, which dotted the Russian landscape from west of the Urals to eastern Siberia. Travelling in boxcars meant for animals, the prisoners were also treated like animals. During winter, when temperatures regularly dropped to –22° Fahrenheit or below, the ride became so dangerous that many prisoners died.[33] Since the boxcar doors were kept locked, the prisoners were compelled to defecate in a corner of the car. They travelled for days in proximity to their own excrement and the dead bodies of their comrades.[34] When the train doors were opened at intervals, the survivors pushed out the dead to be left on the ground. The way they were forced to dump the bodies of their dead comrades, in less than humane ways, certainly made a great impression on them. At least one American diplomat, who was in Russia to observe the conditions of the German and Austro-Hungarian POWs before those countries were at war with the United States, observed that the transport conditions for the Ottoman POWs were much worse than what the Germans and Austro-Hungarians had to endure.[35] Because there was no neutral country looking out for the interests of the Ottoman prisoners, Russians probably figured they could get away with mistreating them.[36] Captive Ottoman doctors and officers in Russia estimated that at least 27 per cent of the Ottoman prisoners died during transport. Hilmi Erbuğ, an officer, remembered that each day four to five prisoners died during transport.[37] The men who managed not to become a statistic during transport knew all too well that death was always near.

The permanent Russians camps in Siberia were only a little less lethal than the boxcars. The Russians had turned long-abandoned factories, partially open to the elements, into permanent camps. Although they were not fit to house humans, they did. Other camps in Siberia, such as garrisons left empty by the mobilised Russian units, were significantly better. In European Russia, the prisoners were sometimes placed in commandeered or possibly 'rented' Russian houses in populated towns. Even in very large camps like Krasnoyarsk, where the prisoners were interned in a Russian garrison, all Central Powers prisoners quickly felt the consequences of overcrowding. As thousands of captured prisoners continued to arrive (mostly Austro-Hungarians), the shortage of beds, mattresses, blankets and firewood became even more acute.[38]

Making things even worse, the winter weather confined the prisoners inside the overcrowded camps for lengthy periods. Each prisoner had only 18 to 21 inches of personal space, which often resulted in tensions among prisoners.[39] The long winter months, combined with such limited personal space, produced a condition known as 'hatred of the near', the feeling of fatigue and morosity that resulted from being in constant close company with the same persons. Psychoanalysts such as Sigmund Freud have observed that every long-lasting relationship between two people contains feelings of aversion and hostility, which only escapes perception as a result of repression. He was referring to long-lasting intimate and emotional relationships, including friendships and marriage.[40] While the relationships developed in prison camps were not voluntary or deeply felt, they involved more than two people at a time and lasted through several years of captivity where the parties involved saw each other around the clock. In such a situation, repression became impossible to maintain. At some point, most prisoners lashed out at their barrack- or room-mates or became sullen, depressed and catatonic.[41]

A poem by an anonymous Ottoman prisoner, written for a camp newspaper in Krasnoyarsk in Siberia, starkly illustrates the painful conditions and the sense of depression he saw all around.

In Captivity (*Esaret'de*)

People [who have become] emaciated and pale-faced
from the wrath of unbearably cold temperatures,
burn from inside out with the desire for freedom
inside these damp and deaf walls.
[They] weep quietly in some dark corner,

> as if sorrow is their eternal love.
> Their hopes freeze in the falling snow.
> Sitting on a rotten bench in some corner,
> a young brave man never lifts his head
> as he sits on dirty and worn-out matting,
> not heeding the winds that make him shiver.[42]

The lines above capture a number of feelings and harsh conditions experienced in the Russian prison camps: cold, lack of food, isolation and dirty camp conditions.

Overcrowding in the Russian camps also fostered the quick spread of contagious disease. Once a contagious disease appeared in the camps or was brought in by infected prisoners, it became impossible to stop its spread since the men in overcrowded camps 'slept always in actual personal contact'. Although other diseases killed numerous prisoners, typhus was the most deadly. By the late summer of 1916, at least 64,000 German, Ottoman and Austro-Hungarian POWs in Russia had already died from disease.[43] Other diseases such as tuberculosis also spread more readily with overcrowding. Whatever the reasons, sources show that Ottomans died at a significantly higher rate than prisoners of other nationalities.[44]

Deadly diseases often claimed their victims in the winter, when the ground was frozen solid, making burial of the dead impossible. The frozen corpses were stacked like firewood next to the prisoners' barracks, waiting for the ground to thaw. These scenes deeply shocked American inspectors, prompting them to exclaim that the 'dead were piled like sticks of wood and carried away to be thrown in a ditch when there is no longer room for more'.[45] Such gruesome scenes drew only passing comments from the prisoners; their descriptions read as if they were just remarking on another sight in the Siberian landscape. Were they really indifferent to the frozen corpses of their dead comrades? Even if they were, which is unlikely, their silence about the death that surrounded them makes an impression. The prisoners may have become numb to such situations, but it did not mean that these frozen and stacked up corpses did not bother them subconsciously. Repression may have been the only choice if they wanted to make it through psychologically. As soldiers, they certainly expected death, but the deaths here were not the result of fighting. The psychic damage was generated by the realisation of how these deaths had occurred and how the bodies were subsequently mistreated. Spring thaw, which softened the ground to make grave digging possible, created another ghastly spectacle. There would be no graves, no markers, only large pits for mass burials of 200–300 dead prisoners at a time.[46] Not wanting to touch the corpses, the Russian guards used the points of their bayonets to roll the bodies like logs into the pits. Such scenes reminded the prisoners of their own mortality, even as they passively watched how the corpses of their comrades were treated.

Cold, hunger, fear and the spectre of death all contributed to the prisoners' sense of helplessness and frustration, but there was another ever present purveyor of misery: lice. Russian captivity narratives, both Ottoman and European, contain myriad references to the men's endless battle with lice.[47] While they devised various ways to kill them – drowning, spearing with needles, burning and squashing between fingernails – their battle was only ceremonial, for it always ended in defeat. One prisoner remembered, 'even though I cleaned my bed and clothes numerous times every evening . . . these creatures would still fall off from my eyebrows into my eyes'.[48] An officer of higher rank confessed that he now found truth in the Anatolian folk phrase 'drowned in lice', which he had regarded as a silly saying until he and his boxcar-mates understood the futility of their fight against lice.[49] Frequently, prisoners passed months without a bath, but even when they could take a bath, they had no choice but to wear the same lice-ridden clothes and sleep in the same lice-ridden beds. 'Verminousness breaks a man's spirit more completely than any other affliction; he loathes himself, and from self-loathing quickly falls into despondency and despair', remarked a European prisoner. An Ottoman prisoner could have made the same observation.[50] Overtaken and defeated by these tiny creatures, these former warriors now felt nothing but a sense of futility and powerlessness.

The Ottomans who had been taken captive by the British and imprisoned in Egypt complained in their memoirs and diaries of brutal treatments at the time of their capture, which ranged from the withholding of water and food[51] to bayoneting[52] of captured men, especially by the non-Muslim Indian units.[53] In general, the Ottoman prisoners in Egypt complained more about their treatment during capture and transport to permanent camps, but less about the conditions in the permanent camps. Once they arrived in the permanent camps, their complaints about treatment subsided.

For one, the Egyptian camps were markedly different from the Russian ones in terms of their cleanliness. Although many soldiers certainly complained of lice prior to capture because they could not bathe and did not usually have a change of clean clothes, their general hygiene seemed to improve after capture as the British put them through a more effective delousing process and their clothes were cleaned before they entered the permanent camps. Some initial logistical problems occurred in the British camps, but soon enough the prisoners were usually well-supplied with water and baths. Despite the relatively better conditions in the camps in Egypt, reaching the permanent camps did not remove the danger of death, which was rampant in Egypt as well. The major difference between the two locations was that the dying did not happen 'publicly' in Egypt as it did in Russia.

Unlike those produced in Russia, Egyptian captivity narratives rarely mention death.[54] The reason is that, in British camps, sick prisoners were admitted into POW hospitals. Therefore, most deaths, if not all, took place out of sight of the rest of the prisoners. The Ottomans in British captivity who were lucky enough to stay healthy and out of the hospitals did not see the wasting of human life that Ottomans in Russian captivity witnessed.

Ultimately, over 10,000 Ottoman prisoners died in British captivity of various causes. In Egypt, thousands of Ottoman prisoners fell victim to pellagra, a deadly nutritional deficiency resulting from inadequate B3 or niacin in the diet. This death rate in the Egyptian camps was more than twice that of the Austro-Hungarian and German prisoners who were captured along with the Ottomans. Instead of merging the groups of prisoner, as the Russians did, the British decided to keep the European prisoners of war in nearby but separate camps. The British had two reasons. If they had to separate the large number of prisoners, division based on some difference made sense. However, the more likely reason was that other prisoners were Europeans and Ottomans were not. Since the camp authorities provided different diets to Europeans and 'non-Europeans', as will be discussed in Chapter 4, separate camps made that process easier to manage.

Food in captivity

Food, or the lack thereof, adversely affected the day-to-day experiences of the prisoners in Russia. Even before capture by the enemy, Ottoman soldiers on all fronts complained of being underfed as they fought the enemy. Intermittent hunger kept them in a weakened condition.[55] Once in captivity, their food complaints shifted, referencing monotony, small portions and poor quality. While the POWs in Egypt complained primarily about the quality of the food, those in Russia encountered inadequate quantities in addition to poor quality food. However, their problems were compounded by the irregular timing of when they could eat; that is to say, they did not regularly receive three or even two meals a day. Foreign diplomats who inspected the Russian prison camps confirmed the prisoners' complaints about 'insufficient food'.[56]

All Russian captivity narratives frequently mention food supply and quality problems. Interned in the town of Varnavino in European Russia, Lieutenant Mehmet Arif noted: 'We all seemed to be starving to death. The so-called meat that was given to the garrison was ox and water buffalo heads that had been preserved under the snow. They were covered with maggots'. Somehow managing to overcome their disgust with this sight, the prisoners 'boiled them in water and ate them' anyway. However, Mehmet Arif noted that 'the odour upset our stomachs and made us vomit'. At the same time, their bread ration had been further reduced to just six ounces a day.[57]

Mehmet Arif, like all prisoners in Russia, regarded the pre-November Revolution days as the 'good days', as far as food was concerned. After the Revolution, the situation became significantly worse.[58] In some places, when the guards walked away, the prisoners were left to find their own food. Rotten or not, meat of any kind became a distant memory for many. Lieutenant Halil Ataman, captive in Krasnoyarsk, remembered hearing a rumour about the possibility of meat being distributed to the prisoners: 'There were all kinds of conversations and jokes among the prisoners about the possibility of getting meat, perhaps there were even those preparing a *selamlık* ceremony in honour of the promised item'.[59] *Selamlık* was the weekly picturesque imperial ceremony held with great pomp on the occasion of the Sultan's going to the mosque for Friday prayers. However, it is clear from all accounts that while *selamlık* was a weekly event in Istanbul, meat in a Russian prison camp diet was not.

Even though there were differences across time and place among the prison camps in terms of severity of food shortage, every Russian captivity memoir contains various references to the inadequacy of food. At another point, Mehmet Arif described the art of sharing a bowl of thin potato soup among thirteen prisoners:

> The thirteen of us gathered around it. We had only one spoon that we began to pass around. Each person ate one spoonful and then gave the spoon to the man next to him. I had carried my own spoon . . . [but] it was small and I wouldn't be able to get much soup with it. . . . As we ate, the soup began to disappear from the tin and turned thicker darker as it did. Tiny pieces of potato began to appear at the bottom of the tin. We reached the point where we could no longer use the spoon. A residue of soup remained at the bottom. We then decided to share the pieces of potato. Each man in turn was going to put a corner of the tin to his mouth and swallow some pieces. This action required a certain skill, including a little shake, to keep the soup from spilling out.[60]

Although this episode takes place in a prison in which Mehmet Arif found himself when he tried to escape, frequently, the camp conditions were not significantly better, as attested to by his comments about maggot-ridden ox heads. Under such dehumanising conditions, the fact that these men were able to hang onto their humanity was an achievement in itself.

In a similar vein, tea drinking, a national and cultural ritual for Ottomans, required both skill and imagination in captivity. Imprisonment and sugar shortage turned this simple social act into an 'art form'. One could drink tea with sugar in three different ways – *kıtlama*, *gözleme* and *umma*. *Kıtlama*, drinking tea while holding a piece of sugar in the mouth, required an abundance of sugar. As someone remarked, 'If you had only a single sugar cube, drinking *kıtlama* style would mean having only one cup of tea. But, if you put this single cube of sugar in front of you and stared at it imagining its sweet taste you could enjoy many cups of tea'. This method of tea drinking was called *gözleme* (watching, observing). In the absence of any sugar, a prisoner could always resort to *umma* (imagination) by 'closing his eyes and imagining a piece of sugar as he drank his tea'.[61] Some prisoners reportedly savoured a single sugar cube over six cups of tea.[62] Tea-drinking as an 'art form' while in captivity was about the power of imagination among men who could not control much about their lives. In the face of dehumanising experiences, such as endless and ineffective delousing and the omnipresence of death, eating and drinking rituals became forms of psychological resistance for the prisoners. As long as there was tea, which was plentiful, imagining that one's cup of tea contained sugar was comparatively uplifting in the face of the other difficulties they encountered.

Despite their creativity, prisoners could not do anything about the inadequate food that generally resulted in scurvy or other nutrition-caused diseases in Russia.[63] Although there is no statistical data on how many people suffered from such diseases, it is reasonable to assume that such diseases were common. Moreover, Ottoman prisoners generally had less to eat than other Central Powers prisoners; this is partially attributable to the fact that Ottomans never received food parcels from home as the German and Austro-Hungarian prisoners did. In addition, the Ottomans were not willing to eat pork because they were Muslims, nor would they eat domestic animals, such as dogs, which their foreign comrades enjoyed as 'delicate and scrumptious' dinners. What was 'delicious' to his Austrian friends, who had invited him to a 'special dinner', was enough to turn Halil Ataman's stomach, even though men like him had been served, and had eaten, maggot-ridden ox heads. When he discovered that the special dinner consisted of a small dog that had been running around the barracks, lieutenant Halil politely excused himself because 'his stomach could not handle fatty meat', and quickly departed from the table.[64] For him, there was a limit to what he was going to eat even when he was not well-fed. He likely refused because he regarded dog meat as unclean.

Compared to the Russian camps, food was relatively plentiful in the British camps. The most persistent complaint was about the monotony of the diet.[65] The prisoners generally found the amount of food sufficient or even 'abundant' once they settled in the permanent camps.[66] Some prisoners made the monotony of the camp diet into a source of wit in the camp newspaper:

Let me tell you about a curious occurrence. The other day I looked to see what was listed for lunch menu. The list read: bean stew with hamburger and stew meat and rice pilaf with vermicelli cooked in beef consommé. When the food came, I noticed that it was nothing more than the rice pilaf and bean stew we have always known ... I told myself that perhaps a new literary movement in food description had started.[67]

The gallows humour visible here reveals that prisoners in Egypt felt confident enough in their food supply to joke about it. Halil Ataman, though, appalled by what he and his fellow prisoners had been reduced to, could not bring himself to make a joke about almost having made a meal of a dog.

Minor complaints aside, officer prisoners in Egypt, unlike those in Russia, rarely had to worry about whether or not they would have a meal. The brief periods of shortages almost always occurred not in the permanent prison camps, but during transportation of the prisoners.[68] The British cited the unexpectedly high number of captures as the source of shortage, but some prisoners were convinced that the insufficient and disagreeable rations they were initially given was a British ploy to break their morale.[69] Once in the permanent camps in Egypt, however, the prisoners' complaints about British cruelty vanished almost entirely. Because food was sufficient in quantity and palatable enough, the prisoners did not fully realise the long-term consequences posed by a lack of nutrients. While many among the enlisted men started to suffer from diarrhoea and other gastrointestinal problems, the signs of a somewhat advanced stage of pellagra, they did not associate their problems with a nutritional deficiency; to them, their sufferings resulted from improperly cooked food.[70]

While the prisoners' food situation improved over time in Egypt, it declined in Russia. Prisoners in Russia frequently had to agonise over how to secure their next meal; this sometimes required creativity. Halil Ataman remembered that he and four friends managed to buy about three kilograms of flour, 'a real treasure', from a Russian peasant. Hiding 'that precious and blessed' flour from other prisoners, they browned it in some butter. Every morning 'we would get a cup of boiling water, mix two teaspoons of browned flour and a little salt, and drink this delicious soup'.[71] While the prisoners in Egypt might have found the flavour of their meal disagreeable at times, they did not really have to worry about their next meal. For example, some prisoners in Egypt felt secure enough about the flow of food to attempt individual or collective hunger strikes to get the attention of their captors, which would have been unimaginable for those in Russia.[72] There was a clear connection between the relative absence of hunger and the proliferation of cultural productions among prisoners in Egypt. That is to say, because the basic needs of the prisoners in Egypt were met, they could occupy themselves with other activities to pass time.

Cultural productions and recreation in the camps

Once established in the camps, the prisoners looked for ways to deal with the boredom, difficulties and uncertainties of their lives, while also attempting to establish some semblance of normality. The one thing they had plenty of was time. They exploited recreation time to keep their sanity and briefly distract themselves from their uncertain situation. The prisoners wanted not only to pass time, but also to do or learn something useful for the future, both for their individual good and for the good of the nation.

The most popular intellectual activity among the prisoners was to learn foreign languages; clearly, this applied almost exclusively to the officers since most enlisted men had to perform physical labour during the day and tended not to be literate in their own language. Although rudimentary schooling systems were established in some of the larger camps in Russia by a united effort of all prisoners, most Ottoman officers sought the personal assistance of their fellow foreign prisoners in learning German, French, Hungarian and Russian. Rich linguistic diversity among the prisoners – ranging from Albanian to Hungarian to Hebrew to Esperanto to Turkish – provided many languages and teachers for those interested. For example, the camp school in Novonikolaievsk offered courses in fourteen different languages.[73] Ottoman prisoners of all ethnicities were eager to teach one of the languages they knew in return to European prisoners. Because prisoners of all ethnicities in Russia shared barracks or were allowed easy access to each other, they had the opportunity to collaborate with and learn from each other even without establishing a formal school. The Egyptian camps, though, were not as linguistically rich as those in Russia for a number of reasons. Since the British had separated Ottomans from 'European' prisoners of war for both political and racial reasons, there was far less linguistic diversity in the camps in Egypt. Therefore, the number of teachers and languages taught depended completely on the availability and willingness of multi-lingual Ottoman officers to participate.

Despite the relative paucity of language instruction possibilities for Ottoman prisoners in Egypt, they did have a greater variety of options open to them for passing time than did those in Russia. For instance, they established musical and theatrical groups that put on shows for their fellow inmates. In 1920, a single camp alone featured a play every three to five days; theatre and music flourished among the Ottomans in Egypt. A number of prisoners were involved in writing and others acted in or produced these plays; in fact, even the enlisted men took part in them. The camp newspapers reviewed some of these productions.[74] The larger number of Ottoman prisoners in each of the several large Egyptian camps more easily lent itself to a fuller development of cultural productions. Larger numbers meant more actors, directors, ideas and, of course, a larger audience, which kept the plays going. As the image below shows, in the evenings, prisoners in Egypt had the choice of their own theatre productions or American or British movies – some featuring Charlie Chaplin and other early motion picture stars – shown by the camp authorities[75] (see Figure 1.1).

In Russia, the dispersal of Ottoman POWs among the numerous camps meant that Ottomans were always in the minority. Therefore, they did not have the 'man power' or the audience to get similar projects off the ground. In addition, they faced larger problems related to survival, which probably left little mental capacity for creative endeavours. For all these reasons, they produced only a handful of plays. Krasnoyarsk, one of the largest camps with about 400 Ottoman POWs, was perhaps the most culturally active. Ottomans here staged several plays and formed a musical group (with violins and *saz*) which performed several times.[76] The presence of only a small number of prisoners from one nationality did not completely impede other kinds of cultural activity. One example is that of Aref al-Aref, an Arab Ottoman and subsequent mayor of Jerusalem under the mandate, who translated Ernst Haeckel's *Das Welträetsel* into Ottoman Turkish; he also produced a camp newspaper in Arabic for his twelve other Arab Ottoman comrades in the same camp.[77]

Sports, soccer in particular, proved to be another popular activity among the prisoners. The warm Egyptian climate allowed for soccer as a year-round sport, one that could be enjoyed either as a participant or spectator. Some Egyptian camps had two organised league matches a day.[78] In addition, gymnastics, wrestling, boxing, fencing and billiards proved popular in Egyptian camps. In Russia, even in the large camp of Krasnoyarsk, the number of willing Ottoman officers in each camp was not enough to form a separate Ottoman soccer team, but several played on Austrian and Hungarian teams. On Sunday afternoons, the game day in Krasnoyarsk, other Ottomans came out to support their compatriots from the side-lines.[79] However, Ottomans in Siberia had a limited window to participate in outdoor activities. Most were not equipped to ice skate with their European comrades during winter. European prisoners either received cash from home to buy such things as skates, or had their families send them by mail.[80]

In Egypt, although the heat could be unbearable, and the prisoners certainly risked sunstroke, nature was less of a hindrance to everyday life. Some large Egyptian camps were near the Mediterranean shore or another body of water; after extending part of the barbed wire campgrounds into the water, the authorities permitted the prisoners to swim.[81] In Russia, though, only a very few who

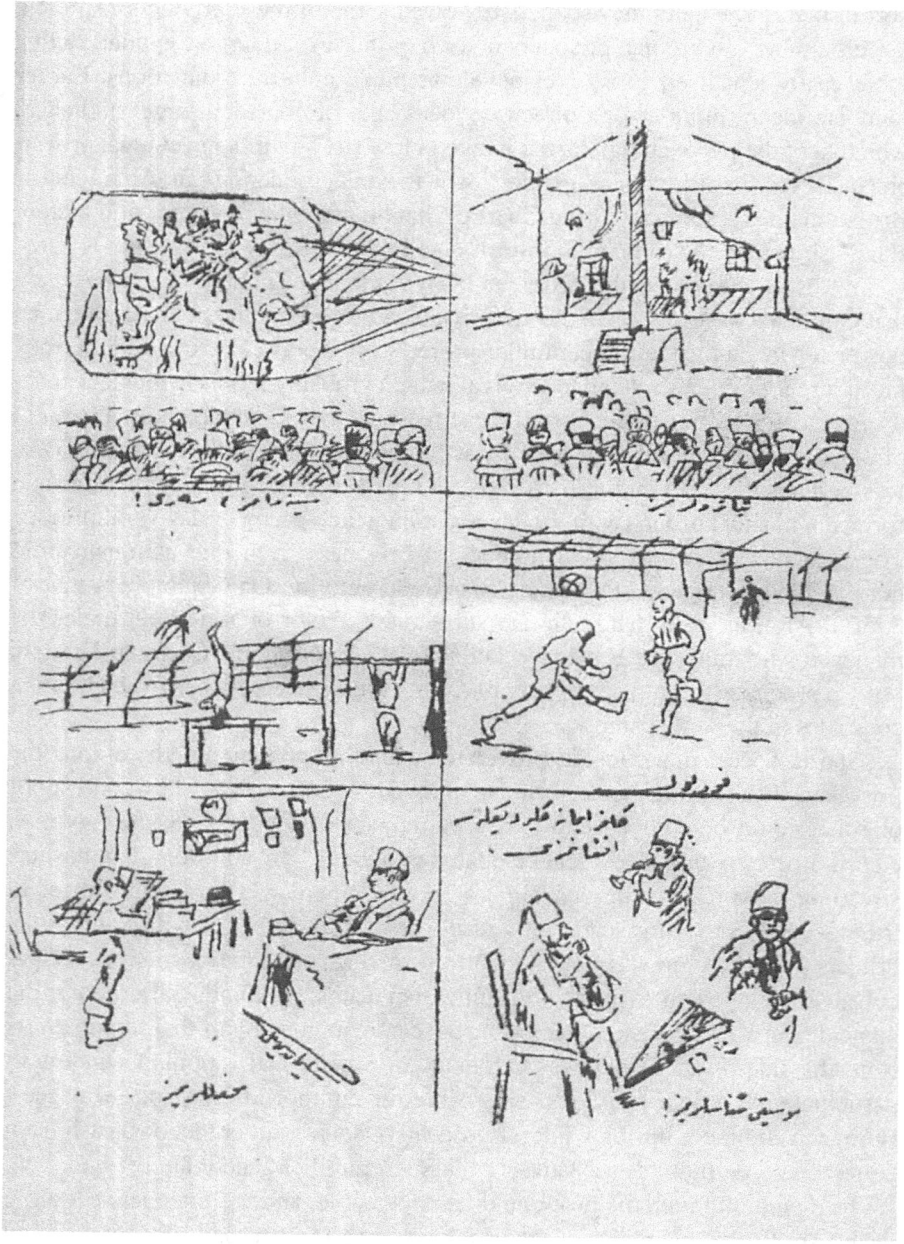

Figure 1.1 Prisoner activities in Egypt as reflected in the camp newspaper *Hatıra-yı Esaret*, Egypt
Source: Courtesy of Atatürk University Library, Erzurum (22449/SÖ)

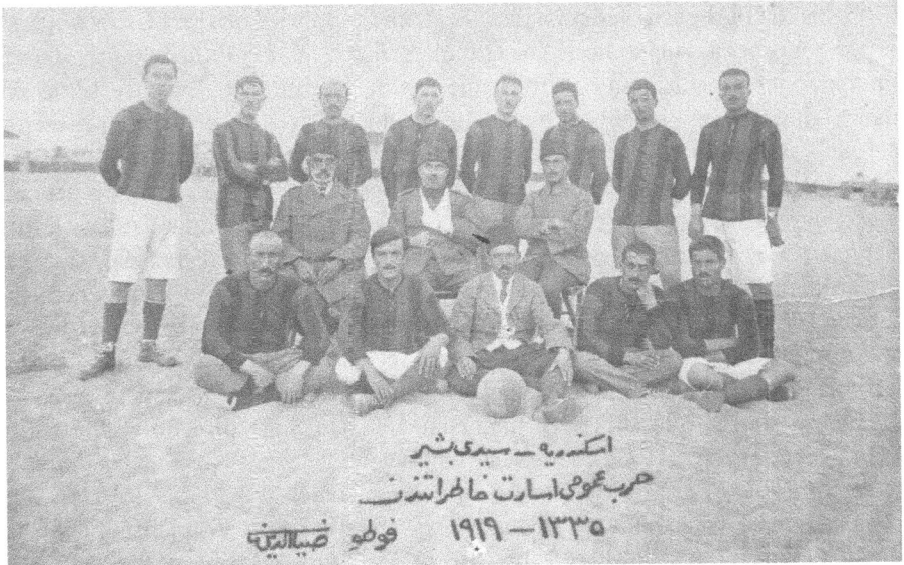

Figure 1.2 Alexandria – Sidi Bishr [Camp], captivity memento from the General War, 1335–1919
Source: Courtesy of Atillâ Ertürk

lived in commandeered houses in small towns located on a river could petition the *nachalnik* (superintendent, commander of Russian guards) for permission to swim. Only the prisoners in the town of Varnavino mention swimming in the river; no one in the much larger Krasnoyarsk camp located on the Yenisei mentions anything similar.

Comparatively better climate and larger numbers of prisoners in Egypt were certainly important factors in starting and maintaining the interest in cultural activities, but there were other considerations as well. Because the basic physiological needs of the prisoners in Egypt were met, they could devote their attention to cultural matters.[82] By comparison, in Russia, those physiological (food, water, homeostasis) and safety (security of body, resources, health) needs were not adequately secured. If they managed through one day, there was always the worry about the next. Moreover, the worry about tomorrow became more pronounced during the period of the Revolution and civil war in Russia. For example, if the large number of Ottoman officers in Krasnoyarsk could not form a soccer team, one contributing factor might have been the unwillingness to destroy the only pair of shoes (or boots) they could expect to possess until repatriation or some foreign aid agency donated supplies to them.

Whereas European prisoners received some supplies from Red Cross organisations or other aid institutions, the Ottomans received very little help from these international organisations or from their own government. Because some of their families might have been worse off than the prisoners, Ottoman prisoners certainly could not expect any help from them. In fact, many gave up on writing letters home when they did not receive responses. There were also more practical reasons for giving up on correspondence. For example, Dr Adnan [Adıvar], the Secretary General of the Ottoman Red Crescent, complained that the Russian government regularly required that the Ottoman POWs write their letters in French.[83] Surely, this disparity in all regards, accompanied by a slowly growing sense of abandonment by their own state, caused further anxiety among the Ottomans. In observing that 'Europeans had a passion for amusement; we were always in sorrow and anguish', Lieutenant Halil did not directly connect the German prisoners' passion to the fact that they received aid, parcels and letters. However, it is clear from his other entries that when the European prisoners regularly received letters and packages from families or aid organisations, and the Ottomans did not, Halil and others were especially unhappy.[84]

Moreover, the infrequent aid intended for the Ottoman prisoners, either from their own government or from a European agency, did not always make it to them. For example, in Stretensk on Lake Baikal, Hereward T. Price, an Englishman captured while fighting for the Germans, witnessed and recorded at least one instance of aid intended for Ottoman prisoners being embezzled by a certain Dr Kallenbach, a German prisoner. The Swedish Red Cross gave money to Kallenbach to be distributed 'to the Turks, who were worse off than any of us; most of this money he kept for himself, and then falsified his accounts so as to make it appear that the Turks had received everything'. This was only begrudging empathy from Price for he hated 'Turks'. In his opinion, Turks 'were not [even] worthy to unloose' the shoe-laces of 'their subject races, the Greeks and Armenians'.[85]

Resisting the captor

Ottoman prisoners in Egypt and Russia resisted their captors both openly and covertly. The prisoners in Egypt could get away with openly expressing their resistance individually and, on occasion, also collectively. Those in Russia could not engage in either kind of resistance; however, even in times of near total control by their captors, the prisoners were able to devise secret plans to resist. Occasionally, this resistance was displayed publicly.[86]

Finding strength in numbers and taking for granted the steady food supply, the prisoners in Egypt openly expressed their resistance, whether it was individual or

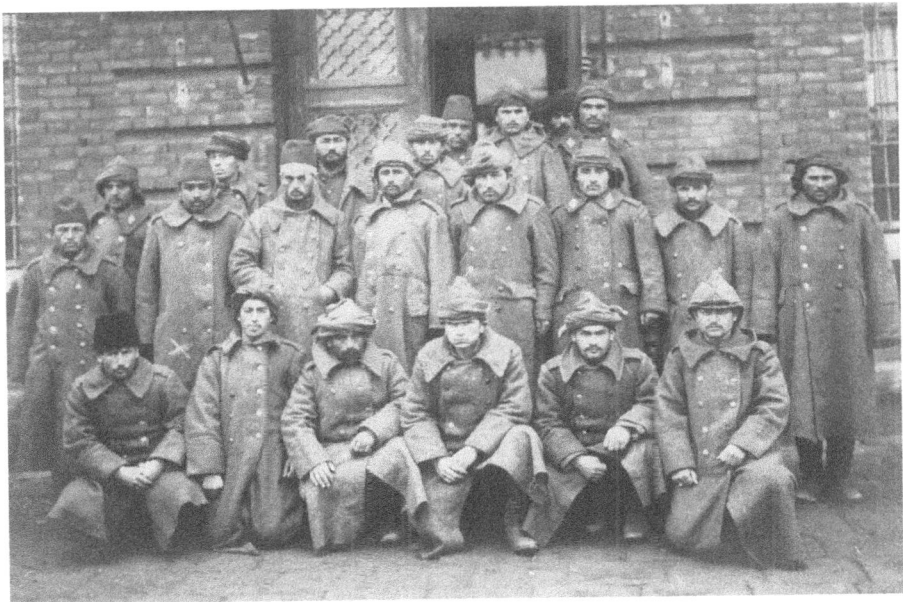

Figure 1.3 Captured Turkish cavalry patrol – lower ranks
Source: Courtesy of Russian State Archive, Krasnogorsk, Album 1087, Photo 4

collective. When these rebellions were individual, the captor could more easily crush them, as was the case for Rahmi Apak, an officer in Egypt who, after repatriation, became a high-ranking member of the Republican People's Party during the early years of the republic. While in the prison camp, Rahmi Apak decided to go on a hunger strike to protest against what he believed was personal ill-treatment by the camp commandant; after a few days, he was force-fed by camp guards.[87] On another occasion, Emin Çöl reported that in one of the camps for the enlisted men, a small protest turned into a large-scale hunger strike because the strike organisers coerced the reluctant to join the demonstration.

> Since we did not go out for the roll call ... or for food, food was brought to us; ... we openly threw the food into a ditch ... The twelve organizers of the movement were going to embarrass those who ate the food and spit in their faces as punishment for not having kept their promise ... When the British attempted to separate those they believed were the leaders, a fight started ... The British were using their fists, we were kicking, slapping, tripping, and even biting them ... [The fight] ended when a British major whistled and yelled 'finişe ... finiş' [finish] and they simply left defeated.[88]

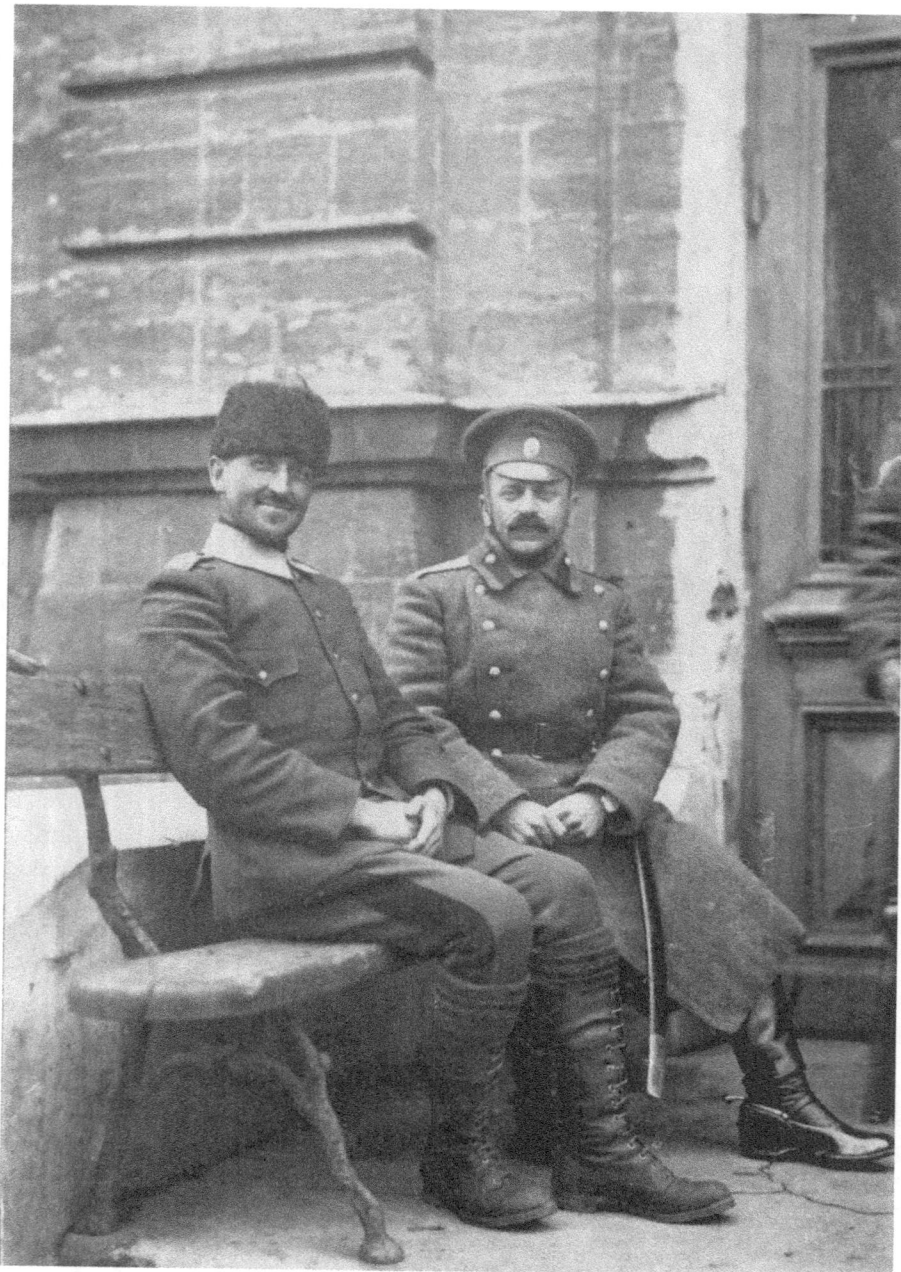

Figure 1.4 Prisoner Lieutenant Mehmet Hüseyinoğlu with a Russian officer
Source: Courtesy of Russian State Archive, Krasnogorsk, Album 1087, Photo 1

Even with some likely exaggeration, this episode highlights the fact that prisoners in Egypt, still possessing emotional reserves, could resist their captors, even with physical force, and still expect to remain alive. Aided by their numbers, they were able to form a collective front even if the instigators had to coerce the less willing.

As in the case of Rahmi Apak, even individual prisoners in Egypt did not fear for their lives if they acted alone. The case of Beykozlu Kel Ali, who was a recaptured escapee, is also instructive in this regard. The camp commandant attempted to make an example of him in front of his comrades by putting him in a one-metre-square isolation chamber. According to a post-repatriation report by an Ottoman officer who had been in the same camp, Kel Ali surprised his two guards when he was released from the isolation chamber. Reportedly seizing a rifle from one of the guards, 'he knocked out the soldiers one at a time with the butt of his rifle' before they could do anything to him. 'He then used the bayonet to cut the barbed wire and passed through the first set of wires before he was confronted by nearly 30 or more British soldiers with bayonets facing him. "Come on, I will kill you all", he said to the approaching soldiers', but he was outnumbered and eventually surrendered.[89] The author reported this not in a memoir, where some literary license might be expected, but in a semi-official report. Even taking into account some possible exaggeration, these relatively bold actions in the confines of an Egyptian prison camp show that some prisoners, while compliant most of the time, did not shy away from open rebellions and public acts of resistance. Being in a prison camp designated for tens of thousands of Ottomans no doubt allowed these prisoners to find some safety in numbers.

With the exception of a few meagre verbal protests regarding food and overcrowding by those POWs confined in European Russia, there are no known acts of open collective defiance against the Russians.[90] A few reported accounts of individual acts are rare and they almost always occurred when a guard was drunk, or under cover of night when identification would be difficult. However, in Russia, prisoners defied the captors in hidden ways, the most common of which was to engage in planning an escape. The enlisted men did not leave written records, but almost every officer prisoner made plans to escape. These plans took months or even years to develop. Despite the lengthy amount of time devoted to planning, they were surprisingly straightforward and simple affairs.[91] The prisoners kept their resistance hidden until they felt themselves ready to declare it openly. Interestingly, none of these escape plans included digging tunnels, disabling guards or cutting barbed wire fences, or any other of the time-consuming strategies we might associate with prisoner escapes.

In Russia, the initial escape was the easy part. As the camp commandant predicted, the real deterrent was not the camp walls or the guards, but the vast

Siberian distances between the camps and safety. Something else that deterred the prisoners from escaping was the rumours, or sometimes actually witnessing, of other escapees reappearing in the camps from which they escaped in a barely alive state or even dead.[92] With all those deterrents, the captors regularly allowed the prisoners to make unsupervised visits to nearby towns because they did not think the prisoners could escape because of the harsh and unfamiliar landscape, and the incredible distances involved between the place of captivity and the Ottoman Empire. However, on such excursions, especially in Siberia, some prisoners established contact with local Turkic peoples who were willing to help them escape.[93] The camp commandants did not always realise that such contacts often encouraged escapes. If the prisoner decided to escape, he would seek permission to go into town, or merely bribe a guard. If things went well, his local contact would provide him with civilian clothes, a little money or food, and directions.[94]

Prisoners took their time planning these simple escapes for several reasons. Devising and reworking even the simplest plan was a good way to deal with boredom and keep the mind busy and away from the depressing conditions of their captive lives. Escape planning also gave them hope of freedom, and allowed them to exercise their imaginations. And imagination – ranging from making plans to escape, to daydreaming about food, or mentally savouring the taste of sugar – was the thing the captor could never control. Escape-planning, even as hidden acts of defiance, made the prisoners feel as if they were still struggling against the enemy; the devising of plans made escape possible, and that possibility gave them back a fragment of their pre-captivity psychological make-up as humans, and men with dignity.

Another reason for the prevalence of hidden defiance in Russia was the lack of trust in fellow prisoners. The harsher conditions of captivity and even occasional competition for resources made many prisoners feel they could only rely on themselves and a few of their closest friends. Especially in large Russian camps, some Ottoman prisoners believed that Russians had placed spies among them. Hüsamettin Tuğaç, for example, believed that two Ottomans in his camp, one of whom was a civilian who 'passed himself as an officer', were working for the Russians. He identified them as Albanian-Ottomans.[95] Yet another prisoner expressed a similar sentiment in a poem he composed for the camp newspaper. In one line in particular, he lamented that he felt 'surrounded by spies from all sides'.[96] The prisoners in Russia were preoccupied with ensuring their own individual survival in the face of all the other obstacles that threatened their lives. Afraid to share information with people they did not trust fully, they could not conspire to support one another and thus were reluctant to challenge the captor. They could not forge a collective identity for any collective action because of their reluctance to share their thoughts or coordinate any means of resistance.

While nearly all prisoners in Russia made plans to escape, there is little evidence of escape planning in Egypt. Security around the British camps was tighter: surrounded by barbed wire, the camps also had sentries posted at intervals with orders to shoot prisoners who came close to the wire. Some exceptions aside, prisoners probably found the probability of successful escape unlikely.[97] Just as important, however, was another factor. Life was tolerable and they were at least safe from the fighting while the war continued. In contrast to the prisoners in Russia, those in Egypt were visited on a couple of occasions by the Red Cross and American State Department inspectors until 1917. Therefore, the prisoners in Egypt felt that at least someone was looking out for their welfare. They would survive the war and return home alive.[98] Furthermore, if escape planning was a mental activity or hidden defiance for the prisoners in Russia, those in Egypt had other opportunities to occupy their minds and express their defiance against the captor.

CONCLUSION

Clearly, there were significant differences both in the way the war was experienced by those fighting on the Eastern front against Russians and those fighting against the British and Commonwealth forces in the region of Palestine and Syria. These differences continued into captivity both in the way the captors treated the Ottoman prisoners and the physical environment in which the prisoners had to survive. Comparatively speaking, the war against and captivity in Russia were more trying and precarious in terms of clinging to life. The next chapter continues this comparative method to examine how the Russian experience created challenges in other realms as well.

NOTES

1. '*Hatırat*' is an unpublished work by M. Feyyaz Efendi (1893–1919), a prisoner of war in Kostroma, Russia. The poem was written as he was dying of tuberculosis immediately after repatriation to Istanbul.
2. Mustafa Aksakal, *The Ottoman Road to War*.
3. Mustafa Aksakal, *The Ottoman Road to War*, chapters 4 and 5. Both the date on which the Ottoman navy bombarded the Russian coastline and the battle cruiser that led the Ottoman navy, *Yavuz*, would seem ironic in later years. Exactly nine years after the bombardment, the Turkish republic was proclaimed, on 29 October 1923, and after his death, the body of Mustafa Kemal Atatürk, the founder of that republic, was carried on the same battle cruiser, *Yavuz*, from Istanbul to Samsun.
4. Mesut Uyar and Edward Erickson, *A Military History of the Ottomans*, pp. 242–3.
5. Ibid. pp. 242–3.
6. Ibid. pp. 243–4.

7. On railroads and transportation problems, see especially Erik Jan Zürcher, 'Between Death and Desertion', pp. 250–3.
8. Linda Schatkowski Schilcher, 'The Famine of 1915–1918 in Greater Syria', pp. 229–58; Elizabeth Thompson, *Colonial Citizens*, pp. 15–27.
9. Uyar and Erickson, *A Military History of the Ottomans*, p. 273. See also Zürcher, 'Between Death and Desertion', pp. 253–4.
10. Uyar and Erickson, *A Military History of the Ottomans*, p. 274. See also Hikmet Özdemir, *The Ottoman Army*; and Zürcher, 'Between Death and Desertion'.
11. While Muslims accounted for 60 per cent before 1878, they represented 72 per cent in the 1880s, and 74 per cent in 1906–7. Carter V. Findley, *Turkey, Islam, Nationalism, and Modernity*, p. 175.
12. Hüseyin Hüsnü Erkilet, *Yıldırım*, p. 346, cited in Edward Erickson, *Ottoman Army Effectiveness*, pp. 129–30.
13. Erickson, *Ottoman Army Effectiveness*, p. 129.
14. Erik Jan Zürcher, 'The Ottoman Conscription System', and 'Birinci Dünya Savaşında', pp. 201–14.
15. The report does not indicate what ethno-linguistic groups were included in the 'other'. War Office, *Statistics of the Military Effort*, p. 633.
16. Edward Erickson, *Ordered to Die*, p. 211. See also, Zürcher, 'Between Death and Desertion', pp. 235–42; Zürcher, 'The Ottoman Conscription System', pp. 447–8; Erik Jan Zürcher, 'Little Mehmed in the Desert', pp. 230–41; Maurice Larcher, *La Guerre Turque*, p. 590.
17. Askeri Tarih ve Stratejik Etüd Başkanlığı (ATASE), World War I Collection, K18/D18/F1-1.
18. Miralay Baki, *Yurt Müdafaası*, p. 132.
19. Uyar and Erickson, *A Military History of the Ottomans*, p. 248.
20. On health related issues of the Galicia expedition unit, see Oya Dağlar Macar, 'Galiçya Cephesi'nde', pp. 35–58.
21. Taşkıran's estimates of dead and wounded seem to cover 1915–18 only (pp. 47 and 51). Erickson's prisoner estimates do not include '1918 returnees from Russia', which he seems to put at about 9,000 only. His wounded includes wounded and permanent loss. 'Official Turkish histories' are cited in Erickson, p. 189. See also Ahmet Emin [Yalman], *Turkey in the World War*, pp. 252–3, 262; and War Office, *Statistics of the Military Effort*, p. 357.
22. War Office, *Statistics of the Military Effort*, p. 638.
23. Erickson, *Ordered to Die*, p. 189.
24. Cemalettin Taşkıran, *Ana Ben Ölmedim*, p. 51. Earlier parts of Taşkıran's chapter 7 are remarkably similar to my article that appeared in *Journal of Contemporary History* in 1999.
25. War Office, *Statistics of the Military Effort*, p. 631, note at bottom of page.
26. Ibid. pp. 630, 635.
27. Two Australian newspapers reported contradictory numbers on the Ottoman prisoners in Russia. *The Argus* (Melbourne) reported that by mid-February 1915, 49,600 Ottomans had been captured by Russia, while *The Northern Miner* reported a much lower number of 16,016 for the later date of March 1915. *The Argus*, 16 February 1915, p. 7; and *The Northern Miner*, 11 March 1915, p. 3.
28. Although there were sizeable groups of Ottoman prisoners in India or Burma, this book

focuses only on those in Russia and Egypt. This is for two reasons: want of evidence from the other two locations, and prisoners from these locations were eventually sent to Egypt after the end of the war. 'Turks' Stronghold in Transcaucasia', *The Times* (London), 15 February 1915, p. 7, column B.

29. For 'General Winter' see Halil Ataman, *Esaret Yılları*, pp. 48–9. Initial and most destructive fighting between the Ottoman and Russian armies took place during the winter months. Many of the prisoners who found themselves in Russian captivity were captured relatively early in the war – some time before the spring of 1915. For an overview of the Ottoman soldiers' experience of war, see Zürcher, 'Between Death and Desertion', pp. 235–58.
30. A. Hilmi Erbuğ, 'Kaybolan Yıllar', p. 203.
31. This particular example involves an old woman who had come to watch the Ottoman prisoners being marched through her town; she noticed that one of the soldiers had no shoes at all and holes in his socks. She took off her own shoes, made of rubber, gave them to the soldier and yelled at the Ottoman officers for his sad condition: Ziya Yergök, *Tuğgeneral Ziya Yergök'ün Anıları*, p. 140. Another similar example is in Erbuğ, 'Kaybolan Yıllar' (p. 203); he observed Russian women offering bread to the Ottoman soldiers.
32. On the issue of shame, see Yücel Yanıkdağ, '"Ill-fated Sons" of the Nation', chapter 1.
33. ATASE, K2841/406/ Fihrist 1-1.
34. ATASE, K313/Fihrist 1; K313/Fihrist 8. While some cars had buckets in a corner for this purpose, other cars reportedly had a small hole on the floor; some probably did not have either as A. Hilmi Erbuğ remembered seeing enlisted men trying to relieve themselves through the tiny window high on the side of the boxcar (p. 202).
35. ATASE, K2482/406/Fihrist 1-8; K313/Fihrist 1; K313/Fihrist 1-1; A. Hilmi Erbuğ, p. 202; US Department of State, 763.72114/622, 'Report on Condition of Military and Civilian Prisoners of War in Siberia', 14 June 1915. Also for a fuller description of the conditions of transport, see Yanıkdağ, 'Ottoman Prisoners of War in Russia'.
36. Spain was supposed to be looking after the Ottoman prisoners, but, having received no advanced funding from the Ottoman government, they did not really do anything in this capacity.
37. ATASE, K313/Fihrist 1-3; Erbuğ, 'Kaybolan Yıllar', p. 202. İhsan Pasha, who was also captured by the Russians, estimated that nearly 50 per cent of the Ottoman prisoners died during transport. ATASE, K313/Fihrist 15.
38. US Department of State, 763.72114/1526, Peking to Washington, D.C., April 15, 1916, p. 5; ATASE, K313/Fihrist 1-1; Başkatipzade Ragıp Bey, *Tarih-i Hayatım*, p. 110.
39. US Department of State, 763.72114/1487, 'Report on Camp for Military Prisoners at Stretensk, Irkutsk Military District, Siberia, January 20, 1916', pp. 5–7; see also 763.72114/1702, 'Report on Prison camp Conditions in Eastern Siberia, 1915–1916', p. 4.
40. While length of the prison-camp relationships may not have been as long as Freud had intended, their around-the-clock nature makes up for some of the difference. Additionally, because the relationships in the prison camps were not intimate as in marriage, the act of repression became more difficult and outbursts less 'impolite' as repressed feelings surfaced. For more on Freud see David S. Werman, 'Freud's "Narcissism of Minor Differences"', p. 452.
41. Ataman, *Esaret Yılları*, p. 147.
42. 'Esaret'de', *Vaveyla*, 31 Mart 1333/31 March 1917, number 67, p. 4. Obviously,

captivity, boredom and ill health also affected the prisoners in Egypt, but no similarly moving protests of this sort exist in their writings.

43. ATASE, K313/Fihrist 1-3; and 763.72114/1702, 'Report on Prison camp Conditions in Eastern Siberia, 1915–1916', p. 4. Thirteen hundred prisoners of all nationalities died in Krasnoyarsk alone during the winter of 1914–1915. Another great epidemic with deadlier results came in 1920. Gerald Davis, 'Prisoner of War Camps as Social Communities', pp. 149, 154. For a brief account of Ottoman doctors who also succumbed to typhus see M. Rıza Serhadoğlu, *Savaşçı Doktorun İzinde*, p. 116.

44. One Austrian source estimated the death rate among the Ottoman prisoners as 20 per cent, a significantly higher rate than the prisoners of other nations: Hans Weiland and Leopold Kern, *In Feindeshand*, pull-out chart. On the TB cases see US Department of State, 763.72114/1702, 'Report on Prison camp Conditions in Eastern Siberia, 1915–1916', p. 4.

45. US Department of State, 763.72114/1487, 'Report on Camps for Military Prisoners at Stretensk, Irkutsk Military District, Siberia, 20 January 1916', p. 50. Tahsin İybar, *Sibirya'dan Serendib'e*, p. 36; Edwin E. Dwinger, *Prisoner of War*, pp. 144, 215; Aziz Samih, *Büyük Harpte Kafkas Cephesi*, pp. 9–10.

46. ATASE, K313/Fihrist 1-3.

47. Hereward T. Price, *Boche and Bolshevik*, p. 125; Hüsamettin Tuğaç, *Bir Neslin Dramı*, p. 89; Mehmet Feyyaz Efendi, *'Hatırat'* (unpublished manuscript), pp. 23, 30; Erbuğ, 'Kaybolan Yıllar', p. 202; Dwinger, *Prisoner of War*, pp. 247–8.

48. Mehmet Feyyaz Efendi, *'Hatırat'*, p. 23, 30.

49. The phrase is *'bitten boğulmak'*, in Yergök *Tuğgeneral Ziya Yergök'ün Anıları*, p. 136.

50. Price, *Boche and Bolshevik*, p. 125.

51. ATASE, K313/Fihrist 13; K313/Fihrist 13-1; K313/Fihrist 6-1; K313/Fihrist 7-1; Türk İnkilâp Tarihi Arşivi, 91/29/29/1-2; US Department of State, 763.72114/2311, Constantinople to Washington, D.C., enclosure, 8 December 1916, p. 2.

52. ATASE, K1486/Fihrist 1; K313/13; Nureddin, 'Mısır Çöllerinde Türk Gençleri, 21', *Vakit*, 2 June 1924, p. 4. Several testimonies by Ottoman POWs confirm charges of bayoneting; they reported that the British soldiers finished off all those Ottomans who were seriously wounded. One further stated that the bad treatment continued until Kut al-Amara fell to the Ottomans and the 13,000 British and Commonwealth defenders of the garrison were made prisoners. It was only then the Ottoman POWs observed a noticeable change in the British attitude towards the prisoners. US Department of State, 73.72114/2311, Constantinople to Washington, D.C., enclosure, 8 December 1916, pp. 2–4.

53. ATASE, K313/Fihrist 7; ATASE, K3437/Fihrist 6-2. This issue is confirmed by at least one British soldier though he blamed it on the shortage of supplies resulting from capturing unexpectedly high numbers of Ottoman prisoners. Imperial War Museum, Lt J. F. B. O'Sullivan Papers, pp. 10–12.

54. War Office, *Statistics of the Military Effort*, pp. 630, 635. One exception to this is the memoir of Cemil Zeki Yoldaş, who mentions that 'some young friends who went insane committed suicide' in the camps. *Kendi Kaleminden Teğmen Cemil Zeki*, pp. 26–7.

55. References to lack of food, especially during the latter years of the war, are rather common in the war narratives and doctors' post-war histories of the supply problems. These will be examined in greater detail in Chapter 4.

56. Erbuğ, 'Kaybolan Yıllar', p. 211; Mustafa Fevzi Taşer, *Cepheden Cepheye*, p. 77. An American diplomat reported that all prisoners in Russia complained of insufficient food:

US Department of State, 763.72114/1513, 'Report on the Internment Camp of Military Prisoners at Skotovo, Priamur District', 17 February 1916, p. 4.
57. Mehmet Arif Ölçen, *Vetluga Memoir*, p. 101.
58. Ölçen, *Vetluga Memoir*, pp. 112–13, 116; Mehmed Âsaf, *Volga Kıyılarında*, p. 82; Başkatipzade Ragıp Bey, *Tarih-i Hayatım*, pp. 98–9.
59. Ataman, *Esaret Yılları*, p. 155–56.
60. Ölçen, *Vetluga Memcir*, p. 192. Although similar events took place in prison camps, this particular episode takes place in a Cheka prison; Mehmet Arif and his six friends were thrown in there briefly when they were intercepted while escaping.
61. Mehmed Âsaf, *Volga Kıyılarında*, p. 81. For another description of creative ways of drinking tea without sugar, see Faik Tonguç, *Birinci Dünya Savaşı'nda*, p. 150.
62. Erbuğ, 'Kaybolan Yıllar', p. 213.
63. US Department of State, 763.72114/2548, p. 7; and 763.72114/1702, p. 5. Scurvy is caused by lack of vitamin C. Pellagra was another deficiency disease encountered especially among those in Egypt.
64. Ataman, *Esaret Yılları*, 161; Mehmed Âsaf, *Volga Kıyılarında*, p. 80.
65. Although it may have been expanded to include additional varieties of foods on the occasion of Red Cross prison camp inspection, for the 'typical' diet of the Ottoman prisoners in Egypt, see Red Cross, *Turkish Prisoners of War in Egypt*, pp. 15–17, 19, 28–9, 50; see also US Department of State, 'Report on the Treatment of Turkish Prisoners of War in Egypt', 26 April 1916, 763.72114/1257; US Department of State, 'Diet Sheet for Turkish Officers', 8 November 1915, 763.72114/1021.
66. Emin Çöl, *Çanakkale – Sina Savaşları*, p. 129.
67. 'İaşe ve Edebiyat', *Nilüfer*, 3 Şubat 1336/13 February 1920, number 2, p. 4.
68. Hidayet Özkök, *Çanakkale'der. Hicaz'a Harp Hatıraları*, p. 54
69. Sokrat İncesu was especially critical of British cruelty. Sokrat İncesu, *Birinci Dünya Savaşında*, pp. 29–30.
70. As Chapter 4 will show, not knowing that they were suffering from a horrible disease likely caused by British racialism, the men thought the culprit was the kind of oil used in their food. What they thought was '*hint yağı*' (castor oil) with its 'disgusting taste and green colour', must have been cottonseed oil. Çöl, *Çanakkale – Sina Savaşları*, p. 133.
71. Ataman, *Esaret Yılları*, p. 160.
72. Ironically, one prisoner who was on a hunger strike complained of being force-fed. Rahmi Apak, *Yetmişlik Bir Subayın*, pp. 165–6; Çöl, *Çanakkale – Sina Savaşları*, p. 133.
73. Some of the schools were much more sophisticated than others. For more on the Novonikolaievsk camp school, established by the German and Austro-Hungarian POWs, see the Report of Donald A. Lowrie, 11 June 1917, *Donald A. Lowrie Papers*, University of Illinois, University Archives, Box 1. One officer in Krasnoyarsk estimated that about 60–70 per cent of the Ottomans learned at least one language; some then moved onto a second language. Tuğaç, *Bir Neslin Dramı*, p. 29; Ataman, *Esaret Yılları*, pp. 122, 140; Dwinger, *Prisoner of War*, p. 213; Ölçen, *Vetluga Irmağı*, pp. 88, 90; Mehmed Âsaf, *Volga Kıyılarında*, p. 39; Başkatipzâde Ragıp Bey, *Tarih-i Hayatım*, p. 94; Yergök, *Tuğgeneral Ziya Yergök'ün Anıları*, p. 154; İybar, *Sibirya'dan Serendib'e*, p. 37.
74. One prisoner tells us that 'Prison camp C' alone had a play every 3 to 5 days. Asaf Tanrıkurt, *Yemen Notları*, p. 135; 'Bizde Temaşanın Geçirdiği Safahat', *Yarın*, 13 Şubat 1336/21 February 1920, number 11; 'Tenkid', 'Diken' Piyesi', ibid. p. 7.
75. Red Cross, *Turkish Prisoners of War in Egypt*, p. 46.

76. Mehmet Feyyaz Efendi, *'Hatırat'* (unpublished manuscript), p. 50; Ataman, *Esaret Yılları*, p. 143; Tuğaç, *Bir Neslin Dramı*, pp. 58, 123; İybar, *Sibirya'dan Serendib'e*, p. 37. Germans and Austrians were very active in Russia in their theatrical productions. See Alon Rachomimov, 'The Disruptive Comforts of Drag', pp. 362–82.
77. Ataman, *Esaret Yılları*, pp. 143–4; Aref al-Aref, *Aref al-Aref*, p. 2; Salim Tamari, 'With God's Camel in Siberia', pp. 31–50.
78. Hüseyin Aydın, *Acı Hatıralar*, p. 45; US Department of State, 763.72114/1257, enclosure, 'Report on the Treatment of Turkish Prisoners of War in Egypt', p. 2.
79. İybar, *Sibirya'dan Serendib'e*, p. 37.
80. İybar mentions running and 'parallel bars' (*barfiks*) during the winter months; it was generally the Hungarians who jogged: *Sibirya'dan Serendib'e*, p. 37.
81. For example, Sidi Bishr (Seydi Beşer in Ottoman Turkish), a neighbourhood in the Montaza district of Alexandria on the Mediterranean, became a summering location for the middle classes after the 1952 revolution.
82. Here, I refer to Abraham Maslow's hierarchy of needs in 'A Theory of Human Motivation', pp. 370–96.
83. US Department of State, Istanbul to Washington, 763.72114/2275, 28 December 1916 notes that very few parcels were sent out of Turkey to Ottoman prisoners. The British government threatened that they would instruct Russia to stop giving any parcels to the Ottomans in Russia. Dr Adnan to American Embassy, 763.72114/1935, 12 August 1918; see also 763.72114/820, p. 8 for prisoners' complaints.
84. Ataman, *Esaret Yılları*, p. 151. I should add that other Ottoman prisoners found the Germans way 'too serious' and soldierly, whereas the Austrians and Hungarians were seen as fun-loving and friendlier.
85. Price, *Boche and Bolshevik*, pp. 143, 173. The author was a professor of English at Bonn when he was conscripted to serve in the German army. It is clear from his memoir that Price liked 'Jews' even less than he liked 'Turks'.
86. Here I am using James Scott's terminology from *Domination and the Arts of Resistance*.
87. Apak, *Yetmişlik Bir Subayın*, pp. 165–6.
88. Çöl, *Çanakkale – Sina Savaşları*, pp. 133–5.
89. Beykozlu Ali's story is very interesting. After the initial escape, which must have been in 1917, he actually worked in two separate places in Cairo – perhaps to save money for his return trip. However, some Egyptians turned him in to the British in 1919. Once Ali was in the chamber, the other Ottomans attempted to help him. They threw cigarettes, bread and other necessities in the direction of the small opening between the roof and the walls of the chamber as they casually walked by it. 'When the wind was blowing in the right direction', some of these things would fall inside the chamber, others outside of it': Türk İnkilâp Tarihi Arşivi, 91/29/29(1-4).
90. Ölçen, *Vetluga Memoir*, pp. 88, 122.
91. Ibid. p. 111.
92. While many of the charges of executions are based on rumours, there are some eyewitness accounts as well. Two particular examples are Başkatipzade Ragıp Bey, *Tarih-i Hayatım*, p. 83 and Mehmed Âsaf, *Volga Kıyılarında*, pp. 77–8. See Süleyman Tevfik Harputlu, *Hayat Tarih Mecmuası*, v. 7, number 3 (Nisan 1971), p. 24 for rumours of such things. There are also a few references to escaped prisoners' corpses being returned to the prison camps. See, for example, Tuğaç, *Bir Neslin Dramı*, p. 121. Even if charges against the

Russians were not true, what matters more here is how the prisoners thought the Russians would respond, not actually how they responded in reality.

93. Examples of Turkic or Muslim peoples providing various help to the Ottoman POWs are numerous. Tatars everywhere helped the prisoners in all kinds of ways: Tuğaç, *Bir Neslin Dramı*, pp. 77, 129–30; Chechens in Grozny provided emotional support: Ataman, *Esaret Yılları*, p. 159. It was the same even farther east. In Krasnoyarsk, a Tatar named Abdurrahman helped Raci Çakıröz escape (Raci Çakıröz, *Çarlık ve Bolşevik Rusya'da 10 Yıl*, p. 28). In Harbin 'Türk-Tatar Cemaati İslamiyesi' donated money to Ottoman POWs who were stranded there awaiting repatriation: Ataman, *Esaret Yılları*, p. 202.

94. Of course, this was one way of escaping; not all escapees asked for help from local peoples. One should add that occasionally German civilians who had been exiled to distant parts of Siberia offered help to all Central Powers' prisoners including the Ottomans. See for example, Taşer, *Cepheden Cepheye*, pp. 82ff.

95. They were Ömer Selim, the civilian, and Captain Rıfat. Tuğaç, *Bir Neslin Dramı*, pp. 118–19, 126, 175. For other examples, see Ataman, *Esaret Yılları*, pp. 100, 110, 119.

96. 'Gayz', *Vaveyla*, 31 Mart 1333/31 March 1917, number 67, p 4. Full text of the poem is in Chapter 2.

97. Nureddin, 'Mısır Çöllerinde Türk Gençleri – 21', (2 Hazirar 1924)', p. 24. For a brief mention of some of the most creative ways to escape from a British camp see my 'From Cowardice to Illness', pp. 205–25.

98. Although Ottomans in Russia occasionally received help from the Swedish Red Cross or the YMCA, no inspection team travelled to Russia during the war specifically to listen to their problems. One exception is the mission of Yusuf Akçura in 1918, which came after the end of the war with Russia, although he was not able to visit the Siberian camps because of the Civil War and the Czech Legion's control of those areas. See also, Ölçen, *Vetluga Memoir*, pp. 214–16.

CHAPTER

2

IMAGINING COMMUNITY AND IDENTITY IN RUSSIA AND EGYPT: A COMPARISON

The last joke I heard of him [Sheikh As'ad Shuqueiri] is this: At the time of the armistice, the English arrested the Sheikh [As'ad] and took him to Sidi Bishr prisoner of war camp. Dressed in a blue shirt and a blue garment (*don*), the old man was living a sad life. One day, as he again was sitting cross-legged on the hot sand and thinking, he heard the voice of an Arab prisoner of war:

– O Allah! O Allah! . . .

– Don't my son, don't summon him [Sheikh As'ad said]. If Allah were to have a sudden desire to come down to rescue us, He will not be able rescue Himself from the hands of the English. Moreover, you will be the cause of leaving Muslims without Allah.

Falih Rıfkı Atay, *Zeytindağı*, p. 59

Chapter 1 demonstrated that the circumstances of capture, conditions of captivity and experiences of Ottoman prisoners in Russia were significantly worse than in the British camps in Egypt. This chapter investigates how those differing circumstances influenced construction and understanding of identity, identification, tradition, culture and nation. In so doing, it argues that the inferior conditions of life in the Russian camps contributed to a contentious sense of community among Ottoman prisoners. However, the presence of German and Austro-Hungarian prisoners, in close quarters with the Ottoman prisoners, was another significant reason for the hardening of boundaries around the concepts of nation, culture and tradition. Even the relatively easy access to Russian civilians became an important factor in this regard. Those Ottomans concerned with staying true to these sources of identification worried that some of their compatriots, those who did not seem to be aware of the cultural danger their imprisonment posed, had already begun to uncritically imitate and emulate European prisoners and Russian locals. Accordingly, Ottomans, rather than bonding together in the face of the captor, frequently turned to policing each other's behaviour, criticising those who did not work to preserve the imagined nation, its culture and traditions. However, the concerns that caused in-fighting among Ottoman prisoners in Russia did not even become issues in Egypt. It was not that the prisoners in Egypt did not care about nation, religion, culture and tradition, as they surely did. The main difference was that the conditions that created the 'narcissism of minor differences' in Russia did not exist in Egypt.

When encountering different cultures and practices, people gain the opportunity to reflect critically upon their own beliefs and practices.[1] Such encounters with different cultures produce critical reflexivity towards significant differences and heighten the sense of awareness of even every day, banal actions and practices. Consequently, even as banal actions and quotidian practices become markers of identification, they also serve to distinguish the nationals who do things properly from both the strange foreign Others and the domestic Others who do not do things properly. Because nationalist discourse authorises particular formulations of nation, culture and tradition, it also delegitimises other formulations, actions and behaviour as against tradition and nation. The purpose of this legitimation is to conceal divisions, differences and fractures within the nation. Under different circumstances, these processes may not be readily apparent, but prison camps function as ideal sites for observing the uneasy process of 'performing the nation'.[2]

IMAGINING THE ENEMY OTHER

European scholars have argued that few front-line troops in the Great War shared the 'hysterical' enemy-phobia which propaganda cultivated among civilians on the home front. Most soldiers developed a rather grudging respect for their opponents. They judged the enemy by the yardstick of his tenacity and courage under fire. According to Audoin-Rouzeau, 'It was this, which forbade the latter [enemy] to be denigrated. Self-respect and respect for the enemy were inseparable'.[3] The British enlisted men used terms like 'Johnny', 'the Allemand' or more affectionately, 'Old Fritz', to refer to the Germans, while their officers may have preferred the more sinister 'Bosche', originally a French slur meaning rascal.[4]

What did the Ottoman prisoners think of their adversaries? The Ottoman image of the British was ambiguously negative. As for the Russians, their image was unequivocally negative and dehumanised, with only occasional expressions of affinity. Moreover, how Ottoman prisoners viewed and imagined their enemy also tells us a great deal about the Ottomans who were doing the imagining. The following discussion will examine Ottoman prisoner soldier representations of the Russians, then the British.

In some ways, the nature of the war on the Caucasus front played a role in the Ottomans' image of the Russians. Because the war there had moving fronts, Ottoman civilians sometimes could not escape quickly enough and became victims of war and violence. After discovering the corpse of a young victim of brutal warfare in a village newly evacuated by Russian forces, one Ottoman officer exclaimed: '8–10 [Russian] soldiers raped and killed a young girl. [We] understood that there was no discipline in the army of these savage enemies of [sexual] honour and life'.[5] A captured officer reported witnessing Cossack soldiers beheading some lightly wounded Ottomans who fought under his command, while Russian officers failed to put a stop to this 'natural savagery' that characterised Cossacks.[6]

Sometimes the hatred of the captor was so overpowering that it became difficult for an individual prisoner to suppress it any longer. On one such occasion, an anonymous prisoner in Krasnoyarsk openly admitted to his hatred for his captors. In a poem, written for a camp newspaper – rather than for a private diary or a later memoir – the author graphically expressed the rage and humiliation felt by many Ottoman prisoners, as well as their collective image of the Russians.

Rage (*Gayz*)

In front of the angels who witnessed my perseverance,
Suddenly I became a prisoner in the claws of the *muzhik*s [Russian peasants].
It is difficult to become a prisoner of an army
that has been the religious, national, historical enemy of my nation since before the dawn of time.
If I were not surrounded by spies from all sides,
I would have revealed the hatred and rage that burn in my brain.
Bloody infidel! Phantasm injecting rage and hatred
into my forbearing heart, with that baseless conceit of yours.
Go on; seize the rule of every land . . .[7]

After establishing the Russians as the enemy of all those things the prisoner held dear – his religion, nation and history – he revealed that his revulsion extended to everything Russian. The experience of battlefield, capture and captivity created this savage image of the Russians for the poet, who depicted them in dehumanised terms, as clawed animals.

As the above poem also revealed, Ottomans regularly ascribed bestial qualities to Russians, which served to dehumanise them.[8] One prisoner, vowing never to forget the voice of his captor, labelled him a 'yellow-bearded, small, blue-eyed northern bear'.⁹ Another described one of his captors as 'a young officer . . . who was not much different from a little yellow [blond] piglet'.¹⁰ Russian soldiers stealing belongings of the captured Ottomans became 'carrion crows'.¹¹ In the heat of the battle, a quickly moving Russian enemy in an encirclement movement was a 'rabid hyena'¹² coming in to kill the wounded army. Noticeably, the species Ottomans selected to characterise Russians were animals that their culture considered to be of a lower order. Pigs were unclean and proscribed. The hyena and carrion crow are scavengers who feed upon the dead or dying. They are associated with gluttony, unseemliness and cowardice. While these dehumanising terms are evidence of a deep animosity or even hatred, it is important to remember that these were men who were vulnerable and at the mercy of their captors. Because they were completely at the mercy of their captors and had witnessed the inhuman behaviour of some Russians soldiers, their dehumanising of the Russians was an acknowledgement of the possibility that their life was dependent on the will of another.

There were, however, occasional moments when the prisoners could briefly identify with the enemy. An Ottoman officer who on another day might well have called the Russians 'demons from hell', was taken aback on hearing his guards singing as he was being sent to a prison camp after capture.

> A song rose from the throats of the Russian soldiers . . . It was so moving and beautiful that we [the Ottoman POWs] listened in silence. We were carried away by the sad melody of the song. The voice of an old and bearded Russian soldier in particular bewitched us. We didn't want him to stop.¹³

While the Ottomans did not understand the meaning of the Russian song, they were quick to sense the feelings and sadness of the words and the soldiers' behaviour. The captives were familiar with similar sad melodies and laments of Anatolia and here it seemed to them that they were hearing the Russian versions of those kinds of songs.

After the Ottoman prisoners became more exposed to Russian culture, they developed more feelings of affinity for Russian civilians. A change was noticeable in the way they talked about the Russian populace. When a POW convoy to Siberia stopped in a small Russian town to camp briefly, one prisoner commented, those 'unclean and awful smelling' Russian town-dwellers ran away from 'us like the devil running away from the recitation of *besmele* (pronunciation of the name of God and his attributes)'. Yet, two pages later, he went on to say that, upon hearing some young Russian peasant women singing at another small town used as a rest stop, 'the singing of the attractive girls penetrated our souls and for the moment made us forget the bitter pain of captivity'.[14] Perhaps in these Russian women – whose husbands, sons and brothers had gone off to the front – the prisoners saw their own loved ones whom they had left behind.

Russian authorities unwittingly facilitated closer relationships between the prisoners and the local populations. Much like in other places in Russia, the camp commandant in Vladivostok, for example, assigned enlisted Ottoman men to work for, and sometimes live with, local families whose eligible men were at the front.[15] The prisoners' assignments were to perform farm and household labour as directed by the women or elders of the house. İrfanoğlu İsmail Efendi, appointed to the unofficial position of camp imam in Vladivostok by the Russian commandant, initially viewed the Ottoman enlisted men helping the locals as a good policy. However, he quickly changed his mind when he discovered that, in a number of cases, sexual relationships had developed between the prisoners and the women whose husbands had been conscripted for the Russian army. The imam warned that such behaviour was against religious doctrines, but received the mocking response of 'What can I do? The young woman demands it! I am her prisoner; I must do what I am told, I just follow the orders'.[16] The situation the men found themselves in might best be described as one of mutual sexual opportunism. As some were willing to stay behind and marry these women, it becomes clear that these prisoners did not view civilian and female Russians in the same light as their captors and jailers.

Despite his criticism of the men's behaviour with Russian women, the imam himself was no acrimonious ogre. Allegedly, when one of the prisoners reported that a child had died in the house where he worked, and the bereaved mother could not afford the cost of an Orthodox funeral, the imam collected money among the men to donate to the woman. He also offered to conduct the child's burial with Islamic rites at the local Muslim cemetery free of charge, so that the mother would keep the money collected rather than giving it to the local priest. However, the men chastised the imam for this idea. 'How does this make sense?' they demanded. Though culturally chauvinistic and paternalistic in his answer, the imam explained: 'Everyone is born a Muslim and stay[s] a Muslim until they are seven years old. Up until that age, we treat the child as such. But after that, if he does not become a Muslim [consciously], that's a different story'. The mother agreed. With numerous Ottoman and other foreign prisoners in attendance, the child was buried in the Muslim cemetery. Muslim burial of a Christian child created a conflict with the local Orthodox priest when he discovered what had happened, but eventually the matter was resolved.[17]

Although we are not sure whether the men's unease resulted from the possibility of committing a sacrilege or from the possibility of offending the locals, the imam explained his behaviour. For him, soldiers having sexual relations with

Russian women and burying a Christian child with Islamic rites were completely separate issues. Extra-marital sexual relations represented a 'dilution of faith', while the burial represented a 'concentration of faith' because no part of Islamic faith was compromised.[18] 'Concentration of faith' strengthened the community of Ottomans, Muslims or Turks by gaining a possible convert, but the other meant losing followers as Turks and Muslims behaved like Russians. Russians might be 'bloody infidels' as enemies and captors in adulthood, but they could also be 'nominal Muslims' in childhood. Furthermore, the prisoners did not view the child or his mother as responsible for their captivity or any ill treatment suffered at the hands of the authorities.

Most Ottomans of all ranks viewed the Russians as the principal enemy, followed closely by the British.[19] However, the same colourful language and bestial imagery used to describe the Russians does not appear in descriptions of the British. In the words of a number of Ottoman prisoners, all British people, but especially the camp guards, were 'simple and vulgar', who 'had not taken their share from civilization'.[20] Eşref Kuşçubaşı, a member of the secretive *Teşkilat-ı Mahsusa* (Special Organization), expressed a similar sentiment while he was interned in Egypt:

> We used to think of the English as having the greatest respect for laws ... Yet I have come across many individual Englishmen who have punched and kicked the law in such a manner that I am now convinced that their respect for law and their vaunted humanity are pretty flimsy and useful only for show ... After the treatment I received at their hands, my love for the British turned to hatred. There is more respect for human dignity and rules of humanity among the Bedouins of Amir 'Abdullah[21] than one could find among the pseudo-civilized British.[22]

Kuşçubaşı's statement serves double duty; his disdain for the forces of 'Abdullah, who had rebelled against the Ottoman state along with his father Sharif Husayn in 1916 and later became king of Jordan, served as a measuring stick for his recently acquired dislike of the British.

Generally, the alterist discourse about the British revolved around the issues of 'civilization' and 'humanity'. Even when one encounters more strongly worded statements, they tend to be about ill-treatment, humanity and barbarity. Therefore, Sokrat İncesu put it this way: 'The inhumane and unethical treatment shown to the prisoners by the British soldiers is still fresh in my mind ... I leave to the [judgment of] our leaders and Turkish history the terrible, hateful, disgusting episodes I witnessed'.[23] Some disliked the British so much that, despite their boredom in captivity, they pointedly refused to learn English, although they were quite willing to learn other languages.[24] Despite the certainly offensive comments about the British, they seem almost harmless in comparison to those said about the Russian captors. Thus when the British soldiers took away the belongings of the captured Ottomans, they were not carrion crows or hyenas as the Russians became, but merely thieves at worst or just enemy soldiers looking for trophies and memorabilia from the war. Viewed in this way, British 'trophy collecting' became a more 'natural' activity.[25]

Why the significant difference between the images of the Russians and the British? For one, Ottoman prisoners did not share the positive attitudes the British- and French-front soldiers had for their German enemies. Moreover, capture changed the relationship between the two opposing sides; the Ottoman prisoners were no longer facing their enemies as equals in battle, but as victims in a vulnerable position vis-à-vis their captors. The moment they lost their status as warriors, their image of the enemy changed as well. Prisoners experienced anxiety and fear at the time of capture, and grappled with their change in status from warrior to prisoner. While all prisoners felt a sense of misfortune and loss of freedom at that point,[26] those who were captured by the Russians expressed more powerful rage and angst than in accounts from those captured by the British.

One example comes from Başkatipzade Ragıp Bey, a former madrasa student, captured on the Russian front. He skilfully illustrates the anxiety and fear that accompanied the moment of capture:

> What we saw was the point of a sword or a bayonet against our chests; what we felt was the chill of a rifle or a pistol against our necks. I could not comprehend anything; I lost my nerves; my body felt gelatinous. The only thing I could think of was that at the slightest wrong move I might have a sword or a bayonet piercing my heart or a bullet blowing my brains out.[27]

Başkatipzade Ragıp Bey described his fear in a way that was honest and real. Soldiers were expected to be brave and sacrifice themselves; therefore, it follows that a soldier would not exaggerate fear just to make a literary flourish. In fact, if anything, one would expect the opposite – an inclination to dismiss and downplay such feelings. But Ragıp Bey was entitled to his feelings, based on what he witnessed in fighting and experienced in being captured on the eastern Anatolian front.[28] This fear of being killed by the enemy also shaped the way Ragıp Bey and many others like him imagined the enemy. If the enemy was already depicted as dehumanised into a hyena or a carrion crow, then it was reasonable to expect him to behave in such a way. Interestingly, the Ottomans captured by the British did not leave any evidence of fearing for their lives. Certainly, they might have felt anxious and saddened, but no similar descriptions to that of Ragıp Bey exist.[29]

Imagining Community and Identity

Psychiatrists argue that, in stressful situations, members of groups become preoccupied with one another. In such situations, the process of dehumanisation occurs in stages; first, the enemy is demonised but retains human qualities, until he is eventually dehumanised.[30] Thus, in the more precarious wartime and captivity situation in Russia, Ottoman prisoners responded by completely dehumanising the Russian enemy. Later, as their situation became more stable, the prisoners re-assigned human qualities to the enemy, especially the civilians. In contrast, those prisoners captured by the British forces, who experienced a less hazardous situation, were content with simply demonising the enemy, viewing him as evil, calculating and uncivilised, but still human.

Of course, there is another explanation for the difference between how the Ottomans depicted their Russian and British captors. How the Ottoman prisoners viewed the captors was also a reflection of how that particular captor viewed and imagined Ottomans and the Ottoman Empire. For example, in the Russian imagination, Ottomans ranked third on their traditional enemies list.[31] Similarly, as some of the encounters between the Ottoman prisoners and local Russians revealed, Russians had a demonised and dehumanised image of Ottomans themselves, expecting them to have tails and horns or other dehumanised qualities.[32] How did the Ottomans imagine the Russians? Ottomans similarly dehumanised the Russians into beasts. Many contemporary British travel narratives and political works on the Ottoman Empire treated it as backward and lacking in civilisation. Accordingly, then, Ottomans thought the British were barbarous and lacking in civilisation.

ETHNIC RELATIONS AMONG THE PRISONERS

Different captivity conditions also influenced inter-ethnic relations among prisoners, especially among Turks and Arabs. The former formed the majority of the army, followed by Arabs. As per the captivity narratives, Arab and Turkish officer prisoners had comparatively cordial relations until the Arab rebellion against the Ottoman state in 1916. From an ethnic Turkish perspective, the rebellion was the discursive point of origin for the crisis, and all had been well up to that point. Of course, the Arab perspective was different. It is not that the two groups did not get along, but there was certainly a souring of relations after the rebellion, although from the Turkish perspective much more depended on how Arabs 'acted' in captivity. For example, a British document noted that when Shia and Christian Arabs in an Egyptian camp joyfully celebrated the news of the fall of Baghdad in March 1917, ethnic Turks were visibly bothered.[33] The note makes no mention of how Sunni Arabs received the news. The point of the discussion below is not to give a platform to resentful and even hateful statements about Arabs by Turks, but to examine how dislocatory events – points of crises such as captivity, rebellion or losing a war – led to blaming and scapegoating, which served as aspects of identity claims.

A significant proportion of Turkish captivity narratives from Russia have something disparaging to say about the Arab-Ottomans, either in general or by identifying specific individuals. While some of these comments are not friendly, they are also not hateful in spirit. They range from questioning Arab understanding of Islam to questioning their loyalty to the Ottoman state.[34] The quote below comes from a memoir that is especially critical of Arabs. Imprisoned in a commandeered house in the town of Varnavino, near Vetluga, Lieutenant Mehmet Arif wrote: 'there were those who were against some innocuous musical entertainment, mainly Arab officers. They declared that musical instruments were forbidden by Islamic canon law'. Mehmet Arif identified those who complained about the music as 'mainly Arabs', which therefore probably includes Turks as well, but singled out Arab officers for criticism:

> Among those who opposed [playing music] . . . was a[n] [Arab] captain who had married a [Turkish] girl . . . in Istanbul. After a year of marriage, however, he left her and went back to his [family] home in Baghdad . . . This man who said that playing musical instruments was religiously forbidden was able to intimidate people even though he had left his wife and new born child hungry and destitute in Istanbul.[35]

The fact that the abandoned wife was a 'Turkish girl' was important, but it also mattered to Mehmet Arif because the act raised the question of what constituted the bigger sin: playing music to entertain oneself in captivity, or abandoning one's wife and child in an impoverished situation. Mehmet Arif's statement had multiple layers of meaning. Although the Arab captain might have spoken as if he possessed authoritative religious knowledge, from Mehmet Arif's perspective he certainly did not have proper knowledge of Islam to recognise the hypocrisy of his own actions. Of course, Islam was assumed as the religion of Arabs, but one that was not understood by Arabs.

While Mehmet Arif did not say it directly, Lieutenant Faik [Tonguç], in Vetluga, boldly voiced this attitude:

> In terms of religion, Turks are probably more religious and more devoted to their religion than Arabs . . . In terms serving for the maintenance of religion, Arabs are well behind [Turks] . . . It was Turks who took Islam, born in the deserts of Arabia, to the interiors of Europe.[36]

Imagining Community and Identity

In this way, Arabs not only failed to understand Islam properly, but they were also not sufficiently devoted to it. Therefore, they were thought to be incapable of defending it and the job had fallen to Turks. Both Mehmet Arif and Faik had clear secularist tendencies. They criticised Arabs' misunderstanding of Islam, but they also had scorn for those who used religion to manipulate people and to suppress activities they did not like. Mehmet Arif may have singled out the Arab officer from Baghdad, but there were non-Arabs in the group who also pronounced music as offensive to the sharia.

It seems that for relatively small places, Vetluga and Varnavino witnessed more than their share of conflicts between Turks and Arabs. In the Turkish accounts, Arabs were always to blame for one reason or another. For example, Lieutenant Faik wrote that when all but a few of the Arab Ottoman POWs in his camp volunteered for British-Sherifian service to fight against the Ottoman forces, the Turkish officers became very agitated. Finally, they

> gave the necessary lesson to these insolent (*küstahlar*) [Arabs] . . . These traitors (*hain*) . . . [who] made clear their contempt for Turkishness sank so low as to volunteer to fight against us who were their comrades in arms only a short while ago. They were not even bothered by their insolence in declaring their hatred and feelings [for us] in these lands of the enemy.[37]

Having already excluded Arabs by referring to Turkishness, rather than to Ottomanness, as a nodal reference point of common identity, Faik blamed Arabs for their disloyalty to Turkishness. In his view, the Arab 'treachery' became an even worse offence because of where this event unfolded. This public display of 'lack of loyalty' to Turkishness by Arab officers in front of a more hated enemy was the bigger affront for Faik because it proved what already did not exist: Arab commitment to Turkishness. The Turkish response to Arab 'insolence' was an important moment of identification, in which the subject, the Turkish prisoner, is produced by identifying with an object 'external' to itself, Turkishness and the Turkish nation. At the same time, this object, the Turkish nation, achieves a social existence through being identified with it by the subject, the prisoners who claimed themselves to be Turkish as distinct from those Arabs.[38]

Certainly, not all Turkish prisoners viewed all Arabs in this way all the time. Moreover, in some cases, it was not necessarily and exclusively the ethnicity of Arabs that created a problem for the Turks. Rather, it was the 'questionable' behaviour of some people who were Arabs. Clearly, though, more Arabs exhibited 'questionable' behaviour than any others. Still, one could suggest that, in these instances, they were blamed for 'not acting like Turks'. Some of the animosity towards both the ethnic and domestic Others emanated from conditions of war, captivity, and the seemingly inevitable defeat as some prisoners searched for someone or something to blame. Sometimes being a Turk or an Arab mattered less than one's actions.

Lieutenant Ahmet's account of an event which took place in a prison camp near Arkhangelsk, northern Russia, illustrates this dynamic nicely. A group of Ottoman officers, consisting of Turks and Arabs, were peacefully chatting about the war, when an 'Arab' colonel, a battalion commander during the war, revealed something shocking about the night they were all captured by the enemy. The colonel said that even though he had received orders from headquarters to increase the number of sentries because of an expected Russian attack, he purposefully removed the regulation number of sentries, clearing the path of the enemy and thereby 'avenging his race', as Lieutenant Ahmet remembered it. 'Suddenly, there was [a moment of] eerie silence because no one [immediately] grasped the gravity of the situation'. The silence ended when Ahmet shouted 'you scoundrel!' as he launched himself toward the colonel. 'Instinctively, other Arab officers [also] attacked the colonel', just as other Turkish officers became involved.

This moment was about Turks and Arabs attacking someone who was directly responsible for their captivity. Yet, immediately after this story, Lieutenant Ahmet launched into another about an Arab captain from Baghdad to show that not all Arabs were like the colonel. This captain 'fought like a lion day after day'. In the end, 'this native son of [our] land threw himself upon an enemy machine gun as his body was nearly mowed down in half by bullets; [as he died], he became the commander of all martyrs (şehitlere serdâr)'.[39] Two Arabs: one treacherous, one a selfless martyr, from Ahmet's perspective. One 'avenged his race', the other sacrificed himself for '[our] land'. In this context, one could suggest that the conflict was less about ethnicity, but more about behaviour and actions. In this case, for Lieutenant Ahmet, an ethnic Other who behaves like 'us' becomes 'one of us' and of 'our land'.

Similarly, sometimes the ethnicity or religion of those whose actions were questioned mattered little even at the time of conflict; they were simply 'others' causing 'us' harm. In reporting an egregious event during a period of significant food shortage, Lieutenant Mehmet Arif only noted that the offenders were non-Turks. He was irritated with a group of Ottoman prisoners-turned-profiteers who had been collaborating with Russian guards.

> We noticed that the opportunists [who had joined the Russian soldiers to charge us exorbitant prices for basic food items] were those who had joined the Turkish army from the various ethnic communities belonging to the Ottoman state. We

stopped them from cooperating with the Russian soldiers. They were a minority. There was a strong reaction against their behavior. They were prevented from exploiting their fellow prisoners by cooperating with the Russians. Cicero, the famous Roman orator, began a speech by saying, 'O bastard children of the Romans! There are no longer real Romans among you, for a bastard generation has appeared from the Romans who mixed with the foreign people of the countries they conquered'. Those who cooperated with the Russian sergeant were the bastard children of Turkey.[40]

His ethnicist – or even racist – tone is unmistakable, but two other things are noticeable in Mehmet Arif's words: first, the collective action of aggrieved prisoners, presumably Turks, in the face of price gouging by fellow prisoners of other ethnicities; and secondly, the 'Ottomanness' of the state, but 'Turkishness' of the army. While the 'collaborators' were Ottoman because they lived within the empire, they could be discursively excluded from the military, which some Turks clearly saw as their domain. In order to determine whether a well-pronounced ethnic dislike towards Arabs was prevalent among Turks, it is instructive to ask whether these kinds of physical conflicts also occurred in the Egyptian camps.

Although not completely free of friction or arguments that turned physical, Arabs and Turks in the Egyptian prison camps fared better. Given that the British had fomented the Arab revolt and were coordinating it from Cairo, this may seem surprising. More aggressively than the Russians, the British had also recruited Arab volunteers from among the prisoners to fight against the Ottoman armies, but accusations of treachery did not immediately follow in the Turkish captivity memoirs.[41] In comparison to many significant fights recorded in the Russian camps, only one fight between the Arabs and Turks in Egypt stands out. This fight involved about ten to fifteen officers on each side, including Rahmi Apak, the officer who went on a hunger strike, described in Chapter 1. He noted that the confrontation started when an Arab-Ottoman 'captain from Baghdad and an Armenian-Ottoman doctor at the rank of lieutenant colonel started to criticize Turks in loud voices'. Rahmi decided that they were intentionally loud because they meant for him and other Turkish officers to hear the criticism through the reed-matting screen which separated them. A derogatory response from Rahmi to the two non-Turkish officers was enough to start a fight.[42] Yet, despite Arabs attacking him immediately, Rahmi Apak chose to blame the fight on being 'instigated' by the British camp commander.[43] In this only reported occasion of a physical ethnic confrontation in an Egyptian camp, Rahmi feared that a hidden hand had instigated the fight. Arabs who collaborated with the enemy in Russia were 'lowly' and declared their 'hatred' for Turks and Turkishness, but

Arabs who directly attacked Rahmi and others in Egypt were only pawns in the hands of the British. The difference in the imagery is significant, but only up to a point. Turks in Egypt did not seem to 'dislike' Arabs or find them to be 'lowly', as those in Russia did, but in the end Arabs were still painted as those who collaborated with the enemy.

If the physical fight just described was an exception, then the relations between Arabs and Turks in Egypt can best be described as mutual gradual disengagement. A story told by another prisoner, Emin Çöl, illustrates this well. Born in Mersin, he had gone to a military school in Beirut and graduated as a non-commissioned officer of the second rank. Just prior to capture by the British in Beersheba, Emin lost his eyesight in action because of an explosion. In Egypt, his captors placed him in the camp for enlisted men and assigned Tahsin Efendi, a classmate and friend of Emin from Beirut, to be his guide. Being friends, the two got along well, but Emin thought whenever Tahsin went to chat with other Arabs in the camp, he always came back with an 'aggravated attitude'. Emin wrote: 'Because my friend's [maternal] grandmother was an Arab, he took after his family [in temperament]'. That temperament made possible what came next: 'In the Ottoman army, [Arab] officers and NCOs, the likes of Tahsin, once they became a prisoner, discovered their Arabness. These types were trying to get out of captivity [by volunteering for the forces of Sherif Hussein]'. Did they want to join the Sherif because they wanted to fight for the Arab cause, or was this merely an opportunity to escape captivity? Finally, things came to a boiling point after Tahsin came back from another visit with his Arab friends. Suddenly, he said, 'We suffered for centuries under the oppressive regime of Turks, but now we are liberated'. Emin responded: 'Are you liberated from us, or we from you?' Although Tahsin did not respond, both knew their friendship was over. Emin asked the camp authorities for someone else to assist him.[44] Had an Arab in Russia made similar comments, it would have been enough to turn the confrontation violent. Because prisoners in Russia were already on edge, such a slight often resulted in physical fights. But here, there was no physical violence, only a separation of ways. The parting statements from each side, but especially from Emin, signal something worth examining in more detail.

The issue of who was 'liberated' from whom, or a variant of that theme, came up in many other instances. In fact, insofar as the topic of Arabs comes up at all in other Egyptian captivity narratives, it was often in regard to the Arab rebellion, not the Arab-Ottoman prisoners in the camps. Many saw the rebellion as one of the main reasons for the Ottoman defeat, and thus one of the reasons for their captivity. Another prisoner in Egypt, Captain Sokrat (Socrates) İncesu, a Greek-Ottoman, originally from Kayseri in central Anatolia, expressed resentment of the Arab rebellion. His attitude on the rebellion is emblematic of many others:

> The role of the British spy Lawrence in the Arab rebellion is an undeniable fact. We came from central Anatolia to fight and rescue the integrity and honour (*şeref ve namus*) of the Arabs from being trampled by enemy boots; history will never forgive them for stabbing us in the back.⁴⁵

The imagery here is instructive. The rebellion could not have happened without T. E. Lawrence, and the Arabs did not recognise that 'Turks' were there to protect Arab honour and dignity. Thus, they committed the unforgivable act of stabbing the Turk in the back. Hüseyin Aydın, an ethnic Turk imprisoned in Egypt, shared the sentiments of Sokrat and Emin that Arabs lived comfortably for centuries while Turks fought to save those lands for Arabs or in defence of Islam.⁴⁶ In this way, undeterred by the attraction of a comfortable life, Turks felt obligated to sacrifice themselves for causes other than their own. In highlighting the role of Lawrence or the British government in general, these statements also attempt to delegitimise the rebellion as well.

Something else stands out. Surely, one could make a military case that the Arab rebellion certainly made the defeat of the Ottomans more possible; however, the discourse about Arab 'comfort', while Turks alone fought to defend them or Islam is a nationalist mythology. It paints Arabs as unconcerned about defending themselves and Islam, and therefore, lazy or aloof. These sentiments about Arabs were fully shared by the Turkish prisoners in Russia. Mustafa Fevzi proudly claimed that Turks had turned Islam from a tribal religion into a world religion. In the process of defending Islam and Arabs, Turks made enemies of the European Christians. The price of this sacrifice was high: 'We exchanged our Turkishness [and Turkish culture] with Muslimness and Arab culture' and 'became concerned' about them, not about ourselves.⁴⁷ Thus, many Turks believed that their nation and homeland of Anatolia was poor because all the wealth went to Arabs. By adopting Arab religion and culture, Turks denied their true identity. In the end, all this Turkish sacrifice was 'awarded' by a rebellion, which they regarded as a stab in the back. Turks' innate altruism and Arab perfidy (*hıyanet*) were convenient shorthand explanations as to why Turks found themselves poor, helpless, defeated and disordered during the Great War. These all helped to explain why the nation, the empire and Anatolia were in their current state. This line of reasoning also preserved the faith in the Turkish nation and its future as a united and powerful nation undeterred by those who take advantage of Turks' altruism.

As the foregoing showed, there were certainly some conflicts and disagreements between Turks and Arabs in Egypt, but they were not as common and certainly not as frequently violent as those in Russia. Given the reported frequency of poor inter-ethnic relations in Russia, could this be attributed to something in the nature of captivity there? So that contingency can be ruled out, the chapter will now turn to examine daily encounters among ethnic Turks.

GENERATIONAL AND INTER-RANK RELATIONS

Yet another visible dividing line among the Ottoman prisoners was based on military rank, which takes the form of generational conflict as well. Perhaps it is no surprise that frequent references to unfriendly relations between junior and senior officers in Russia pepper their captivity memoirs. Rather than naming individuals in their writings, junior officers often used the term *ümera*, literally, high ranking officers, to collectively refer to those more senior in rank, or to ranks of major and above.

The junior officers' resentment of their seniors reached such a level that nearly every Russian memoir abounds with complaints, accusations and even expressions of abhorrence for superiors. The kindest term prisoners in Russia used in reference to *ümera* was 'obstructionist', but the language was often a lot stronger than that.

Ümera in Russia could be considered obstructionist, dull and callous for a number of simple reasons. Although they all realised that they were required to abide by the military power structure, the junior officers sometimes questioned the motivations and decisions of their higher-rank officers. One account from Krasnoyarsk related that whenever the junior officers wanted to organise theatrical and musical groups, or even to have the Qur'an recited on religious and national holidays, the senior officer in charge invented one excuse after another to deny the requests. Hilmi Erbuğ noted that Colonel Arif Baytin, the highest-ranking Ottoman prisoner, always used the same paternalistic excuse – that anything smacking of religion and nationalism would anger the Russians and, as a result, put the Ottoman prisoners in danger.[48] Without much success, junior officers reminded Arif Bey that German and Austro-Hungarian POWs in the same camp used every occasion – Franz Joseph's birthday, Christmas and even the Ottoman victory in Gallipoli – to organise large gatherings without incurring the Russians' anger. The juniors' request to establish a theatrical group was repeated numerous times until Arif Bey and other *ümera* finally authorised a one-time performance. With no negative reaction from their Russian captors, the floodgates opened, and Arif Bey no longer stood in the way of other plays being produced.[49] Perhaps because the *ümera* feared a backlash and the juniors did not want to beg continually for permission, they decided to organise other activities without seeking 'official' approval from Arif Bey. Even then, the disapproving behaviour of 'our dull, callous and insensible superiors' might have always been there, but it did not stop those who wanted to make something of their time in captivity.⁵⁰ For instance, in 1919, after the Russian Revolutions when the prisoners' salaries were cut off and chaos in Siberia made life even more difficult, Arif Bey, the highest-ranking Ottoman in Krasnoyarsk, opened a 'teahouse' in the camp, which he called '*HayLayf*' (High Life).⁵¹ Clearly, by then, even Arif Bey had to realise that he had been overly cautious – if his cautiousness was the real reason why he initially turned down requests about theatrical plays.

The complaints of the junior officers about their superiors ranged from mild to severe. For instance, on one occasion, Ragıp Bey accused the seniors of unfair division of the supplies – blankets, coats, hats, boots, etc. – provided by the Red Cross, a rare event in itself. The junior officers and the more needy enlisted men had to share what the higher ranks did not want: 'It was only after the *ümera* had the first pick of the supplies, the remaining was divided by lottery among the junior officers and men', he noted.⁵² Since a lottery system was used to divide the remainder, it meant that not everyone received anything, while the *ümera* had their choice.

Ragıp Bey also provides a more egregious example of *ümera* corruption. When the invalid prisoners in Krasnoyarsk heard that those who were sickly and invalid would soon be repatriated, they rejoiced. But according to Başkatipzade Ragıp Bey, their happiness did not last very long. He noticed a conspiracy arising in response to the policy, one that bothered him deeply. He reported, 'unfortunately, in reality the poor infirm soldiers could not take advantage of this right'. As it turned out, the *ümera* and Ottoman doctors in the camp colluded to declare the senior officers invalids, even going so far as to provide invented diseases and conditions, rather than helping those who had actual medical justification for repatriation. Ragıp Bey continued, noting that 'the senior officers turned out to be invalids!!! They wanted to go back to the homeland as soon as possible!!! . . . This was the biggest crime committed by doctors [and *ümera*] in captivity'. Another senior officer's recording of this event corroborates Ragıp Bey's charges. This angry lieutenant, graduate of a madrasa education, fell shy of calling his superiors derogatory names, but he was not bashful as he accused them of unethical and selfish behaviour.⁵³

Junior officers in Egypt also complained about the *ümera*. However, the relationship between the groups was not nearly as troubled, nor was trouble as common and as continuous as in Russia. For example, when the junior officers in Egypt griped about the senior officers arranging to have themselves listed as invalids and elderly to allow for early repatriation, they did not have to confine their reaction to their personal memoirs and diaries. Rather, they turned to their camp newspapers, and expressed their derision with satire and wit. One of these pieces, titled 'Prayers for Youth and Old Age', actually poked fun at the *ümera* and their efforts, rather than expressing contempt. Other criticism appeared in the form of caricatures in the camp newspapers. Even in memoirs, where some criticism appears about the *ümera*, it was always mild in nature.[54]

While junior officers in Russia were offended at the *ümera*'s objections and perceived obstructionism to their efforts, those in Egypt were offended by something else. They grumbled about the *ümera*'s lack of interest and participation in camp activities, like taking part in anything useful or educational. As Rahmi Apak put it, in Egypt, the Ottoman 'colonels, lieutenant colonels, majors stayed in the barracks and did not get involved in anything; they were awaiting the armistice'. Junior officers thought that there was so much the *ümera* could be doing – such as teaching languages to officers, or reading and writing to the enlisted men.[55] In other words, the junior officers in Russia denounced the *ümera* as obstructionists, unethical and selfish, while those in Egypt found them to be unmotivated and uninvolved. From the junior officers' perspective, the latter was much better.

In Russia, signs of a growing lack of respect for the senior officers appeared over time. It was one thing to be critical of the *ümera*, but it was another to openly defy or ignore them. They were still, after all, superior ranking officers. For example, Lieutenant Mehmet Arif reported on disrespect for authority and superiors in Varnavino. He observed that some superiors were requesting clearly personal favours in the form of an order, and he was not reluctant to turn them down, because it amounted to an abuse of power.[56] However, he also thought that some young officers were not making an ethical distinction between a legitimate order given by a superior and one that was personal. These people simply turned to open defiance of their superiors: 'We were confused. No one listened to anyone else. We often heard such words as "You are a prisoner here and I am a prisoner here. You have no authority to intervene"'.[57] It seems that the some junior officers regarded captivity as a levelling experience, one that wiped out distinctions of rank once they all became prisoners. Mehmet Arif implied that the disrespect against authority and hierarchy was partially the result of psychological factors. However, on occasion, it probably was also the result of conscious effort to deny deference and respect to senior officers for their real and perceived inequitable behaviour. Whatever the reasons, it is important to underscore that these conflicts all occurred in Russian camps. Due to the dire physical conditions, senior officers may have clung more defiantly to their power, however meaningless in the camp, to preserve their own sense of power. If the accusations against the *ümera* are at least partially true, we might interpret their behaviour both as selfish and uncaring, as the junior officers saw it, but also as the *ümera*'s way of attempting to maintain a distance between themselves and the junior officers.

TRADITIONS UNDER THREAT: MAINTAINING 'NATIONAL' IDENTITY

A number of factors – the physical layout of the places of internment, the senior officers' involvement and authority, easy access by prisoners to townspeople – worked to undermine unity and the sense of community and cooperation among Ottoman prisoners in Russia. Relations between junior and senior officers posed one set of issues, but the junior officers also quarrelled amongst themselves. In a number of these quarrels, concern over issues of cultural and national identification and tradition seemed to be the cause of disagreement and resentment. Comparatively speaking, the more stressful and anxiety-ridden Russian prison camps resulted in more noticeable breakdown of social, cultural and even military norms.

Most junior officer conflicts in Russia were verbal confrontations, but some turned violent. Lieutenant Mehmet Arif reported a disturbing event in Varnavino, where prisoners had been placed in commandeered large houses. A young junior officer, who lived in the same house as Mehmet Arif, and the daughter of the family across the street had established a relationship. From the attic window of the prisoners' house, the young officer could see into the girl's house and communicate with her by use of signals. MehmetArif noted that 'whenever our young lieutenant would find a way to leave the barracks, she and her family would go out for a walk as well'. The officer planned, somehow, to meet up with the girl and talk to her. Despite the reputed innocence of the whole affair, some other Ottoman prisoners, presumably older in age and higher in rank than the young officer, had noticed his signals to the girl. They did not see anything innocent about what was going on, as Mehmet Arif reported:

> We were soon to learn that this matter affected the honor of our barracks. The young officer's signals ... supposedly sullied the honor of the fellow prisoners and cast a shadow on their dignity. A few officers took upon themselves the task of defending the honor of the barracks. They seized the young lieutenant and began to beat him in the presence of the women. The crying and shouting of the women and their attempt to explain by gestures that the fists that struck the officer were blows at their own hearts deeply affected a great many of us.[58]

As he ridiculed the aggressors, Mehmet Arif asked sarcastically, 'Was this young lieutenant going to make a cuckold of the officers in the barracks in broad daylight? The barracks had honor. They thought they were defending it. Who was going to defend the honor of the officer who was felled by blows?'[59] While some were 'pleased' with the punishment of the young officer, Mehmet Arif and others were astounded that a few officers took it upon themselves to vindicate the 'honor of the barracks' by committing public violence against one of their own. Any prisoner who raised the issue of reporting the incident to the Russian commander in town was warned not to because 'it would create erroneous opinions about Turkish society in the mind of the Russian captain and further sully our national honor'.[60]

For Mehmet Arif, some demonstrated that they did not understand the connection between the 'honor of the barracks' and 'national honor' by taking the action they did. In the end, the national honour was 'protected' by not reporting the event to the Russian captain, but Mehmet Arif and others resolved to report it to the Ministry of War when they were repatriated.[61] Although he realised that discouraging reporting might encourage the aggressors, Mehmet Arif was incensed about those who got away with horrible behaviour. However, he also had no intention of drawing more attention to their internal problems.

The image Ottoman prisoners projected to townspeople and guards was important to many like Mehmet Arif. He reported another incident that he found more disturbing than waving to a Russian girl across the street. After years of wearing them through war and captivity, winter and summer, day and night, the prisoners' uniforms had started to fall apart. Rather than repairing them, some Ottoman officers decided to put away their uniforms to save them for repatriation. However, instead of finding something appropriate to wear, these officers 'sewed lose robes, like nightshirts, and began to walk about in them' in and outside of the barracks. They did not notice 'how ridiculous they looked wearing robes on their backs, skullcaps on their heads [*takke*], and [wooden] clogs on their feet' in plain view of the townspeople.[62] During favourable weather, they sat outside and 'watched those who passed by but paid no attention to those who looked at them. They did not realize', complained Mehmet Arif, 'that they were exposing the Turkish army and nation to ridicule'.[63]

If the pyjama-wearing officers opened up the army and nation to ridicule, why didn't the rest of the prisoners do something about it? In fact, it turned out that the prisoners in Varnavino were preoccupied with more pressing concerns. Some prisoners had taken advantage of the general reluctance to speak to the Russian commander about internal problems, and exploited that situation to get away with all manner of bad behaviour. 'The prescription "to protect national honor" greatly increased the insolence of some of the prisoners', Mehmet Arif noted. 'They became ruder and more aggressive . . . The actions of those who gambled at night or pulled knives and attacked each other were hushed up . . .' Reluctance to inform the Russian commander or punish the guilty themselves resulted in fourteen serious incidents in two years, mostly 'fights or brawls'.[64] Mehmet Arif noted, 'it was the duty of all of us to protect our honor as the officers of a great nation, but some of us had forgotten this . . . [O]ur uncertainty about our future, combined with the political confusion of the country [Russia], intensified our apprehension. The instability affected all of us'.⁶⁵ The political chaos in Russia after the revolutions and the prisoners' own psychological response to such chaos and uncertainty about their own future further undermined the understood norms about proper behaviour.

While some prisoners responded by turning inward, focusing on their own immediate needs, others became distressed about what they perceived as visible threats to, and disregard for, nation, religion, culture and tradition within the camps. They preoccupied themselves with worries about tears in the national fabric. One such prisoner in Krasnoyarsk was Başkatipzade Ragıp Bey. He was particularly anxious about the threat that European prisoners posed to national culture and tradition. In this case, he remarked on European prisoners' habit of bathing naked, 'without using waist cloth (*peştemal*)'. While the practice certainly offended him, he could dismiss it as 'their custom'. However, when some Ottoman prisoners started to imitate this behaviour, he complained bitterly: 'just when we were criticizing this European habit, an increasing number of mischievous and fickle-tempered Turks also started to bathe completely naked'. Ragıp Bey lamented yet another newly invented impropriety among some Ottoman prisoners. Some officers had 'started to walk about outside bareheaded and naked-legged [*başı açık, baldırı çıplak*]'. That is, 'without hats and in shorts' in the European fashion, during summer time.⁶⁶ Another prisoner, Hasan Basri, agreed, and concluded that these types showed little 'traces' of being Muslims.

Such *alafranga* (*alla Franca*; 'European') behaviour did not end there. Ragıp Bey had noted positively earlier that many Ottoman prisoners took advantage of the presence of German and Hungarian prisoners in the camps and attempted to learn a foreign language. In fact, he had picked up some German in that way. However, he soon noticed a 'threatening' side to this otherwise great learning opportunity. What disturbed Ragıp Bey and a number of other officers was that sometimes this teacher-pupil relationship took on what he described as homoerotic tendencies.

> In fact, any Turkish officer who fancied some young and 'moustache-less' [handsome] foreign officer immediately picked him [the foreigner] as his teacher and thus became acquainted with their 'cursed ideas' . . . This kind of behaviour did not bother Europeans, for they did not put much value in such matters. In fact, [they] apparently did not understand honour in terms of sexual honour.⁶⁷

Even when no such homoerotic situation existed, he was still uneasy because of the very familiar discourse and too close a friendship (*pek çok ülfet etmek*) some Ottoman officers established with European prisoners.

Almost equally disturbed, Hasan Basri noted in his diary in 1916 about another new practice among some Ottoman prisoners. 'Yesterday, the new fashion appeared among friends here: shaving their moustaches. It spread from youngsters to elderly (or juniors to seniors) . . . Since we are not used to it, it presents an extremely ugly scene to one's eye'.[68] In a culture where a moustache was a symbol of virility, this statement was not simply about aesthetics or what was ugly, unsightly or handsome, but about the proper way of looking or behaving like a Turk or Ottoman. What made it improper in his eyes was that the 'fashion' was the result of aping European prisoners in an attempt to look and behave like them. He was more concerned about the evidence that the Europeans were having an influence on his countrymen.

Given his feelings above, Ragıp Bey might have read more into becoming 'moustache-less' like the Europeans than Hasan Basri Efendi did. In Ragıp's case, it was the Europeans who were moustache-less that some Ottomans befriended; here it was a case of Ottomans becoming moustache-less. Differences between European and Ottoman-Turkish culture, honour and codes of behaviour were clear to Ragıp Bey and others, but as he saw it, not to all Ottoman prisoners – and this posed a threat to the future of the nation, especially if these prisoners took these strange, European practices home.

Threats to culture, tradition and proper ways of behaving could come from anywhere, even from those theatrical plays some junior officers so badly wanted to organise in Krasnoyarsk. Colonel Arif Bey, as the highest-ranking Ottoman, had first opposed plays with the excuse of such cultural activity possibly angering the Russians. For Ragıp Bey, also in the same camp, the problem was of a different nature. Plays often reflected home life, everyday interactions and families in which women were present. Who performs the female roles in a prison camp play? Ragıp Bey reported about the first play: 'the first clownery [play], something called cabaret, was produced by Gabaracı Halil in which some Turkish officers played like girls'. This was bad enough, but there followed plays in which 'Turkish officers performed belly dancing'. Moreover, other officers watching the plays 'got drunk in the theatre and tossed bottles, danced, and resorted to all kinds of charlatanry'.[69] Both the officers in drag and those who sought the close company and tutoring of handsome Europeans were a threat to cultural traditions according to Ragıp Bey. For him and other like-minded officers, that kind of behaviour was a source of anxiety as it challenged the respectable gender identities they believed were dictated by tradition. From some Ottomans preferring moustache-less Europeans as teachers to others dressing in drag for entertainment, it might have seemed to Ragıp Bey as if many Ottomans or Turks had simply abandoned all tradition and custom as they copied the European prisoners in the camps.

Prisoners in Egypt also performed in plays, and comparatively many more of them; did they get the same kind of reaction as provided above by Ragıp Bey in Russia? In 1920, after a double-feature theatrical play, the camp newspaper, *Yarın*, reviewed both in its pages. While expecting to see Hüseyin Rahmi's *Mürebbiye* (*Governess*), a national satirical play that attacked the prevalent elite custom of entrusting children to the care of domineering governesses from Europe, the prisoners, once in their seats, realised that they would see a '*Frenk* [French or European] comedy' in addition. The *Yarın* reviewer found the young 'mademoiselle' in the play riveting. 'As she played with her skirt and moved about flirtatiously, she was, to tell the truth, more woman than [a real] woman'. He went on to praise 'her' further before moving onto the second play of the night. Given the subject matter and critique of using European governesses in *Mürebbiye*, the British camp authorities only approved a censored version of the play. The reviewer could not help but compare Angel, the French governess in *Mürebbiye*, to the mademoiselle in the first comedy. It was a close call, but the mademoiselle was apparently much more impressive with her feminine charms than Angel.[70] Why was there such glaring difference in the way Ottoman officers in drag were perceived by Ragıp Bey, on the one hand, and the reviewer in *Yarın*, on the other?

Other prisoners in Krasnoyarsk mention the plays only in passing; they provide neither glowing reviews like those in Egypt, nor firm disapprovals like Ragıp Bey. Perhaps they saw the theatre simply as an activity that entertained them while interned in a prison camp. Rather than disapproving of theatre as a cultural activity in general, Ragıp Bey detested at least two things about theatre in Krasnoyarsk. These officers were the representatives of the state and the nation in this foreign land. For Ragıp Bey, they did not take their role seriously. Instead they turned to swishing around in skirts and dresses in this moment of crisis. However, Ottoman officers in Egypt also dressed in drag without attracting a single criticism of their behaviour. What made the crucial difference was that whether in drag, or bathing naked, or walking around without a hat, or engaging in 'homoerotic behaviour', these Ottoman prisoners were, at bottom, guilty of imitating European prisoners with whom they shared camps and whose plays and activities they watched and participated in. In short, the problem was the emulation of European prisoners and customs. 'Naked bathing' never became an issue in the Egyptian camps because there were no European prisoners to copy. Therefore, the prisoners used their *peştamal* (wrap cloths) as they would have at home. Some prisoners in Egypt wore shorts as supplied by the British, but no one called them 'bare-legged', and the donning of shorts was certainly not interpreted as an affront against national culture and tradition.

Blind imitation of European behaviour by fellow Ottomans, therefore, represented a danger to the fabric of the community for the likes of Ragıp Bey. Yet Ragıp Bey was no xenophobe. He conversed with, established friendships and learned German from Europeans. He believed that he and other Ottomans had much to learn from them. He was certainly friendly enough with them, but if he maintained a certain distance, this was not clearly apparent in his captivity narrative. In fact, in some instances Ragıp Bey saw himself in full agreement with Europeans, and against some of his fellow Ottoman prisoners. For instance, late at night and in the dark, an Ottoman prisoner tripped over Ragıp Bey's jerry-built wooden prayer 'rug' while going to his bed. Immediately, he started to berate Ragıp Bey about the requirement (*farz değil* – not required) of performing prayers while in captivity. A few others joined in the criticism, telling Ragıp Bey that his 'rug' took up too much space in the crowded barracks. Awakened by the loud exchanges, some European prisoners observed the incident. Soon after, at Christmastime, according to Ragıp Bey, the senior German officer in the barracks publicly presented Ragıp Bey with a gift. 'Ragıp Bey', he said, 'we [Germans] collected some money among ourselves and bought a real prayer rug for you from one of the Tatar merchants in town'. Both embarrassed and elated by the gesture, Ragıp Bey did not miss the opportunity to note, 'in comparison to us, Europeans were more devoted to their religion. Among us many tended towards irreligiosity, May God Protect Us . . .'[71] Using the foreign Other to criticise the domestic Other was not new, but it served as a more powerful critique in this instance. In one strike, Ragıp Bey turned the Orientalist conception of 'religious and fanatical' Turk on its head and at the same time attempted to achieve cognitive control over domestic Others by constructing a discourse on proper behaviour and national culture. No doubt, he also hoped that Germans coming to his defence and purchasing a prayer rug for him also shamed those Ottomans who were critical of his praying in captivity.

Ragıp Bey and a host of others like him worried over the danger of losing their cultural, traditional and even national specificity as some among them too easily adopted practices of cultures foreign to their own. Another such person was the imam at Vladivostok prison camp, İrfanoğlu İsmail Efendi. Although he came under criticism from the enlisted men for being 'too friendly' with the local Orthodox priests, he responded that there was nothing wrong in establishing friendly relationships with non-Muslim leaders, or with non-Muslims in general. Instead, he pointed to a larger problem. Referring to the sexual relationships some men had with the Russian women in whose houses and farms they worked, he maintained that what mattered more was that one did not adopt a practice that went 'went against Islamic religion and culture'. It was unacceptable, in his view, to ignore 'new conditions and problems' brought by the war. Knowing that some of the men expressed willingness to marry these 'war-widowed' Russian women, the imam cautioned: 'Nations mix with nations. Religions meet with one another; they almost become infused with each other . . . Moral principles, traditions, and customs become confused. These things become so jumbled that if the war lasts much longer, there might not be any difference left among nations!' He implored the men: 'let's not abandon our religion and belief here [in these lands]'. This stark new reality needed to be confronted with moral courage. 'There was no other option but was to ask Allah to keep us from this confusion and disorder'.[72] What is noticeable in these examples is the mutual practice of policing each other's behaviour.

The question of what was culturally appropriate to 'our way of life' arose even at times when one might assume that there was a relatively well-understood norm. One example that perhaps best demonstrates this sort of contention comes again from the town of Varnavino. The occasion of the conflict was the funeral of Lieutenant Gani who had just died in captivity. Since the town did not have a Muslim cemetery, the Ottoman officers agreed to bury him at one edge of a church garden. Then came a simple question that proved to be unexpectedly contentious: how to conduct the funeral. Mehmet Arif wrote that prisoners suggested all kinds of ideas for what should be a simple affair. Some wanted to 'show the Russians how we conduct our funerals'. 'We should', these officers said 'form a procession bearing Gani to his grave. Those who have the best voices and know the Koran should chant it while walking at the head of the procession'. Yet others suggested that 'the formula of *Allahu Akbar* (God is most great) should be recited during the procession'. Some said, 'no, the best thing to do is recite prayers in the procession'. Mehmet Arif claims that he could not convince anybody initially that reading prayers would be no different from the procession the Russians themselves had in their funerals. After extensive discussion and arguments, the final decision was to take Gani to his grave in silence.[73]

The funeral of Lieutenant Gani highlights some issues. Mehmet Arif, and perhaps others as well, noticed the irony in impressing the Russians with how Ottomans conducted funerals by significantly embellishing quietist Islamic funeral rites; this embellishment, as Mehmet Arif put it, would have made Gani's funeral similar to how some Christians conducted their funerals. Before thinking that Mehmet Arif was a traditionalist, we need to see another object of his criticism. Some prisoners, likely troubled by Gani's death and his burial in a foreign land, turned to religion. Reportedly, this group met in a room of the prison barracks and started a several-hour daily session of reciting prayers and pronouncing the names of God in such a loud manner that their chanting could be heard throughout the barracks and even in the streets by those Russians who walked by.[74] Mehmet Arif, who earlier criticised the funeral plans for being too similar to Christian tradition, was now objecting to people who were worshipping in such a loud and 'obsessional' manner. Whether right or wrong, the problem for Mehmet Arif in both cases was the conscious attempt by some to impress or invite the attention of Russians by altering what should be simple, private ceremonies. All this, of course, points to how the presence of the external Other may lead to a re-examination of certain cultural practices, even if in the end they reconfirm the traditional as the only proper way.

Scholars of nationalism have argued that separate from any rhetorical and ideological statements, national culture is also rooted in the 'trivial' or banal aspects of identity and identification. Identifying with practices, traditions and 'things' that are national and traditional – that is, understood to be our own way of life – results in production, reproduction and contestation of social interactions, habits and routines of everyday life in minor and sometimes unconscious ways. Identifying practices as national and traditional informs the shared norms that determine the appropriate ways of behaving, dressing, talking and eating. These practices and behaviours happen unconsciously in everyday life when one is in one's home environment. However, when one is not in one's home environment, especially when you are torn away from your own and thrust into an alien environment, then those everyday acts become more conscious and meaningful. Furthermore, the encountering of 'different cultural codes can reveal that others act differently'. This 'revelation', in turn, induces a 'heightened sense of awareness towards what seemed common-sense' acts in the form of 'our way of life'.[75]

At moments like this, even banal actions such as how to use latrines gain more meaning and become symbolic of the Ottoman and Turkish sense of proper cleanliness. In Russian camps, for example, use of latrines, which were almost always outdoors and open to the elements, created culture clash and conflict with European prisoners who shared the same camps. This was especially the case with the enlisted men. At latrines, European prisoners sat on a plank and conversed with each other as they took care of their needs, but the communal nature of the latrines offended the sensibilities and personal modesty of the Ottoman men. They also did not share European prisoners' standards of cleanliness; neither did the Europeans theirs. Much to the anger of their European comrades, Ottomans insisted on bringing water in earthen ewers to cleanse themselves afterwards, as they did not find the European practice of using small rocks for the same purpose sanitary enough. Unfortunately, the European prisoners considered the water splashed around by the Ottomans to be more unsanitary than their own practice. In protest they resorted to throwing the stones they had at the ewers to either break or to tip them over.[76] Usually in the minority in every large Russian camp, the Ottoman enlisted men, unable to speak any foreign languages, could not voice their protests. Latrine encounters were not confined to the enlisted men, but also occasionally plagued the officers as well. This happened more often at the commandeered large houses of the elite because of the presence of European-style toilets. Conflict erupted when some Ottoman prisoners attempted and insisted on using the *alafranga* toilet in *alaturka* (*alla Turca*) style, or by standing on the seat in their shoes or boots. Naturally, finding muddy footprints on the toilet seat bothered the European prisoners. In the end, something as mundane as latrines marked the Ottomans as different from the other prisoners and created tense encounters with others. However, this realisation of difference was also a moment of realisation of what was 'our' way of doing things, what was traditional and clean.

In Egypt, the latrine 'problem', at least among the officers, was of a different nature than in Russia. Because they did not have to share their latrines with Europeans and no unpleasant encounters were created, the prisoners poked fun at their own awkwardness in attempting to use modern, *alafranga*, toilets. Such awkwardness was common and seemingly funny enough to make it into the camp newspapers in the form of cartoons, where the confused prisoners attempted at first to use the modern toilet in the *alaturka* fashion by squatting with their feet on the toilet seat. However, as the cartoon tells the story, the prisoners eventually overcame the initial awkwardness and discomfort with *alafranga* toilets. In fact, the image suggested that the whole thing was turned into a ritual where the prisoner intending to use an *alafranga* toilet could not do without having some reading material, such as a newspaper, with him.[77] In this way, the prisoners in Egypt slowly adapted to *alafranga* toilets without both the ugly encounters and the moment of realisation about 'our' way of doing things and cleanliness. In short, those in Russia were much more likely to realise their differences and become aware of doing even mundane things in the way they always did.

Captivity and exile away from home allowed the prisoners to see the differences between their culture and that of their captors and reflect critically upon their own. In this comparison, they could learn, borrow and of course, reject what they saw. Critical reflection and defensive borrowing was acceptable and encouraged, but some saw uncritical borrowing as damaging and threatening to 'our way of life'. Along with more precarious conditions of captivity, which made life more disordered and anxious, those prisoners in Russia had access to more cultures and traditions to which they could compare their own reflexively. While this provided a great many chances of comparison, and therefore moments of identification with their own national and traditional culture for some, it also seemed to offer more chances to some others for unconcernedly aping the ways of other cultures and traditions. This then further increased the tensions among the prisoners in Russia, as there were more reasons to police each other's behaviour.

The likes of Ragıp Bey, the imam of the Vladivostok camp and Mehmet Arif, among others, reveal before our eyes in the form of alterist discourse the proper and improper ways of behaving, dressing, acting and identifying. These concerned Ottomans were not necessarily judging the moral values of another tradition, but questioning those other Ottoman prisoners who seemed to copy European practices eagerly and without reflection. This was because some Ottomans started to behave like Europeans in their dressing, or dressing down, and in adopting other 'European' behaviour – from shaving their moustaches to bathing naked – which were perceived as threats to national tradition and culture. None of these men produced a list of what it meant to be Turkish or Ottoman and what behaviour excluded one from belonging, nor could they. However, as various issues and moments came up, they identified with or distanced themselves from acceptable and unacceptable, proper and improper behaviour. Because belonging to a nation, tradition and culture meant belonging to a particular kind of nation with certain characteristics and traits, some outlooks and behaviour could be excluded or invalidated as un-national and un-traditional. As the prisoners decided, as if in a 'daily plebiscite', what was national, traditional, acceptable or the opposite thereof, the process of including and excluding also helped maintain and ground their own identity through identification. It was in this process of identification with an object external to themselves that a subject was produced. Yet, at the same time, through the subject's identification with the object, in this case the nation, it gained social existence and meaning.

The Ottoman prisoners in Egypt did not have access to local populations or to the German and Austro-Hungarian prisoners, who were in separate camps. This meant that they could only compare themselves to the British. However, since they were the captors and lived separately from prisoners, Ottomans in Egypt did not have the same kind of opportunity to observe other cultures as closely as those in Russia, where many ethnicities, traditions and cultures lived together, day in and day out. This also meant that the situation in Egypt did not pose the same kind of threat to culture and tradition. It is not surprising, therefore, that tales of Ottomans imitating the British do not appear in the memoirs, diaries and camp newspapers from Egypt.

NOTES

1. Umut Özkırımlı, *Contemporary Debates on Nationalism*, p. 81; Yael Tamir, *Liberal Nationalism*, p. 30.
2. Özkırımlı, *Contemporary Debates on Nationalism*, pp. 33, 53, 56, 164–9, 175, 191.
3. Stephane Audoin-Rouzeau, *Men at War*, p. 169.

4. J. G. Fuller, *Troop Morale and Popular Culture*, pp. 38–9. The French word *Bosche* was borrowed by the British officers. See also Audoin-Rouzeau, *Men at War*, pp. 165–6.
5. Faik Tonguç, *Birinci Dünya Savaşında*, p. 141.
6. Mustafa Fevzi Taşer, *Cepheden Cepheye*, p. 29. What the prisoner means here is that savagery was natural to them.
7. 'Gayz', *Vaveyla*, 31 Mart 1333/31 March 1917, number 67, p. 4.
8. Demonisation is used to refer to the act of designating somebody as the source or agent of evil. Demon here is at best an extremely wicked person, an evil spirit, or at worst a devil. As such at least some human qualities remain. In dehumanisation, one is deprived of all human qualities and turned into a beast.
9. Tonguç, *Birinci Dünya Savaşında*, p. 220.
10. Sadi Selçuk, *Esaretin Acı Hatıraları*, p. 8.
11. Tonguç, *Birinci Dünya Savaşında*, p. 169. The term used is '*leş kargası*'.
12. 'Sarıkamış', *Vaveyla*, 29 Nisan 1332/ 12 May 1916, number 23, p. 9.
13. Mehmet Arif Ölçen, *Vetluga Memoir*, p. 52. For other positive qualities of the Russians see Mehmed Âsaf, *Volga Kıyılarında*, pp. 138–9.
14. Since the foreign Other is a fantasy figure, one should not be looking for complete consistency in the expressions used to refer to it. Quotation from Taşer, *Cepheden Cepheye*, pp. 58, 60–1, 72.
15. Ahmet Rıza İrfanoğlu, *Allahüekber Dağları'ndan*. This is an unusual source and has been treated carefully. It features the former prisoner's remembrances through the words of his son, who claims to have recorded some of his father's recollections and remained faithful to what İsmail Efendi actually said in relation to unrecorded parts. While this makes the work less reliable in theory, stories told by the former prisoner closely complement those told by the officers. Sometimes, İsmail Efendi brings up issues officers did not. Moreover, without it, we have no information on the enlisted men at all. Since the Russians used the enlisted men for labour, each man had a duty in or outside of the camp. Because İsmail Efendi failed miserably in the several work assignments he was given, the camp commander, appalled by his incompetence, allowed him to become the camp imam (prayer leader), which was his peace-time occupation.
16. İrfanoğlu, *Allahüekber Dağları'ndan*, pp. 91–2. I took some liberties in translating the original text, which reads slightly differently: '*Ne yapalım genç karı geliyor, üstüme çıkıyor, oturuyor, benim elimeden ne gelir, ben onun esiriyim, ben bir emir kuluyum*'.
17. Ibid. pp. 101–3.
18. Ibid. pp. 101–3.
19. Rahmi Apak, *Yetmişlik Bir Subayın Hatıraları*, p. 133; ATASE, K 313/ F15.
20. See Sokrat İncesu, *Birinci Dünya Savaşında*, p. 31 for the quotation; other similar comments can be found in Hüseyin Aydın, *Acı Hatıralar*, pp. 41–2; İncesu, *Birinci Dünya Savaşında*, pp. 29–30; Apak, *Yetmişlik Bir Subayın Hatıraları*, p. 176; İnkilâp Tarihi Arşivi, 91/29/29/1-13.
21. 'Abdullah I (1882–1951) encouraged his father to negotiate with the British and rebel against the Ottomans.
22. Eşref Kuşçubaşı, *Turkish Battle at Khaybar*, pp. 128–30.
23. İncesu, *Birinci Dünya Savaşında*, p. 32.
24. Hüseyin Mümtaz, 'Bir Mülâzım-ı evvelin harb ve esareti', p. 32; Apak, *Yetmişlik Bir Subayın Hatıraları*, p. 169.
25. Emin Çöl, *Çanakkale – Sina Savaşları*, pp. 123–4. See also Hidayet Özkök, *Çanakkale'den*

Hicaz'a, p. 53; Muhiddin Erev, 'I. Dünya Savaşında bir Yedek Subayın Hâtıraları: 4', p. 59; Ernest Pye, *Prisoner of War, 31,163*, p. 130. Items usually mentioned in this regard are watches and other similarly valuable items.

26. See Yücel Yanıkdağ, '"Ill-fated Sons" of the Nation', Chapter 1.
27. Başkatipzade Ragıp Bey, *Tarih-i Hayatım*, p. 80.
28. Niall Ferguson, *The Pity of War*, chapter 13, would seem to support Ragıp Bey's fears of being killed by his captors.
29. In terms of fear of being killed by the British, one possible exception is the account of Bedros Sharian, an Armenian-Ottoman soldier captured in Palestine. When captured, Sharian was in 'an extraordinary state which it is impossible to explain', for the British 'had a right to kill me because I was in Turkish uniform'. Although the book is 'based' on Sharian's recollections, it was written by Ernest Pye, president of the School of Religion in Athens. It is difficult to distinguish Bedros's impressions and words from that of Pye, especially when he begins to editorialise and moralise. It is, of course, possible that Sharian felt exactly as stated in the text. Furthermore, what either Sharian or Pye says above is more about Turks than about the British because the British had 'a right to kill' someone in Turkish uniform. Pye, *Prisoner of War, 31,163*, p. 129.
30. Vamık Volkan, *Blood Lines*, pp. 111–13.
31. Richard Stites, 'Days and Nights in Wartime Russia', p. 20.
32. Yücel Yanıkdağ, 'Ottoman Prisoners of War in Russia', p. 78.
33. PRO, CAB 21/60/100, 'Mesopotamia Administration Committee', specifically notes the joy of the Shia Muslims (from Kerbela, Najef and Kadhimein) and Christian Ottomans and the cautious indifference of the Jewish Ottoman POWs at the news of the fall of Baghdad.
34. For criticism of Arab 'treachery', see Ölçen, *Vetluga Memoir*, p. 105.
35. Ölçen, p. 100; for another example of a Turk questioning Arab commitment to Islam, see Tonguç, *Birinci Dünya Savaşında*, p. 210.
36. Tonguç, *Birinci Dünya Savaşında*, p. 210.
37. Ibid. p. 209; Taşer, *Cepheden Cepheye*, p. 53, tells the same story in the same camp. For another occasion of near physical fight, see idem, p. 250; also Halil Ataman, *Esaret Yılları*, p. 110 for further statements about the loyalty of Arab officers.
38. On Žižek, see Alan Finlayson, 'Psychology, Psychoanalysis', p. 157.
39. Ahmet Göze, *Rusya'a Üç Esaret Yılı*, pp. 77–8.
40. Ölçen, *Vetluga Memoir*, p. 108.
41. The British military authorities believed that with the exception of 'a good number of low Baghdad types . . . [who] would not have been of much military value', 80 per cent of the Arab Ottoman POWs would be willing to join the Sherifian army. However, they found that many Arab POWs were not willing to fight again. These Arab POWs, whether out of some kind of loyalty or distaste for fighting, stated that they could not fight against their own government: British Library, India Office, L/PS/10 Political and Secret Department Records, 'Correspondence for Arabs fighting for the Sherif', P 1165, February 23, 1917, p. 2; and India Office, L/PS/10, 'Report by Lt. Colonel Parker', P81, 1917, p. 3. However, one finds various messages that announce the departure of varying number of Arabs leaving the Indian and Burmese POW camps for Egypt to join the Sherifian forces: India Office, L/PS/10, 3763/1918; L/PS/10, 1351/1918; L/PS/10, 452/1918; L/PS/10, 3660/1918; L/PS/10, 3122/1918.
42. Apak, *Yetmişlik Bir Subayın Hatıraları*, pp. 168–9.

43. Ibid. pp. 168–9.
44. Çöl, *Çanakkale – Sina Savaşları*, pp. 131–2.
45. İncesu, *Birinci Dünya Savaşında*, p. 39. I realise that the 'stab in the back' theory might have been internalised by Sokrat İncesu in the later 1920s and 1930s and incorporated into his memoir.
46. Aydın, *Acı Hatıralar*, pp. 34–7.
47. Taşer, *Cepheden Cepheye*, p. 53.
48. Baytin was the highest-ranking officer after an Ottoman general managed to escape from Krasnoyarsk. He was otherwise respected for his skills on the battlefield. Hilmi Erbuğ, 'Kaybolan Yıllar', p. 220.
49. Başkatipzade Ragıp Bey, *Tarih-i Hayatım*, pp. 100–1.
50. Erbuğ, 'Kaybolan Yıllar', pp. 220–1.
51. Clearly, the motivation behind this was the loss of POW salaries during the Civil War; the prisoners were now forced to make a living on their own. Başkatipzade Ragıp Bey, *Tarih-i Hayatım*, p. 108.
52. Ragıp Bey uses *kansız* (spineless, cowardly) or *mayası bozuk* ('lacking proper character [from birth]') to refer to people he does not respect. On the occasion of the Red Cross supplies, see Başkatipzade Ragıp Bey, *Tarih-i Hayatım*, pp. 102–3.
53. Başkatipzade Ragıp Bey, *Tarih-i Hayatım*, pp. 102, 106. General Ziya Yergök, who was a *Kolağası* (a rank between a captain and major) at the time, remembered this event slightly differently. He claimed that the invalids were to be selected from 'those who were captured early in the war, those well-advanced in age, high-ranking officers, and those for whom the doctors invented an ailment . . . I received a report certifying that I had *Chute de Rectume*'. *Chute de Rectume*, which as an 'ailment' baffled the Russian officials and doctors, could only be glorified and exaggerated haemorrhoids invented by the doctors to make Ziya Bey's repatriation possible (Yergök, *Tuğgeneral Ziya Yergök'ün Anıları*, pp. 167, 175). I think the passive reporting of the event by Ziya Bey, complete exclusion of real invalids from the list and doctors' efforts to invent diseases give great credibility to Ragıp Bey's charges. This does not mean Ziya Bey was personally involved but only benefited from it.
54. 'Gençlik ve İhtiyarlık Duası', *Yarın*, 6 Şubat 1336/6 February 1920, number 10, p. 1 (cover caricature); and 'Alem iş-ü-nuş'dan', (caricature), *Yarın*, 16 Kanun-i Sani 1336/16 January 1920, number 5, p. 5. For criticism in a memoir, see Aydın, *Acı Hatıralar*, pp. 40–1.
55. 'Albay, yarbay, binbaşı rütbesindeki esir Türk subayları, barakalarına çekilmişler, etliye sütlüye karışmıyorlar, barışı bekliyorlar'. Apak, *Yetmişlik Bir Subayın Hatıraları*, p. 167.
56. I should mention that we are not talking about a direct disobeying of orders, but instead a resisting and ignoring of orders or requests that amounted to drudgery (*angarya*) in the minds of the junior officers. For example, Mehmet Arif relates a number of such requests by superiors ranging from asking him to draw a picture of the scenery around the place of internment so that the officer can remember it after repatriation to fixing and mending their hats. Ölçen, *Vetluga Memoir*, p. 106.
57. Ibid. p. 106.
58. Ibid. pp. 117–18.
59. Ibid. pp. 117–18, 106.
60. Ibid. pp. 117–18, 106.
61. Ibid. pp. 106, 118.

62. I switched here between the Turkish and English version of this memoir. I changed 'no one' in the English version to 'they did not' in the Turkish version; the original Turkish version indicates 'no one among them noticed' that they looked ridiculous. Ölçen, *Vetluga Memoir*, p. 106; Ölçen, *Vetluga Irmağı*, p. 115.
63. Ölçen, *Vetluga Memoir*, pp. 106–7; Ölçen, *Vetluga Irmağı*, p. 115.
64. Ölçen, *Vetluga Memoir*, p. 118.
65. Ibid. p. 106.
66. Başkatipzade Ragıp Bey, *Tarih-i Hayatım*, p. 96; Hasan Basri Efendi, *Bir Gemi Kâtibinin Esaret Hatıraları*, p. 129.
67. Başkatipzade Ragıp Bey, *Tarih-i Hayatım*, p. 96. I have taken some liberty in translation to make it more comprehensible. The literal translation is: 'In fact, [the Europeans] apparently did not connect [understand] honour in terms of the "wretched organs of the body" [sexual organs]'.
68. Hasan Basri Efendi, *Bir Gemi Kâtibinin*, p. 149.
69. Başkatipzade Ragıp Bey, *Tarih-i Hayatım*, pp. 100–1.
70. 'Temaşa', *Yarın*, 19 Mart 1336/19 March 1920, number 18, pp. 6–7.
71. Başkatipzade Ragıp Bey, *Tarih-i Hayatım*, pp. 97–8.
72. İrfanoğlu, *Allahüekber Dağları'ndan*, pp. 76, 92, 93. Ragıp Bey would have agreed with the imam in a number of ways. He had romantic feelings for a local Russian girl, Taisa (Tayse in text). In the end, despite her imploring him, he decided to leave her behind in Krasnoyarsk. He cited reason such as not wanting to mix 'national customs and traditions' as well as 'blood'. However, the decision was probably more practical as he was about to escape by way of Afghanistan. Taisa even offered her willingness to a polygamous marriage arrangement and likely conversion. Başkatipzade Ragıp Bey, *Tarih-i Hayatım*, p. 117. Dr Şehidullah Fikri Altan married his woman friend and brought her to Turkey, see M. Rıza Serhadoğlu, *Savaşçı Doktorun İzinde*.
73. Ölçen, *Vetluga Memoir*, pp. 101–2.
74. Ibid. p. 102.
75. Tim Edensor, *National Identity, Popular Culture*, p. 89; Özkırımlı, *Contemporary Debates on Nationalism*, p. 175.
76. İrfanoğlu, *Allahüekber Dağları'ndan*, p. 98.
77. *Esaret Albümü*, Sidi Bishr, 1336/1920, no pagination. Some Egyptian POW camps were built near the Mediterranean, which allowed the prisoners to swim.

CHAPTER

3

SAVIOUR SONS OF THE NATION: INSIDE THE PRISONERS' MINDS

This chapter examines the hand-written prison camp newspapers in which the prisoners of war discussed, at length, the weaknesses in their nation, state, society and culture while they awaited the end of the war, and then their long-delayed repatriation. Their literary efforts were nothing less than an earnest self-examination of their society with its shortcomings and mistakes. In the prisoners' formulations, these weaknesses had brought the nation to the brink of imminent destruction at the end of the Great War. As they diagnosed the causes of neglect, slumber and decline, they also offered hopeful suggestions for fixing those problems. The prisoners' views were remarkably candid and passionate, not only because these writings were not meant for public consumption, but also because they were produced under difficult circumstances when apprehension about being direct likely disappeared. Given their personal situations as prisoners of war, the fact that they did not resign themselves to their own and their nation's fate is remarkable in itself.

In the process of self-examination, the prisoner-authors identified a number of problems they deemed to be causes of the weaknesses in their nation, state, society and culture. These problems included the ignorance of the majority of the Ottoman population; a misinterpreted Islam, where the misinterpretation discouraged people from working for a modern world and materialistic achievements; and an educated and politically important elite engaged in self-aggrandisement, rather than acting for the common good. In their writings, as the officer prisoners identified problems and offered solutions, they constructed a national community by 'performing' the nation. This performing was accomplished through 'a daily plebiscite' of both inclusion and exclusion as the officer prisoners determined the borders, or criteria, of what it meant to belong to the nation.[1]

The prisoners argued that the nation could overcome the difficulties it faced if only various segments of the population could become enlightened enough to agree upon a common national goal.

HISTORICAL BACKGROUND AND TURKISH NATIONALISM

During the eighteenth century, Europe's scientific, military and technological ascendancy put the Ottoman Empire on the defensive. While earlier generations of the Ottoman political and intellectual elite were well aware of the shift in the power relationship, it was in the nineteenth century that the question of 'How can this state be saved?' became increasingly urgent among three main groups: high-ranking bureaucrats of the *Tanzimat* reform period (1839–76), the Young Ottomans of the 1860s and finally the Young Turks from 1889 on. In many ways, the Ottoman prisoners became part of the educated class's long search for a means to 'save the state', but they were also different in some important respects. These men were neither state bureaucrats nor were they members of the intellectual or political elite.

The Young Ottoman movement can be summed up as a critique of the *Tanzimat*, drawing inspiration from three sources: the *Tanzimat*, European political thought and Islamic tradition. The Young Ottomans represented a substantial advance over the leaders of the *Tanzimat* in their mastery of European thought, but in other ways, they were more conservative than the *Tanzimat* leaders. They criticised the leaders of the *Tanzimat* for having moved too quickly towards Westernisation, thus cutting themselves off from the resources of their own tradition and culture. The Young Ottomans wanted to create a new Islamic cultural synthesis by selectively borrowing from the West in order to strengthen the Ottoman state. Aiming for a balance between Islam and Western civilisation, they regularly made reference to the Western practices they could associate with or justify in terms of early Islamic practice or the Qur'an. This method came to be known as Islamic modernism. The end of the 1870s brought political 'neutralisation' of the Young Ottomans by Sultan Abdulhamid II, who dissolved the Ottoman parliament, which had met for fewer than two years (1876–8).[2]

By 1889, growing resentment against the autocratic rule of Abdulhamid II (r. 1876–1909) triggered the re-emergence of a resistance group in the form of the Committee of Union and Progress (CUP), which became known as the Young Turks. The Young Turks became familiar with current European thought, especially in the emerging social sciences, notably psychology and sociology. They lacked the Young Ottomans' Islamic engagement; the intellectuals among them responded to European 'scientific materialism', positivism and social Darwinism.[3] Among their favourites was Gustave LeBon, whose elitist theory influenced the Young Turks, who had at first advocated the education of the masses only to discard it by 1906. Following scientific and elitist ideology, the Young Turks described the masses as despicable and senseless.[4] Believing in the value of the superior individual while condemning the people, the Young Turks dedicated themselves to the creation of an elite class.[5]

They generally viewed Islam as a means of mobilising and manipulating the people, but their principles were resolutely secular. The Young Turks' writings linked materialism to Westernisation, which was portrayed as being the driving force behind the material progress of the West. Although there were early ideological differences, the Balkan Wars created deeper divisions within the CUP, resulting in factions that can be characterised as modernist and Westernist. The modernists promoted defensive Westernisation while opposing Western imperialism, whereas the other advocated wholesale acceptance of Western civilisation.[6]

Both factions recognised that a fundamental difference existed between the declining East and the powerful West. However, they differed on the nature of the West's superiority and the solutions needed to cure the ills of Ottoman society and save the state. The modernists attempted to prevent wholesale Westernisation by promoting a single-minded Westernisation policy: the development of technology that was deemed necessary to catch up with the West. However, the Westernist Young Turks, while paying lip service to Islam in public, privately denounced those trying to reconcile Islam and Western civilisation. They dominated intellectual life in the Ottoman Empire. The Westerniser intellectuals regarded Ottoman Islamic culture as old-fashioned and unresponsive to contemporary problems.[7] In short, members of these groups were convinced that the old society had to be reformed or changed in order for it to cope with the modern world, but agreeing on the extent of change was the crux of the problem. This work suggests that the writings and actions of the junior officers provide a fuller understanding of the nature and extent of nationalism that existed among a larger segment of society than the writings and actions of the Young Turks or other political elites.[8]

Similar to anti-colonial nationalisms as theorised by Partha Chatterjee, some Ottoman prisoners divided the world of social institutions and practices into two broad domains: the material, or the outer, and the spiritual, or the inner.[9] The material domain was the sphere of science, technology and economy. The spiritual, also called the inner or moral domain, bore the marks of cultural identity, or what made the nation different from Others and other nations. Accepting the superiority of the West in the outer domain – that is, in science, technology and love of progress – the prisoner-writers advocated Ottoman adoption of those aspects they thought had made Europe powerful. However, in the inner domain, they aimed to remain true to their culture. Thus, the national movement was founded on both identification with, and distinction from, the West.[10]

PRISON CAMP DEBATES: CAUSES OF OUR MISERY AND DANGERS OF NATIONAL EXTINCTION

Once they were settled in permanent prison camps, the officers had time to reflect on a number of problems that faced the nation. One of the most visible problems they identified quickly was the ignorance of the people as represented by the peasant soldiers. Prison camp surely was not the first time the officers had to grapple with the peasant soldiers' ignorance. However, away from dangers and distractions of the front, captivity provided the time to observe and reflect more deeply about the peasants, while the newspapers provided the platform for exchange of ideas with others as to what the problem was and what could be done. In discussing the peasants in general and peasant soldiers in particular, the officers made no attempt to hide their disbelief and abhorrence for the peasants' ignorance. Some may have felt pity towards their men, but sometimes their attitude was one of contempt. In their writings, the officers discursively excluded peasant soldiers and, by extension, peasants in general, from their vision of the nation, for their lack of education, civilisation and even human qualities. They could be included in the nation after their symptoms were identified, illnesses diagnosed and finally remedied.

The most notable feature of the peasant soldier, as portrayed by the officers, was ignorance, which amounted to something akin to complete lack of interest in the most elementary facts of their daily existence. Sometimes the officers explained this state of ignorance as a simple lack of knowledge, as naivety or as idiosyncrasy. For instance, some officers were struck that a peasant soldier had not bothered to learn the name of the Russian town where he was held captive for over three years. At other times, the peasants' ignorance pertained to subjects that were more important and immediate.[11] Şevket Süreyya, who was never captured, wrote about peasant soldiers under his command on the Russian front. Perhaps assuming Islam to be a monolithic religion among the peasants, he was surprised by what he discovered:

> At first, I thought my soldiers were religious and even fanatical, but found them to be ignorant. Still, I told myself that they might be ignorant, but Muslims nevertheless. However, I understood a little later that despite the word 'Islam' entered in their identification cards under the category of religion, there were incompatible religions or, more correctly, remnants (*tortu*) of religion, denominations, various beliefs, and mystic orders alive and well among them.[12]

The Ottoman peasant soldiers, whom the officers reportedly assumed to be devout Muslims, generally did not even know the basic prescripts of their religion or nationality. Şevket Süreyya, himself a committed nationalist, was astonished when he questioned his soldiers – who were all 'Anatolian Turks' – on their nationality:

[When I said:]

– 'From what nation are we?'
there was a different answer from everyone,
– [when I asked] 'Are we not Turks?'
they answered: 'I ask pardon of God!' ('*estağfurullah!*')
So, they were not accepting their Turkishness.[13]

Why was being a Turk 'offensive' enough to ask for God's pardon? From Şevket Süreyya's perspective, this was a case of a Turk not recognising his Turkishness. How could people who did not know their nation from another be expected to defend that nation? However, from some peasants' point of view, there were other reasons for disavowing one's Turkishness. Shortly before his capture, another officer, Rahmi Apak, questioned a peasant boy who refused to accept that he was a Turk. The boy insisted that he was an Ottoman. In hopes of convincing the boy of his Turkishness, Rahmi insisted that 'even the Sultan was a Turk'. The boy responded: 'Efendi, do not commit a sin, the Sultan cannot be a Turk'. Rahmi Apak learned from these soldiers that in some regions 'the term Turk was used to refer to *kızılbaş* (Alevi Muslim) . . . whereas Sunni [Muslims] were called Ottomans'.[14] According to the peasant boy's definition, religion and ethnicity were defined by each other; in this case his Sunni religion defined his ethnic identity as Ottoman. Still, among the prison-camp authors, the judgment of peasant ignorance held sway: 'These miserable fellows [soldiers] did not even have the faintest knowledge about religion and Islam'. Another officer commented that when they were asked the name of the Prophet of Islam, his men would naively answer, 'Our Master, Sultan Feraşad (Reşad)'.[15] Faced with peasant soldiers who did not know the name of their Prophet, the correct name of the Sultan, or their nationality, the officers concluded that the Anatolian peasant soldiers were even ignorant of the most basic information that identified them – their religion and nationality. Other officers felt awkward among their men because of this ignorance. 'When I was struggling with my soldiers who did not mentally identify with the war, did not know where and why they fought, and were not even aware of their own *existence*', one officer wrote, 'I felt some sort of a mental conflict between feeling pity and strangeness towards them'.[16] If some men were unaware of their own 'existence', then their inability to identify with the war may not have been their real problem. The issue of identifying with the war raises further questions. Were these peasants fighting for the nation, the religion or the sultan they could not properly identify?

Although they did not question the military prowess and bravery of the simple Ottoman soldier with the exception of occasional stories of desertion, the officers' attitude regarding the men's ignorance often turned into outright anger and contempt.[17] Placing the status of the peasants in the context of Ottoman society as he imagined it, an officer in Krasnoyarsk contended in 1915 that there were really only two classes in the empire: (1) the educated, or enlightened class (*tabaka-yı münevvere*) and (2) the 'middle' class (*tabaka-yı mutavassıta*) that contained all the rest, the illiterate – peasants and urbanites alike. The crudeness of this scheme made some sense in the context of what the officer wanted to point out. By using an example or two from the 'state of the Ottoman army', he aimed to 'deduce the nation's moral and ethical competence [or worth]'. The author made it clear that he was writing from his personal observations, which were based on what 'he saw, heard, and felt in his heart'. However, he was sure that other officers shared his views:

> In our country the enlightened class is made up of us soldiers [officers] and civil servants [*memurlar*]. Generally, the rest [of the population] is in a dense state of ignorance and vulgarity ... [During the war] I was subjected to the calamity of witnessing [on many occasions] soldiers huddling around a fire. But even as they could see another soldier of the same army or even the same regiment freezing to death only three steps away, they were not moved to help a fellow soldier. Forget military brotherhood [*uhuvvet-i askeriye*], if these people had even the slightest degree of human sentiment [*hissiyat-i insaniye*], they would not have allowed a doomed to death comrade to struggle against his fate ... With very little effort, they could have brought the [comrade] in front of the fire and ... could have strengthened his fire of life on the point of being extinguished.[18]

He related other examples of lack of compassion, involving a wounded soldier who had collapsed on the snowy ground and resigned himself to his fate. Soon, a convoy of men on mules singing folk songs appeared on their way to pick up supplies. They saw the wounded man struggling on the ground, but 'they shut their ears to the sorrowful moans coming from the unknown depths of his wounded heart and continued on their way'. In still another instance, he saw some men 'lowering themselves to stripping away the great coat [off the victim's back] or taking his money from his pocket. What primitiveness, what callousness'.[19]

We have to admit it. Almost a majority (*hemen kısm-ı azâmi*) of the soldiers that make up our army are psychologically invalid [*ruhen malul*] and are pathological [*marazi*] to such extent. The reason why the members of our nation have such rough and savage (*kaba ve vahşi*) manners is not only the result of a lack of education. There are also collective effects of our army being unable to fully render its duties. Even among the Russian enlisted men, whose level is not considerably above ours, there is so much compassion and tenderness in their dealings with one another . . . Even they saw the lack of compassion among us and they did not hesitate to tell us this to our face.[20]

The officer wanted to draw larger conclusions from his observations. In a society founded upon practice of 'mutual assistance' (*teavün üzerine müesses*), the members of a military 'should be united for above ordinary assignment'. Among them, the sentiments of 'collaboration and compassion must reach its highest levels'. A military is 'a whole which consists of many parts. Even the smallest of incompatibility, or the simplest of lack of union, will shake its unity from its foundation'. For him, this was such a 'picture of catastrophe', that if this 'dark page was not torn away from the army's (book of) code of conduct, we are assured that we will continue to decline more every day'. He did not want to 'put all this responsibility' on the shoulders of the officers, since, he believed, there were larger causes behind such behaviour. He ended his piece with a plea to his comrades: 'If we want to live on [as a nation], we need to imbue the men's hearts with a sense of compassion and assistance by means of explaining' and showing them the errors of their way.[21]

This officer's words of revulsion and shame relegated the enlisted men to the realm of those 'lacking human sentiments'. Even Russian peasant soldiers possessed empathy for each other. In this way, some officers consigned the peasant soldiers to a position somewhere between humanity and inhumanity. The harsh conditions of war, particularly on the Russian front, were a factor in causing the men's bad behaviour. Thus, one does not find similarly harsh sentiments expressed in the Egyptian prison camp newspapers or memoirs; even if some of those officers also felt similarly, their relatively more acceptable conditions did not produce the same feelings of animosity toward their charges.

In confronting the question of whether the peasants belonged within or outside of their idealised notion of the nation, the officers in both locations believed that segments of society 'must be included [gradually] by first declaring them excluded for their lack of civilization'.[22] Thus, the officers prescribed a strategy that first described the peasants as existing outside of the nation – not only because of their uncivilised and ignorant manner, but also because they were thought to occupy a liminal position between humanity and inhumanity.

The officers, by enumerating the negative qualities of the peasant soldiers, at the same time identified the qualities that distinguished themselves as essential parts of the nation. In other words, the men's discursive exclusion served to maintain the officers' identity as enlightened or compassionate nationals. Likewise, the liminal peasants, with their distinctive traits and lacking qualities, whether descriptive or metaphorical, served to mark the limits of the nation's boundaries. Furthermore, by declaring the peasants outside of the nation, the officers claimed the opportunity and the power to intervene and make the ignorant less ignorant, and the barely human, human again.

As the officers reflected on the ignorance and other problems of the peasants, through their captors they also received continually worsening news of the war. The disheartening condition of the peasants and war news combined to create among the officers an enveloping sense of anxiety and fear for the future of the nation. As the war ended and the victors partitioned the empire, the Greeks invaded Anatolia. While Ottoman prisoners still remained in the camps after the war's end, their fear became deeper as it also changed in nature. Given their own situation, the peasants and the partition, many of the officer prisoners started to fear a 'national extinction'. By this, they did not mean the literal extinction of Turks as a people, but complete loss of sovereignty as a nation.[23] Throughout the war, many junior officers shared this fear about the nation's future.

In February 1920, fifteen months after the end of the war, while many thousands of Ottomans still remained behind barbed wire, the following poem appeared in *Nilüfer* (*Water Lily*), a prison camp newspaper in Egypt. The poem reflects openly and self-critically on the political, cultural and even ethical situation.

Us (*Biz*)

Through science, the whole world has superiority today;
As for us, we have fallen, sunken, thrust into misery,
We are hungry, our backs are bare, and we are helpless, trembling
We are lazy, fond of ease . . . really, a slave to comfort.
We do not know a thing, but always pretend high knowledge
And speak up, [as if] always familiar with wisdom.
Virtuous and wise, literary men and scribes, we all are;
but we are always political men, desirous of fame;
To boast is our highest guiding rule;
But our actions still don't agree with smallest of [our] aims.
Exhausted is our sense of compassion, we won't run to assistance.
As a matter of fact, maybe our hearts cannot even handle compassion.[24]

This poem illustrates several issues addressed in this chapter: the West's power and Ottoman misery, laziness. selfishness, empty pride and lack of aim. The poem, written or appearing after the Greek invasion of Anatolia but before the Sevres Treaty of August 1920, is sharply self-accusatory and critical. The author suggests that certain Ottoman social and cultural practices caused the misery of the community. Another piece in a later issue of *Nilüfer* called the state in which the Ottomans found themselves a 'historical tragedy' (*facia-i tarihiyye*) because the nation faced a 'heart-rending situation of extinction of a generation' (*bir neslin izmihlal-i elimi*).[25] Yet another poem in *Türk Varlığı*, also produced in Egypt, was as encouraging as it was ominous. The author suggested that it was no time for begging mercy from the strong West because the West had none to give. It was time for taking direct charge of their own fate and immediate action. Passively expecting mercy from the West would bring only one thing to the Ottoman: a 'bullet and arrow through his heart'.[26]

In their diagnoses of what really caused the ills of the nation, culture and tradition, the officer prisoners did not hold back; as what they wrote about the peasants showed, no one, no group, no issue was exempt from harsh criticism. In trying to figure out their empire's and nation's weaknesses, they needed a point of comparison. Europe filled that purpose.

What happened to the Ottomans that prevented them from achieving a similar level of success as the Europeans? One of them suggested that European advancement had been prompted by the Turks themselves, starting in the fourteenth century with their invasion of Europe. In order to 'hold out against the terrible current of Turkish raiders', he stated, Europeans were forced into perfecting sciences and trades, which allowed them to 'achieve their success of today'.[27] However, he went on, in contrast to Europeans, the post-conquest generations of Ottomans 'did not take seriously scientific, technical, industrial developments'. Instead, he suggested, 'we' chose to live 'lazily and with the attitude of someone who inherited a great fortune'. Characterising their lazy lives as a 'superstitious slumber', he added that this 'inexhaustible, interminable inertia, this endless, unending sleep', finally ended with heartache.[28] And this is where they found themselves at that point.

As the prisoners searched for causes for and solutions to their ills, not all of them distinguished between the symptoms and their causes. A number of prisoner writers identified certain interpretations of religion and religious practice as obstacles to advancement in the modern world; and therefore, the cause of many of their community's current ills. In a piece called 'From West to East', one writer in *Türk Varlığı* noted that religion's influence in more advanced nations was a thing of the past.

> In examining histories of nations, it is evident that every nation firstly followed the path of religion as its goal. In this direction, a lot of blood was spilt, wars were fought. As long as the ignorance of the people continued, that path had full appeal. After that, a period of reformation (*intibâh-ı teceddüd*) started as everyone shook off the nightmare of ignorance ... Learning (and knowledge) advanced, civilization progressed as religion's devotees started to multiply. Hundreds reached millions. As the ability to control all of them declined and every nation was obliged to govern itself; [every nation] was forced to discover the ways to benefit and exalt itself. And finally, religion as a path no longer came to satisfy the psyche and lives of peoples. Ultimately, it [religion] was forced to abandon its place to [the idea of] nation. And this situation [nation as path] has come to our day. Lately, even the fashion of nation has [begun to] pass.[29]

In this crudely summarised human political and religious history, the prisoner asked where Ottoman and Muslims stood on this scale. The short answer was: 'well behind'. Pointing out that since the Ottomans were just leaving the religion phase, fully entering the nationalism (*milliyet*) phase would take some time.[30]

Although this prisoner did not explain why Ottomans and other Muslims were still in the religion stage in this schema, others offered some explanations. Some also broadened their geographical references beyond Ottomans and Muslims as they turned to a comparison of Easterners with Westerners. One author wrote: 'the humankind of Asia and Europe are two masses of peoples who oriented their faith and spirit (*iman ve ruh*) towards two different poles of a spectrum'.[31] Accordingly, he suggested, 'ever since time immemorial while one's [the Asian's] eyes were turned to the heavens, the other's [the European's] were turned to earth'. In terms of religious belief, 'we see that before anything else Asians idolized the celestial universe like the moon, stars, and the sun'. Then, in a clear reference to Jesus and his role in Christianity, he suggested that Europeans instead 'idolized the people they slowly brought up among themselves and finally deified'.[32] In short, Muslims and Easterners worshipped supernatural deities in heavens, but Westerners worshipped mankind who lived in this world even when he was deified.

Apparently, this search for a deity in heaven produced certain cultural mentalities that the prisoner thought undermined material progress by diverting the attention of Muslims and other Asians:

> Instead of using their ideas [and intellect], Asians have used their illusions (*hayaller*) and as a result have fallen into poverty in the face of a materialistic life. Many intelligent peoples of the East have either been exhausted on the endless

roads of divinity or simply sat idly on sheepskin rugs in dervish lodges in order to reach the bliss on the other side of the bridge (*ahiret köprüsü*) from this world to Paradise.³³

On the one hand, this author marked the influence of Islam as playing a role in Asians' and Muslims' poverty and regression; on the other, he pointed out the effect of the choices people made. In other words, the Islamic world or the Ottomans having fallen behind Europe was not due to some inborn characteristics of Islam as a religion, but had to do with the choices Muslims made concerning where to devote their attention. For this author, the path to personal and national success was not to be found in religious education or unanswerable metaphysical questions, but in something else entirely. He wrote:

> The dazzling advances of today's beings have not happened because of means found in worlds far away from our globe, but because of small experiences gained in their own environments ... From now on, for human beings to rely on illusions is as pitiful as an attempt by a bird without wings trying to fly ... Let us not forget, perhaps today's humanity – by distancing itself every day from illusions, from distant truths, and starts – may have found a shortcut to victory, power (*tahakküm*), and even to deity. Why shouldn't we walk through in this [same] simple and natural path[?] [partially illegible].³⁴

Although certainly very harsh in tone, the author was trying to give Turks, Ottomans, Muslims and other Asians one last wake-up call. It was meant to jolt them from their slumber to face reality.³⁵ Instead of living for the 'afterlife', Muslims and Ottomans needed to pay attention to the methods of advanced nations.³⁶

Seemingly directed by religion, living for the afterlife created deep fears and anxieties among the people; this was thought to produce laziness and undermine material progress. Another prisoner noted that this fear and anxiety was the result of 'learned mentalities' related to committing a 'sin' or behaving sinfully, but he argued, these anxieties were all based on 'groundless anxious stories about *jinns* and [other] imaginary beings'. In such an apprehensive state of mind, people adopted a state of 'agitation and avoidance' that produced 'idleness and laziness'.³⁷ The peasants were especially vulnerable to the seemingly opposing demands of these two different worlds: this material world and the afterlife. Caught between two forces and burdened by an 'indolent brain', such people could not handle the 'extraordinarily delicate and uneasy arena of life', and became more 'confused and dim-witted'.³⁸ Accordingly, they never developed 'Love for this World' (*Dünya Sevgisi*).³⁹ To a great extent, the peasants were singled out, but the writer probably meant to include others who were uneducated, and therefore ignorant.

It might seem as if these men were blaming religion as a system of belief, but instead their admonition was for the way Islam was interpreted; for Muslims and Ottomans to survive, religion now needed to be reinterpreted for the modern life. Misinterpretation had created 'distressing decline', under the influence of 'invisible poisons' (*gayri mer'i zehirler*).[40] But, 'with determination and willpower', one prisoner stated, a 'comprehensive and fully-determined sacred religious transformation (*dini inkilap*)', was possible.[41] The religion was sacred enough to deserve a transformation to make it responsive to the times, which would allow for the survival of the nation and the larger community of Muslims. The bottom line was that this transformation really had to be a reinterpretation: 'we need to cure and strengthen (*teşfiye ve takviye*) the real code of laws of the book of religion, not the misinterpreted pages on the next world that blind our eyes and eat away at our determined and steadfast characters'.[42] In the end, the piece targeted the misinterpretation of the Qur'an by those who were said to be obstacles to progress.[43] A deep and proper transformation would make it possible to teach the people 'lights of reality appropriate for our century'. These 'lights of reality' would improve morale for the next generation. 'For any ethnic group (*kavm*), the most necessary thing was [spiritual] morale (*maneviyat*)'. Because without morale any ethnic group was 'without a doubt and misgiving (*bi-la şekk ve şübhe*) destined to decline (*inkiraz*)', the transformation became all the more necessary and urgent.[44]

But who were those who misinterpreted the Qur'an and religion and therefore stood in the way of progress? For some, the answer was simple: madrasas or schools of religion. However, madrasa here seems to have stood for religious education in general, from the lowest in the form of village schools to the highest level. Because they 'do more harm than good', one urged, 'we need to remove our children from . . . thick-headed (*vurdum duymaz*) madrasas'.

According to many of the officer prisoners, these Qur'anic schools produced the peoples' ignorance, even where religion was concerned. Therefore, they argued, children needed to be 'rescue[d] . . . from the hands of village teachers, who did everything but teaching'. To leave Ottoman youth 'to be poisoned in such a manner was nothing short of murder', one officer added.[45] Another remarked ironically: 'We searched for our enemies on the frontiers, but the most gruesome enemy was apparently in the village schools'.[46] Therefore, for the officer prisoners, village schools and their uninformed teachers became the internal enemies who frustrated the efforts of those attempting to create a population that focused on modern and worldly, materialistic concerns.[47]

If misunderstood religion was partly responsible for the poor, ignorant and backward condition of the people, some prisoners argued, then the Ottoman state itself was responsible for the remaining part. Thus the state was implicated in being yet another cause of the poor condition of the peasants. In 'Garb'dan Şark'a' or 'From the West to the East', the author blamed the Ottoman state for deliberately sacrificing the lives and property of Anatolian Turks for the benefit of other ethnic and religious groups (*reaya*) in the empire.[48] Somewhat similar to the discourse we encountered in Chapter 2 about Turks' self-sacrifice for others' benefit, this line of argument went farther. Another essay was more accusatory: 'For this state that supposedly carried the name of Turk, Turkish people became not only strangers to it, but almost its enemy. The state was not even aware that Turkish people was its only support'.[49] For these observers, the people's ignorance kept the nation from achieving its full potential, but the state kept the people ignorant and poverty-stricken by sacrificing them for the benefit of others. The political and intellectual elite might have worried about 'how can this [Ottoman] state be saved?' The prisoners, however, were more concerned about saving the nation while they blamed the state for the nation's deplorable condition.

Thus, according to the officer prisoners, the two most important obstacles facing the nation were the loss of the war, stumbled into by that same state, and the pervasive ignorance among the masses. Nothing could be done about the outcome of the war or the possible sacrificing of the state, but the nation could survive and regenerate if it could find a solution to the problem of ignorance. This would ultimately prepare the nation to deal with its dismal political situation. While the task of overcoming the people's ignorance, given its depth, seemed almost insurmountable, the officers attempted to find a solution anyway.

EDUCATING THE IGNORANT PEASANT SOLDIER

The Ottoman officers' solution to bolstering almost every shortcoming of the peasant soldiers was education. Education could teach the men their religion, nation, humanity and more. They saw that educating the peasant soldiers in the camps could serve as a model for educating and uplifting the peasants as a class after repatriation. At the very least, educated and uplifted enlisted men would bring back to their villages positive lessons. In this way, they could influence their cohort. In the past, the Ottoman ruling elite had always used education to impose their own values on society; the officers would do the same.[50] They decided to get started on the task immediately in the camp schools they established in Russia and Egypt. The officers' informal efforts in the camps pre-dated, and very likely influenced those of the Turkish army of the early republic, which always promoted itself as a place of 'education' for illiterate peasant soldiers.[51]

A typical school for Ottoman enlisted men in Krasnoyarsk, for example, had classes on reading and writing (*okuma yazma*), personal hygiene (*hıfz-ı sıhha*), religion, arithmetic (*hesab*) and civics (*malumat-ı medeniye*).[52] The officers believed that such classes would gradually 'lift' the men from their state of ignorance. Encouraged by comparatively milder conditions and a larger student body, the officers in Egypt also taught a range of classes from Qur'anic readings to agriculture.[53] Courses on agriculture and arithmetic prepared the peasants to be better farmers and managers of their finances. The courses on religion and the Qur'an aimed to erase the traces of pre-Islamic and folk beliefs.[54] While not all prisoners would take advantage of the prison camp educational opportunities, the officers, nevertheless, hoped to teach them the essential basics about their nation, identity, religion and culture, as well as some basic principles of 'civilisation'.

Unfortunately, the voice of the masses of illiterate peasant soldiers did not make it into the written records of the prison camps. However, there are records of two previously voiceless peasants who gained the means to express themselves after having gone through prison camp schools. Of course, this is not the autonomous, unaffected voice of the peasant, but one shaped and moulded through education provided by the officers. These are voices well-worth hearing, nevertheless.

A Bountiful Product of a Few Months of Education!

If I saw the letter 'Alif' [ا] I would have looked at it as if it were a post.
If I saw the letter 'Ba' [ب] I would have laughed as if it were a trough.
They made me read and write, and I did not grow tired.
Whereas I was living like a criminal [or a murderer] in a cage,
Today I now know my history.
My officers, my veterans, my masters
I'll always remember you auspiciously ...
Do not interfere, may my life be a sacrifice for the nation.
Let me die, so that the flag and the nation should live on.
Oh peasants, oh labourers do not wait;
The exalted God (*Yüce Tanrı*) is with us – do not be afraid.[55]

These few lines by Sergeant Hacıkadiroğlu İbrahim Çavuş of the town of Burdur in southwest-central Anatolia, suggest that he learned to read and write in one of the Egyptian camp schools. As the poem attests, this man's whole life was changed by literacy and he expressed his appreciation of his officers' efforts on his behalf. The soldier gives us a good idea of the change that took place. In this way, İbrahim Çavuş becomes the exceptional norm; what he credits the camp school for teaching him, he did not possess previously. The prison camp school not only made him literate, but also instructed him about his history and nationality – the very things that his officers thought the enlisted men were missing. In this way, İbrahim Çavuş was nationalised through education and through identification with an object, the nation, and ideals beyond himself. While religion and God are not missing from his writing, how they appear is important. İbrahim Çavuş affirmed that God was on the Turks' side. Religion and God came into the equation only indirectly, in the form of giving courage to those who fought. Yet, the sacrifice he was willing to make was most directly connected to the nation and the flag.

Yet another 'bountiful' product of prison camp education was provided by a group of enlisted men in a British prison camp. They put together a theatrical production as part of their class work. Ottoman officers, fellow enlisted men, officers and British camp officials attended the play in which the men portrayed the evils of their village schools. Not surprisingly, the play's image of the village schools was identical to that depicted in the officers' writings.[56] According to the dramatic play, after prison camp schooling, the peasant soldiers miraculously developed some understanding of the causes of their nation's ills.

More evidence of the impact of the camp schools could be seen when the prisoners learned of the Greek invasion of their homeland and the resulting War of Independence (1920). The very people whom their officers had repeatedly criticised earlier for not bothering to help a fellow soldier in distress, now collected what little money they could among themselves to send to needy refugees created by the Greek invasion and the War of Independence.[57] This was the kind of change the officers hoped to see in their enlisted men, and to have extended throughout Anatolia after the war.

At least in Egypt, when each camp school term was over, the officers organised a graduation ceremony both to congratulate the graduates, and to encourage participation of other enlisted men in the programme. The best-performing students were given prizes such as undershirts and socks. Their names, along with their grades, were circulated in the camp newspaper for everyone to see.[58] One observer noted that 'courage was visible on the faces of every efendi who appeared [on the ceremony stage]. What struck the eye was the presence of certain vigour in their expressions empowered by their knowledge'.[59] Reflecting the metamorphosis from *efrad* (recruits and individuals) into *efendi*s (gentlemen), 'the appearance of diplomas and presents evoked yet another delight among them. We could see from the distance the flood of joyful brightness in their eyes as they picked up the diplomas extended to them'.[60] (See Figure 3.1.) Joy and brightness in the faces of students proved to the officers that these men, who used to worry only about the afterlife, had learned to enjoy the fruits of

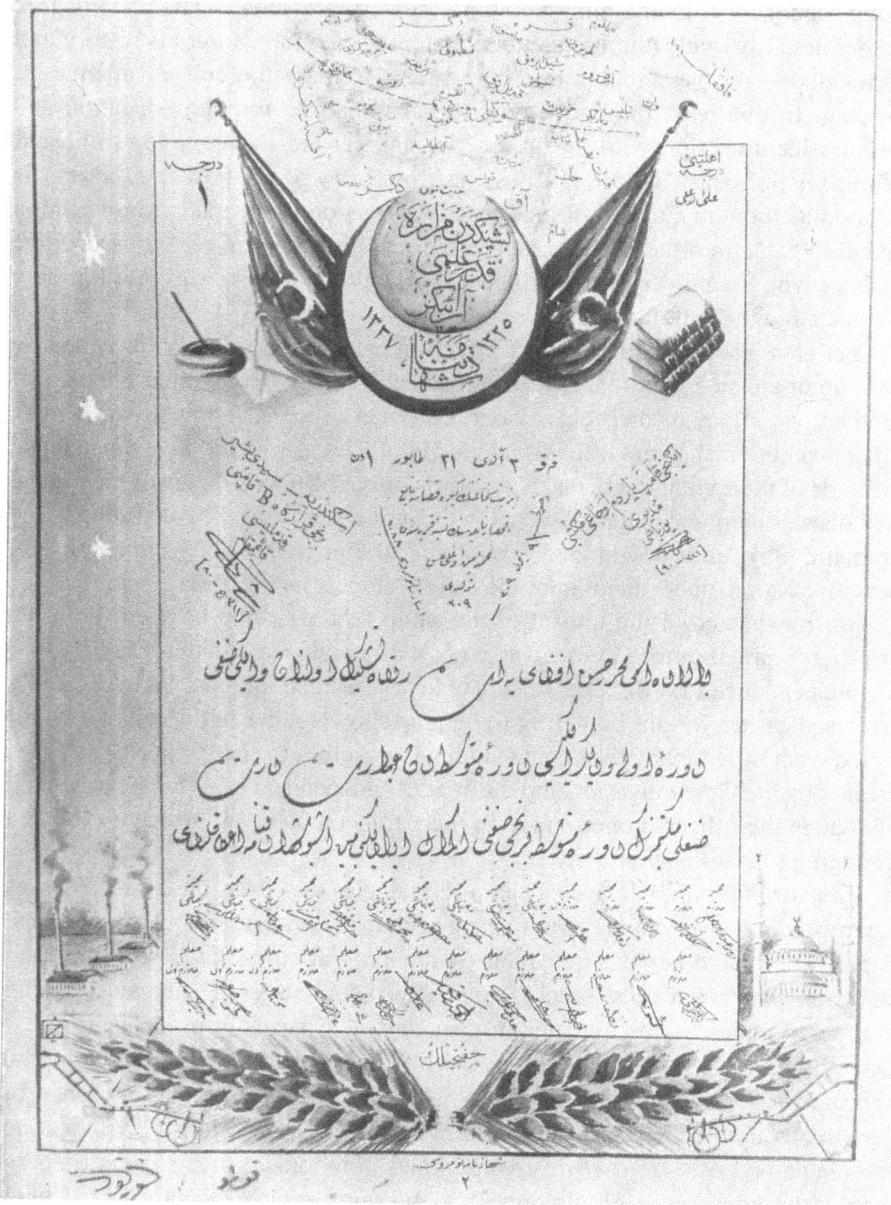

Figure 3.1 Prison camp diploma and recognition of achievement for Mehmed Emin oğlu Hasan Efendi of Geyve, İzmit. Degree of completion: Excellent.
Captivity number: 1088
Source: Courtesy of Atillâ Ertürk

worldly accomplishments. The officers claimed that they had accomplished in a few short months what the village schools had not accomplished after years of attendance:

> Turkish youths, who did not learn a thing even after five years of attendance at village schools of the traditional teaching style, learned enough in the new style inside the barbed wire in the short time of three to four months to erase and change the various sinister signs of illiteracy . . . It will not be too difficult to raise the nation's sons, who were left in the hands of the otherworldly village teachers . . . to the best specimens of the world.[61]

In addition to highlighting the accomplishments of the men and their officer-teachers, this passage also condemns the clearly ineffective traditional teaching style of the village school, which would have employed repetition and memorisation. For the officers and the men, the advantages of the modern style were obvious in the results produced. Clearly, however, where and how this transformation took place was just as important.

The award ceremonies highlighted the role of the officer-teachers. The men's successes were also their own, and it was time to pat themselves on the back for the accomplishments of the peasant soldiers. It is clear from the editorials and bits of camp news in the camp newspapers that while there was a certain sense of pride at their accomplishment, there was also a reminder to those peasant soldiers who could now read and write that it was the officers who had taught them.[62] As one essay noted, 'Happy are the teachers who enlighten the formerly dark hearts'.[63] They were happy for the students, themselves and the nation that they were hoping to rescue and regenerate. Their experiment in the prison camps was a great success, and they were prepared to embark on a similar endeavour upon repatriation.

BEYOND THE CONFINES OF THE CAMP SCHOOLS: EDUCATING THE NATION

While promoting education in the prison camps, officers regularly considered the larger question of how they could initiate the education of the larger Ottoman-Turkish society. Disappointed that the imperial state devoted little attention and even less financial support to public education, one officer revealed what he considered to be an embarrassing situation. He noted that the Ottoman state's education budget was only one-fifth of the education budget of Bulgaria, a former Ottoman colony. That a former colony had surpassed the Ottoman Empire so soon after its independence in 1908 (autonomy in 1878) was seen as evidence of Ottoman backwardness and the state's disregard of such issues. Claiming that attempting to fix such problems through the state, or the state itself, would be incredibly difficult; the author offered an alternative. 'There are many things young people like us can do as part of [our] responsibility to the nation', he said; owning up to it, he continued, these responsibilities have been 'much too neglected'.[64] The time for turning to the government and expecting these things from it 'had long past'. The 'debt' the young 'educated' sons of the nation owed to the people, and to the nation, was considerable and the kind of thing that only they could repay – not 'with empty words, but with actual acts'.[65] The present situation demanded action from the educated types who talked mightily, but did not involve themselves in the actual task of uplifting the peasant and rescuing the nation through education.

By way of talking about the education of the nation, in an essay titled 'Knowledge is necessary to live' in *Türk Varlığı* in Egypt, one prisoner wrote on the issue of who merited this education and who would be counted on as allies in this endeavour. Unlike the officer in the above who divided the community into two basic categories of ignorant and educated classes, this one offered four general categories. His schema identified those who could be counted on to help remedy the situation, as well as those who needed the remedy. The *ulema* class was comprised of those 'who possessed knowledge and knew' things. To the *müdrik* class belonged those people who possessed enough intellect to 'know what they did not know and readily acknowledged' their shortcomings. The third was the 'ignorant class' (*cühela*), or 'those who possessed no knowledge' at all. The fourth in this scheme was the '*humakâ*', or fools and idiots, who had no 'comprehension of what they knew, what they did not know, or even of their own existence'. Foreshadowing the actions and thoughts of the mental health specialists who came to dominate the discourse in the 1920s and 1930s, this writer decided that the fourth class was of no use for his purposes; therefore, he decided to 'leave them to the specialists' for further 'classification, legislation and even possible curing'. The writer chose to focus on the second and third classes, because they possessed enough potential to be educated and refocused. This could be done 'first by creating a sense of awakening, a sense of vigilance', and educating them to reach enlightenment (*nûr-ı maarifle tenvîr*).[66] This, the author imagined, would make the educable masses more useful to themselves, their community and most importantly, to the nation.

Starting the planning while still in an Egyptian prison camp, the author of 'İçtimai Dertlerimizden – Bilgisizlik' (One of Our Social Problems – Ignorance) suggested an agenda to be activated when the officers returned home. The burden of educating the peasants would fall on the shoulders of the repatriated officer prisoners and other like-minded, educated persons. The author proposed that each person focus on an area near where he lived. Of course, their focus would be Anatolia. After identifying villages that did not have schools, the officers would visit the villagers and inform them, 'in a language they could understand', about the benefits of education for themselves and their children. Then, the first task would be to convince the villagers to construct a school building. This, the author believed, would not be as difficult as it might have sounded, because 'villagers who appreciate the harm of ignorance, who have suffered for it most sadly, will surely view such good deeds [and people who do them] as grace', from God. When the villagers were convinced of the benefits of education, the officer imagined, then they would gather all the materials needed and build their own schools rather than expecting it from the state. Once the school building was put up, the rest would be easier:

> The only thing remaining for our educated young men is to educate them [villagers]. As he sees the results of good deeds, the villager will be grateful to those who do the kindness. He will carry the educator on his shoulders. He will feed him and obtain every need he has ... As these young people take care of this particular duty [of education], they can also base villagers' agricultural practices and trading (and finances) on more solid methods ... The young teacher should also become the villagers' mentor (*akıl hocası*).[67]

Connecting what should be done after repatriation to what was just accomplished in the camp schools, the author added that showing the 'virtue and benefits of science and knowledge to our soon to be repatriated enlisted men in a way that will take root in their heart will make our future duty much easier as they propagandize for us', upon returning to their villages.[68] The peasant soldier graduates of the camp schools, instead of being obstacles to progress, would become the vanguards of progress. As the officers' collaborators, the repatriated peasant soldiers would act as agents of civilisation and advancement. With the benefit of camp education, these previously ignorant men had turned into 'contemporary-minded, mature men who would enliven themselves and infect others with the attitude of enjoying life'. The officers optimistically thought that the educated enlisted men, after 'having erased off the signs of pitifulness that is characteristic of ignorance ... would completely grasp the kinds of changes [required] in every village'.[69]

The writer above argued that the advocates of village education must use a language the villagers could understand. What did he mean? Some officers believed that besides a lack of communication, there was also an incompatibility of languages between the educated and the uneducated classes. Europeans had resolved this problem between the 'white folk' (*beyaz halk*) and 'black folk' (*kara halk*), that is between the 'enlightened' and 'unenlightened', but Turks lagged behind: 'We want to ask [and] understand the illness of the people. We want to remedy it, but they do not even understand our language ... Everywhere is a disease of inability to understand one another'.[70] This incompatibility of languages was thus a major cause of the cultural divide between the educated class and the 'unenlightened' peasants.[71] Young teachers and officers had to use a simplified Turkish both to bridge the divide and to explain to the peasants their backwardness. This call to simplification – or 'Turkification' – of the written language was not new, for the likes of Ziya Gökalp, the intellectual father of Turkish nationalism, had spoken of such issues on earlier occasions.[72] For the prisoners, this also meant that they had to talk to the peasants at a level they could understand. The intention was to be able talk *to* them, rather than over them. The camp-educated enlisted men made perfect envoys, as they had the advantage of knowing the language of the peasant and being familiar with that of the enlightened class.

Urging for the education of the entire peasant population, what the officer prisoners were suggesting was a significant undertaking. The plan to promote the peasants' education relied on sending educated people as teachers or trainers to the backward regions and making use of those enlisted men who were educated as ambassadors. The plans they made for the nation's education at the end of the Great War while still in prison camps is remarkably similar to the ones adopted by the Turkish republic in 1940. The Village Institutes, as they came to be called, combined academic, agricultural and technical subjects in the curriculum. These Institutes trained villagers who would then return to their villages to act as teachers and community leaders. They would work to spread new skills and improve rural life.[73]

Clearly, though, what happened in reality was not as ambitious as what the officer prisoners imagined in the camps.[74] When the Village Institutes first came up for discussion in the Turkish Grand Nationalist Assembly in 1940, the deputy for Bingöl, Feridun Fikri Düşünsel, a former prisoner of war in Egypt and a writer in the camp newspaper *Badiye*, said in the chamber:

> We are face to face with the Republic's most beautiful work. Truly, there was a great need for such an organ [of government] to go to the village, to show close interest in the villager, to take care of his every need, and to take into account his every affair ... from consideration of civilization and social progress.

He asked the Minister of Education to ensure that the teachers sent especially to the villages of eastern provinces should make it their mission to 'improve their [peasants'] language and instil and inspire into the soul of the villager all the aims (*gayeler*) of our country, our nation, our solidarity'. Yet, even as he asked

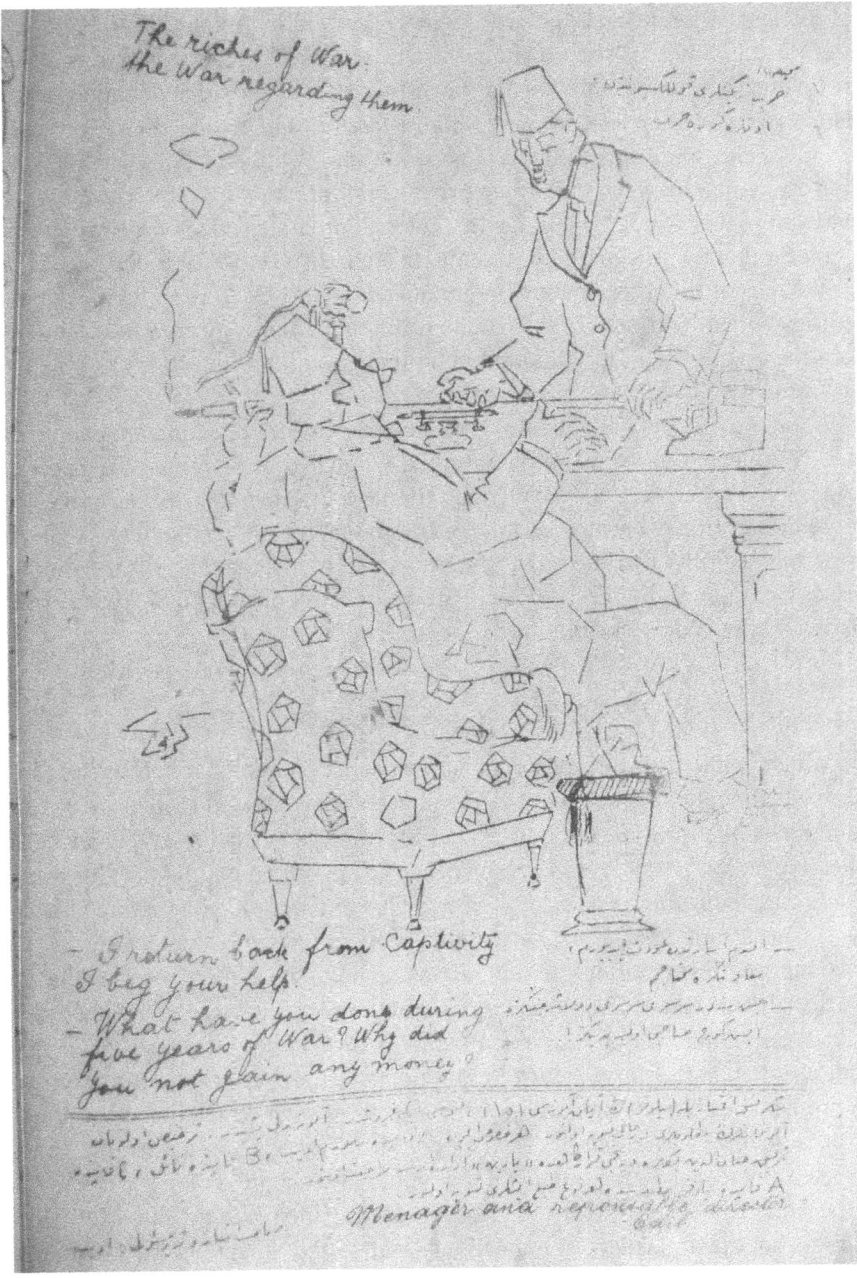

Figure 3.2 Prisoner imagining reception by the 'War Rich' upon his repatriation
Source: 'From the War Rich Collection: the war according to them', in *Nilüfer* (1920)

that the teachers reinforce the sentiment of nationality among the villagers, he never mentioned in his speech similar debates he had had with his fellow prisoners.[75] Nevertheless, despite the significantly earlier discussions of such issues in prison camps, scholars working on Village Institutes have traced their origins to later ideas and sources both internal and external. While this book cannot establish a direct link between the officer prisoners' ideas about 'going to the nation's backward regions' and the Village Institutes of republican Turkey, it will suffice to suggest that the prisoners' promotion of such ideas may have been one stream that flowed into such projects.[76] As in other fields, such as the women's movement in the late Ottoman Empire, the early republican reforms would not have taken the course they did without much pioneer work earlier on by people who have remained invisible and anonymous.[77]

When the officers in the camps took up the issue of educating the people and actually educated the enlisted men, they diverged from the elitist ideologies of the Young Turks, who had abandoned the idea of educating the peasants long before these officers became prisoners. But the junior officers believed that educating the peasants was the most important step to awaken and lift the ignorant masses from their ignoble situation, and to put them on the path of advancement; this would serve the regeneration of the nation.[78]

THE SOLUTION: *GAYE* AND *MEFKURE*

The officer prisoners did not doubt the enormity of the task before them, but they also thought that if they could unite among themselves and agree on a 'common aim', they could educate and regenerate the nation. What made the collective action possible was the existence of an aim among those who wanted to uplift and educate the peasant soldiers. This aim was no simple thing or idea; it was a 'common soul, a common mindset' (*ruh-i müşterek*). Because the task of saving and regenerating the nation was so colossal, many more people than just the officers needed to possess this common soul in order for their 'jihad' against ignorance and possible national extinction to be successful.[79] This 'common ideal' (*mefkure-i müşterek*) among the people was required to give the project consistency and strength.[80] When the nation developed this common ideal, 'a genius [was] more likely to emerge from among us', to lead the people. Otherwise, without a common ideal that united the people, no one 'had the right or the authority to represent the national desire [ideal] as he saw it'.[81] Either behind a national leader or collectively without that genius, a '*seferberlik*' (mobilisation) was needed in this war against ignorance, backwardness, lack of civilisation, and economic and industrial underdevelopment.[82]

Although they did not specifically name him, by using the word *mefkure*, or ideal, in the sense that Ziya Gökalp, the intellectual father of Turkish nationalism, used it, the prisoners showed that they were aware of his ideas. Influenced by Émile Durkheim, Gökalp initially identified this 'ideal' as knowledge of society which developed when human beings became aware of the existence and value of the social group to which they belonged. This realisation sometimes took place during a time of deep social crises, such as war and defeat. Both the prisoners in camps and the people of the nation were facing such a situation. Only by realising its 'ideal', its 'aim', would the society understand its own nature, origin and task as a nation.[83] Before settling on *mefkure*, Gökalp used other words: *Hayal* (phantom), *gaye* (aim) and *emel* (aspiration). In the early 1920s, Gökalp extended the meaning of ideal so that it amounted to something beyond self-knowledge of society. It now encompassed expressions of the 'soul' of society – everything from fairy tales to religious beliefs to legal and economic concepts. The only condition was that they needed to be 'collective ideals, common to members of society', ideas that existed in its 'collective consciousness'.[84] For him, this is what unified a group of people into a cohesive nation.

From the officer prisoners' perspective the problem that the nation faced in this difficult time was the absence of this *mefkure*, or common 'ideal'. They used other words or phrases to express the same idea: *gaye* (aim), *ruh-i müşterek* (common soul), *medeniyet gayesi* (aim of civilisation) and *tevhid-i âmâl* (unity of desires).[85] However, the phrase *gaye* (aim, purpose, intention) seems to have been more commonly used. *Gaye* was necessary to advance and regenerate the nation; however, they realised that they faced a problem: the lack of *gaye*, or *gayesizlik*. Someone without *gaye* was of no use to the nation even if 'he [individually] was donated with the most perfect educational tools and civilization'. Those qualities were useless if not connected to the larger goal of helping the nation. *Gaye* had to be something 'very sacred' and 'much esteemed' so that the 'whole nation could follow it collectively with their hearts and spirits, and use it to inspire (and inculcate) their children and grandchildren'.[86] By being optimistic about the future and teaching and spreading *gaye* to those who were without it, it was possible to arrive at a 'very bright *ruh-i müşterek*', (common soul) with 'our conviction of conscience and faith' (*kanaat-i vicdanımızla, imanla*).[87] Faith in this context referred to faith in the aim. Everyone needed this aim 'more than anything else'.

> From a student in school learning his lesson syllable by syllable to a father practicing his religion among mosque columns to a mother who lives dreams of the past by the hearth to a shepherd whose flock walks behind him to a soldier who stands guard at the border, the whole nation had to possess this *ruh-i müşterek*.[88]

Clearly, the officers who were writing about this aim knew what it meant and why it was important. They wanted to identify those who suffered from *gayesizlik* or those who had not yet recognised how crucial it was, and teach them about its potentials and its role in regenerating the nation. It was no surprise that the ignorant peasants did not have *gaye*, but the officer prisoners believed that there were even educated types who did not possess it or understand its power.

In search of people suffering from *gayesizlik*, one of the groups the prisoners settled on was the state's civil servants. Others, however, could be found in all walks of life. Why would the civil servants of the state be obstacles to what the officers wanted to achieve? For some officers, civil servants were directly responsible for the backwardness of the peasants, and therefore, the nation. In a bold generalisation, one prisoner branded them as self-serving individuals who clung to the security of their government jobs 'like a climbing ivy plant', (*sarmaşık*) and cared for nothing else.[89] Much like an ivy that attached itself to whatever it found nearby, the civil servants were difficult to dislodge from their precious jobs, which they used only for personal gain. Another piece asserted that civil servants had failed to acknowledge that 'they are the servants of [the people] and the nation'. Instead of obeying the laws of the state 'that determined [both] their obligations and authority, they have treated their benefactors, the people, in contemptuous and despicable manner'.[90] Accordingly, the civil servants as a class without a national *gaye* became obstacles to the education and regeneration of the nation. Some even suggested that choosing the civil service as a career would hurt the future of the nation. All it offered was the 'safety' of a job, while other careers would be more useful both to the individual and to the nation. In this way, choosing a career, a livelihood, became not a personal decision as much as one with national importance.[91]

From the officers' point of view the civil servants had lulled themselves into a false sense of security and accomplishment. As it stood, they worked for themselves, not for the people or the future of the nation. Therefore, they presented an obstruction to the realisation of a single-minded *gaye*. These officers viewed other educated but 'aimless' types as belonging to the same category of people who did not contribute to educating the people and regenerating the nation. As difference turned to antagonism and antagonism into threat (or obstruction), these groups were also discursively excluded from the nation the prisoners imagined.

But what did these officers mean when they used the word nation? Were they talking about Turks, Ottomans or Muslims? In the foregoing we discovered that some officers were displeased by their men calling themselves Ottomans but not Turks, or deciding that being a Turk carried denominational meanings. Were the officers more precise in terms of their identification? Given that the officers were suggesting following the lead of Europe and committing to a religious transformation, were they ideologically close to the Westernist wing of the Young Turks who advocated adoption of Western civilisation with its roses and thorns?[92]

TURKS, MUSLIMS AND OTTOMANS

While critical of those who aped Western ways carelessly, for the danger such imitation represented to national culture and tradition, some officer prisoners attempted to diagnose why such behaviour manifested itself. In other words, they asked why some Ottomans imitated Europeans. As he pointed to the dangers of such conduct, one prisoner maintained that the adoption of Western ways could be seen even among those young people who considered themselves nationalists (*milliyetperest*, literally, someone who worships the nation). How could someone who was *milliyetperest* end up acting in such a way? Why would he still be considered a nationalist? The same prisoner then went on to explore a scenario of how this might happen and how it could be prevented.

> Because we have fallen behind the West ... [our culture] seems uninteresting (*yavan*) [even to our own selves] As a result, we feel ashamed to acknowledge as 'ours' the many good qualities we possess ... [This] brings forth a dangerous catastrophe. Unfortunately, a majority of our young people who are deprived of a sound and real national training [and education] become confused and unsuccessful in this sort of situation. Finally, in a state of deep confusion, they ... become Europeanized (*frenkleşmek*) ... This is more [dangerous] than dandyism [*züppelik*] ... It is such an extensive social disease that its damage is seen abundantly among all youngsters ... Currently, this degenerate (*tereddi*) behaviour is even evident among our youngsters known to be convinced nationalists (*milliyetperest*).[93]

Admitting it was true that some of our 'institutions' lagged behind or were seen as 'old fashioned' especially in comparison to the West, he suggested that this was the reason why young people tended to adopt European behaviour and 'institutions' as guides even without necessarily wanting to do so. Describing this 'attraction' to the West as normal as an 'electrical occurrence' (*hadise-yi elektrikiyye*), he suggested some quick solutions:

> Even if it is incomplete, the young generation has [national] consciousness; they have a culture (*hars*) ... This culture is one of the common institutions that constitute the nation. Nation (*millet*) means the whole of the shared institutions of literature, music, architecture, language, letters (*hurufat*), traditions, customs,

and, of course, sentiments. Accordingly, before everything else, it is necessary to establish firmly and reinforce thoroughly those institutions that contain national meanings [and character]. The first institution that needs to be firmed, whose foundation will be strengthened, is '*hars* – culture'.[94]

Since no nationalist would even consider the possible inferiority of his culture compared to a foreign one, this author was suggesting that while some unidentified institutions needed bolstering, the real problem was the failure of the educational system. A better and more proper education could imbue the younger generation with knowledge and awareness of national and cultural institutions and cultural practices that they could be proud to call their own. Providing us with a rare definition, the author suggested that it was those cultural practices in common that constituted the nation.

While the prisoners frequently referred to *millet*, which they used in the sense of nation, as in *milliyetperest*, they rarely defined this or other similar concepts.[95] Definitions of the terms they regularly used were rare because they took their words' meaning for granted. Rather than writing about abstract concepts such as nation and identity, prisoners actually acted, wrote and critiqued with the nation and culture in mind. The concept influenced their actions subconsciously without requiring explanation. They did not consciously define what it meant to be a Turk, Ottoman or a Muslim, but wrote as a Turk, Ottoman or a Muslim. Therefore, we might try to discern what served as points of identification from whatever they left behind.

Sometimes the officer prisoners resorted to metaphors to make a case about the importance of maintaining cultural institutions and practices. In the following, an imaginary dialogue takes place between two prisoners. Ostensibly it is about music. The exchange gives us a sense of what the above author may have been talking about when he referred to the attractiveness of certain Western cultural institutions. As it appeared in a camp newspaper, two views were set up to clash. In this conversation the Europeanised character, *Tepegöz* ('low-browed', or Cyclops), who played Western music, told the other, *Ne Münasebet* ('Of course not' or 'Far from it'), who liked Turkish music that he, *Ne Münasebet*, was backwards because his music is old-fashioned and primitive. To *Ne Münasebet*'s comment that they are all members of the same nation, *Tepegöz* responded: 'true . . . but there is a difference. We are not the men of the same time period . . .'. Offended at being called backwards, *Ne Münasebet*, which is also the name of the newspaper produced in a prison camp in India, responded:

> *Ne Münasebet*: . . . just because you study western music you see yourself as being better than me? Look, look at you! You are one of us, yet you do not like

us. If you are an easterner, then it is necessary that you get your nourishment from eastern music.

Tepegöz: Your knowledge of human society is narrow. Simple and primitive music is enough to satisfy your tastes. For those whose musical tastes are advanced, your style of music is ineffective. All Oriental music does is to put one in a melancholic mood (*hüzün*).

Ne Münasebet: Whatever are you saying? Oriental music does not numb people, you are lethargic on your own! Don't our various melodic styles (*makam*) each have different effects on us? Don't you feel certain grandeur within yourself with *rast makam* (melodic mode) or a stirring in your body with *karcığâr* [*makam*]?

Tepegöz: The difference I see is superficial. If only you understood *alafranga* (European) music . . . [but] like everyone else you will slowly come around![96]

Eventually, Tepegöz asked his companion, 'Do you remember when you said the other day "Please, Tepegöz, this tune (*hava*, air or melody) is very nice, play it one more time, so I can listen again"?' But the answer he received put an end to the conversation: 'How you misunderstood. I enjoyed it because I associated it to *Hüseynî* [makam]'.[97] In the end, *Ne Münasebet* likened European music to a Middle Eastern *makam*, more specifically a mode that is supposed to bring serenity and ease to its listeners. The message of the exchange is that traditional music became national music and, as such, it represented a source of identification and psychological sustenance for the members of the nation. Some foreign music, especially when likened to a national form, could also serve the same purpose. But, the critical point here was that *Tepegöz*'s total abandonment of Turkish or Oriental music, as a source of national nourishment, undermined the rekindling of a unified sense of national purpose.

Earlier we discovered that at least one officer was astonished that his men called themselves Ottomans and did not identify as Turks; were they necessarily exclusionary? The piece that follows called 'Ballad', answers this question and more. It is only a short sample of a significantly longer poem, which appeared serialised in the Krasnoyarsk camp paper, *Vaveyla*, in December 1915. Likely composed by a minimally illiterate man, it gives us a good sense of how various identities might have coexisted unproblematically, especially for the enlisted men. If the author is an enlisted man (or even a sergeant) who was literate prior to captivity, the heroic poem represents the genuine voice of the subaltern – the peasant – with regard to those things with which he identified.[98]

Ballad

Ottomans we are, our soldiers roar [like lions].
My mother and father should not cry; we will come back some day.
If we do not return, we will all die in the path of religion.
It is not a bloody *bayram* (holiday);⁹⁹ this is the Jihad of believers.
My God's paradise was promised in these lands.
Even if we die, the soul of the nation, religion and state will live on.
Whosoever is Muslim will not stay home, but will avenge us.
Listen to me, as long as one Turk remains, let us continue our fight . . .
In the land of the Muscovite, there are many Muslims, let us unite with them.¹⁰⁰
Let us topple the towers that display the Cross above the Crescent.
Ottomans we are, let us plant our flag in the four corners [of the world].¹⁰¹

Clearly, in 1915, the author considered himself and others as belonging to three categories Ottomans, Muslims and Turks, simultaneously without any contradiction.¹⁰² One could suggest from the context that he did not appeal to all Muslims of the world (*umma*) in a broad sense, but to Ottoman Muslims and the Muslim Turkic peoples of Russia. Yet, there is still some uncertainty in that for words like 'believers', or 'whosoever is Muslim', point to something larger than Turkish-Turkic Muslims. Notably, again, the Turkic populations of Russia are referred to as simply 'Muslims' and not Turks, even though the author feels himself to be a Turk, among other identifications. Perhaps even the fact that he used the word '*Islam*' in Turkish rather than the more appropriate '*müslüman*' to refer to Muslims also gives away his rather rudimentary literacy. In many writings, the distinction between Islam as a faith and Muslims as a community disappeared. Evidently, Islam came to refer to a community rather than to a faith even though it was Islam that was the common denominator of that community.

The officer prisoners' writings show only little more discrimination and selectivity in terms of identity markers used than the enlisted men. One officer in Krasnoyarsk, writing in *Vaveyla*, pleaded with his comrades to mind their behaviour, and wrote: 'Let us not forget that we represent the Turkish nation in this garrison. Let us show [others] that we are the inheritors of the great Islamic religion'.¹⁰³ There is no distinction between Turkish nation and Islamic religion. For an officer in Egypt, writing an editorial in *Işık* on the occasion of a religious holiday in 1919, one was more important than the other. He suggested that all prisoners should prepare for

the real holiday (*bayram*), big holiday! This holiday, which will someday be marked on calendars, is more natural, more scientific than Islamic unification (*ittihad-i İslam*) . . . It will be the day of Turk(ish/ic) unification (*Türk ittihadi*). Then history will record this day of Turks' second *Ergenekon*.[104]

While the quotation above might seem to be coloured more heavily with Turkism, identification with Islam is still there even if accorded a secondary role. The feelings and emotions of a person at that moment could also influence their feelings of identification as something familiar and important presented itself. Travelling in a train through a densely forested area of Siberia after escaping from Krasnoyarsk, Ragıp Bey, a madrasa graduate, and devout Muslim, noted: 'I was lost in thought as I was contemplating how Turkish soldiers (*yiğitleri*) [of the past] had galloped their horses around here. I likened the tall trees of the forest to their lances'.[105] There is no '*ittihad-ı Islam*' here or anywhere else in the memoir. A sense of connection to the geography, spurred on by lance-like tall trees, stirred deep emotions.

The poem '*Turan*', dedicated to the author's 'little brother', gives a good mixture of these images, combining Turkism with Islam. It appeared in an Egyptian camp newspaper called *Türk Varlığı* (Turkish Presence/Existence). Turan, of course, was the ancestral homeland of ancient Turks and as such it evokes notions of pan-movements, but this is not a secular nationalist manifesto:

'Turan', What is it? Where is it?
You ask of Turan? It means fatherland, my dear child!
Your ancestors sprung and came to life around here,
By expanding, by battling, they became glorious in these places:
'Büyük Orta', 'Red Apple', 'Beyazid', and 'Karakorum'!

'To populate (and prosper) there . . .' This has to be your ideal
Even if the whole world perished, this is your race (*ırk*)!
Like that of your ancestors: your fame should be heard in Europe;
What you call 'Turan!' is there, your real homeland.

The Turk has two sentiments: One care (*kaygı*) is Turan!
Turk's national sentiments fill and overflow for 'Turan'
The other sentiment is his Quran that inspires [illegible]
Turk lives only for his religious and national tradition!

Never forget these passions (*ışklar*) in your soul, my dear child
These are glories left to you from the Prophet and Oğuz [tribe],
These are excitements left behind by centuries [passing];
Beware, my dear child, never forget this holy tradition![106]

As the poem appeared in 1920, one is tempted to suggest that the reason Ottomanness is not mentioned could be the result of the prisoners' having already given up on it by that date. The author's first allegiance is to Turan and Turkishness, but is closely followed by Islam. In fact, what seems like priority given to Turkism in the first three lines of the third quatrain is reversed in the fourth line, where the Turk lives for his religious tradition first.

As the *Turan* poem above shows, romantic ideas of nationalism had strong appeal among the prisoners. This was a rather new phenomenon among the Turks, who had recently discovered mutual affinities with the Turkic peoples of Central Asia, and thus the idea of a broader pan-Turkism emerged.[107] Given the fact that some of the prisoners had studied the history of the Turks while in school and that those in Russia came into contact with Turkic peoples, this is not surprising. While Turkish history in the civilian schools and textbooks was minimised, the military schools discussed Turkish history in detail.[108] Central Asia was of great importance to those Ottomans who emphasised their Turkishness. In prisoner writings, allusions to the region are more common among prisoners held captive in Russia, than those in Egypt.[109] A significant number of prisoners in Russia felt something familiar in the cities and regions the prisoners' trains passed on their way to different camps or in the locales where they were imprisoned. One of them, stating that the 'city of Krasnoyarsk was part of the land where the Gökturks used to live', made his environment more familiar by connecting to it through ancient 'national' history.[110] There were other such places, as well, that made the POWs feel nostalgic about their Turkish history, homeland and ancestors. Another prisoner who kept a diary recorded the places his train passed:

> We come to the city of Tümen (Tyumen). Our journey continues as we pass the first flourishing city of Asia, this old Turkish city and Turkish civilization located in the heart of this land of our ancestors [*dedeler yurdu*] where now their esteemed (*saygıdeğer*) souls flew and swarmed through the high skies and where we inhaled their delightful odour and kissed their soul ... We came to Manchuria station. This place is a very old Turkish motherland and Turkish city. This is obvious from the people we see, and there is a certain noble quality in their faces. Both their faces and the language they speak are nearly the same as ours.[111]

Turkishness could be expressed just as easily without any reference to Turan and where religion and Islam mixed in with Turkishness much more seamlessly and naturally. In the following lines, there is a clear worrisome and anxious sentiment about the future of the nation that is at the brink of a disaster. However, the defeat of the Turks is not a defeat of Turks alone. This poem appeared in *Türk Varlığı* in Egypt when Anatolia was under Greek and Istanbul under allied invasion.

Don't Mourn!

Our race that established thrones and won glories in all environs,
Is now withered in the face of disasters.
While Anatolia, heaven-like country, is being destroyed
To mourn fell on us; we cried inwardly.
Would you believe the Crescent lost to the Cross and Islam bemoans [?]
...
Surely no single flower is left in gardens
[But] one day, of course, it will sprout again
Do not let it open up the unhealed wound
Let them struggle to plough the hilltop
Yes, it is true, this savagery is too bloody
Surely, one day heavenly God will have pity on us
On that day, will yell 'I am a Turk',
The surviving Turk, shouting to the universe.
Sons of Turks are hopeful; he won't mourn
Will avenge us surely; he won't forget.[112]

Past glory mixed in with some current reality is also clearly evident here. People need a golden age with which to identify and in order to imagine a future golden age, even if current circumstances have left no traces of it. The poem ends with a positive although threatening and vengeful note. The vengeance is not for Islam, but for Turkishness.

Having already found ourselves mentioning places as far away as Karakorum in Mongolia or other parts of Asia beyond Anatolia, we might briefly examine the prisoners' occasional references to the East and Asia. The rescuing and regeneration of the nation was certainly the most important aim for the future, but some also tied their national struggle to something larger. For them, the fate of 'the East' (*Şark*) and the 'World of Islam' also hung in balance. Failure for Turks meant failure for the entire Islamic world. It made sense that they would see themselves as defending Islam or the Islamic world as well, but they referred to the East and Asia. They found similarities in terms of mentalities among Eastern and Asian religious traditions.

Many of these prisoners believed there was much riding on the success of the Turks because 'Turkey was the heart of the eastern world'. Because of this its survival and regeneration was important for all Easterners and eastern nations (*şarklılar, şark milletleri*), who were 'helpless as a child who has fallen and cannot get up'.[113] But Turkey was different: 'I would like to absolve my nation from this eastern characteristic of having fallen into slavery'.[114] After all, another editorial added, 'the dark clouds that wanted to settle on the Islamic world were rising from Turkey. As long as we continue to writhe in hopelessness, we will separate the [people of] the great East from ourselves and ourselves from them'.[115] Not only the ignorant people of the nation were in need of enlightenment and rescue from the despair they were in, but the 'down and out elements of Asia were in great need of a Turkey that achieved [and completed] its knowledge [acquirement] and advancement'.[116]

These men did not feel the need to justify their assertion that Turkey was and would continue to be the leader of the East, because from their perspective it made sense without rationalisation. It was understood that, as in the past, when the Ottomans 'never failed to protect the lands of the East' from Europeans, a Turkey, a 'new' Turkey that escaped the dark clouds of extinction and regenerated itself would become a beacon of hope for the rest of the Eastern world.[117] The claim about 'protecting the lands of the East', was another version of the discourse about Turks protecting Islam from Europeans or Christianity as Arabs watched idly, which was encountered in Chapter 2. This idea served a second purpose. It served as a way to explain how Turks' commitment to others took attention away from themselves and their own problems. Once again, Turkish commitment to others who were different from them, was used as an explanation for the backwardness and belatedness of the nation.

Given the tension between defending Islam and the East against Europe on the one hand, but also wanting to be like Europe in many ways on the other, one prisoner pleaded earnestly with his fellow prisoners in a way reminiscent of the later republican slogans about relations with Europe. He wrote, 'up to now we have been a barrier to Europe; let us now become a bridge'.[118] This metaphor of the bridge was not new and neither would it disappear any time soon. It continues to our day. Commenting mostly on recent Turkish-EU relations, one modern scholar captured the image and meaning of the bridge in the following form:

> Turkey, which has been labelled by both outsiders and insiders as a bridge between the East and the West, has an ambivalent relation not only to the geographical sites of the East and the West, but also to their temporal signification: namely, backwardness and progress. Turkey has been trying to cross the bridge between the East and the West for more than a hundred years now, with a self-conscious anxiety that it is arrested in time and space by the bridge itself.[119]

However, unlike what the later republican leadership might have thought about crossing this bridge, this particular prisoner and a number of others were not suggesting that Turks needed to cross the bridge. Instead he was suggesting that Turkey and Turks needed to serve the function of a bridge between East and West. Since Turks shared with the peoples of the East the illness of backwardness in comparison to the technologically advanced and powerful West, the new and regenerated Turkey would share its guiding light with Eastern peoples. Once it regenerated itself, the nation of Turks would help other Asians uplift themselves. 'As we work in a quiet orderliness within our own homeland, we will always be reminded of the necessity of being an example and a guide to millions of people' of the East. Because of this, 'Turkishness' had to advance quickly, 'leading the East' toward the field of knowledge (*saha-yı irfan*).[120] Another essay noted something very similar in sentiment: 'Ottoman Turks are not only charged with advancement on for their own benefit; at the same time they had the aim of advancing' Eastern peoples.[121] Only in that case, as 'we bring the flames of knowledge to our own people in a way they will accept it and perform it, will the East live and Turkishness be ever-lasting (*payidar*)'.[122] It is noteworthy that even in such a position, these men never let go of the idea of the Ottomans or Turks being the defenders and leaders of the 'Eastern world'.

Because all Eastern or Asian peoples were threatened by the same 'nightmare of ignorance', which at least one prisoner believed amounted to the 'bloodiest of all murderers', Turkey would start the fight by using 'citadels of science and knowledge, trade cannons' and 'lights of science'. These they would learn from Europeans. The fight would go on until the land of Turks became 'a grave for this ancient enemy [of ignorance]. What a victory [it would be]! This is the Greatest Jihad! This is the Holy War! This is the real fight for existence!'[123] Turkey's success would be an example to all Easterners. However, all this would be possible only if Turks understood one another, educated and uplifted the ignorant, and unified around a *gaye* to regenerate the nation. All these represented crucial changes, but only by changing in the interest of the nation would the project succeed. Only when Turkey and Turks succeeded 'would both friend and enemy (*yar-ü-agyâr*) say that 'there is change in Turkey'.[124]

CONCLUSION

As the foregoing showed, the prisoners' concern about the future of the nation was both real and deep as they first waited for the end of the war and then the repatriation that didn't materialise quickly enough. This seemingly obvious observation hides something behind it. Other scholars have pointed out that the intellectual and political elite worried over the question of 'how to save the state?' The prisoner officers examined here did not seem to be concerned about 'saving the state'. In fact, some of them implicated the state in 'destroying' the nation by giving an assumed preference to the *reaya*. The state became 'foreign' to the people and a refuge for those selfish civil servants. However, the prisoners were deeply concerned about protecting and saving the nation. Although they discursively excluded the ignorant peasant soldiers from the nation, they also cared for them enough to attempt to uplift them to a place where they would be worthy of inclusion. We might be tempted to assume that the disregard for the state was more obvious in those essays that appeared in 1918 or after, when the prisoners saw the writing on the wall about the future of the Ottoman Empire and the state. Why bother saving the state when the war's victors were about to destroy it completely? This is probably partially true. Seeing that the state could be rebuilt, saving the nation became their focus. Yet, this assumption does not explain why they ignored the state and focused on the nation as early as 1915 in some cases in their writings, or why they blamed the state and the civil servants for the backwardness of the people. Was it possible that, unlike the political and intellectual leadership, they cared about 'how to save the nation' all along, even if their preference became much more noticeable after 1918? This chapter suggested as much.

We also noticed that while some officers ridiculed their enlisted men for not knowing their identity and refusing to acknowledge their Turkishness, in a number of pieces the officers themselves pointed to their Turkishness, Muslimness and Ottomanness at the same time. Was this hypocrisy? No, for them the problem was the peasants' denial of their Turkishness. Interchangeable use of identity markers without much pointed discrimination among the prisoners points to the presence of broader notions of identity existing at the same time. It is likely that while they were used interchangeably, one or another of them – whether Turkishness, Muslimness or Ottomanness – held a singular importance. Of course, Ottomanness was certainly on the decline at the end of the war.

What is also noticeable here is that identity construction was not merely semiotic, that is symbolic, where people discover their nation through discursive practices. It involved and relied upon construction of 'otherness' and alterity at a number of levels. Those Others could be ethnic Others as well as domestic Others. As Žižek would have argued, these Others undermined the fulness of the nation by being ignorant, selfish, and *gayesiz* (aimless). However, as much as they were a nuisance that undermined the realisation of the nation, they also served two useful purposes in terms of national identification. Their existence explained why the nation was not yet complete, but it made its future fulness a possibility towards which they could all work through educating the ignorant and teaching the aimless about a national *gaye*. Secondly, the exclusion of the ignorant, the aimless, the selfish, and others served to confirm and maintain the identity of those officers who considered themselves the gatekeepers of the nation, those who determined its borders.

NOTES

1. Timothy Mitchell, *Rule of Experts*, pp. 182–83; Timothy Mitchell, 'Making the Nation', pp. 214–15; Homi K. Bhabha, Dissemination', pp. 139–70.
2. Islamic modernism was also practiced by Jamal al-din Al-Afghani and Muhammad 'Abduh in the nineteenth century. Carter V. Findley, 'The Advent of Ideology', pp. 148–9, 157ff; Şerif Mardin, *The Genesis of Young Ottoman Thought*; Şerif Mardin, 'European Culture', p. 18.
3. Findley, 'The Advent of Ideology', p. 157. The foremost scholar on the Young Turks is M. Şükrü Hanioğlu. Among others, see his *Preparation for a Revolution* and *Young Turks in Opposition*
4. Hanioğlu, *Young Turks*, pp. 207–8, 22–3, 32.
5. Hanioğlu, *Young Turks*, p. 206; Fatma Müge Göçek, 'Ethnic Segmentation', pp. 528–9.
6. M. Şükrü Hanioğlu actually uses the terms modernist and moderate, as opposed to my 'westernizers' and 'Islamic modernists', respectively. Berkes's terms for these groups are different.
7. Hanioğlu, *Young Turks*, pp. 14–15, 18, 23, 200.
8. It is useful to consider if only briefly how the historiography on the Young Turks has interpreted their identity and nationalism. M. Şükrü Hanioğlu argued that the Committee of Union and Progress (CUP) gradually converted to Turkish nationalism well before the revolution in 1908; even as early as 1906, CUP propaganda had acquired a Turkish nationalist focus (Hanioğlu, *Young Turks*). Hasan Kayalı argued that political Turkish nationalism was not a viable force until after the Great War. The CUP subscribed to Ottomanist and Islamist political ideals to the end; like Arabs, Turks carried multiple layers of identities (Hasan Kayalı, *Arabs and Young Turks*). More recently, Kemal Karpat argued along similar lines: 'Historical Continuity and Identity Change', pp. 1–28. In the same volume as Karpat, Erik Jan Zürcher ('Young Turks'), looking at actual policies, as opposed to writings, argued that the period of 1918–22 was the zenith of Ottoman Muslim nationalism. In the end, Zürcher may be right in his conclusion, but he does not give due weight to the possibility that the leadership of the National Resistance (*Milli Mücadele*) may have used the term 'Ottoman Muslims' simply as a political ploy to maintain the support of the religious leaders, Kurds and other Muslim peoples who remained within *Misak-ı Milli* after the armistice: Arabs, Circassians and others. After all, stirrings of Kurdish nationalism started during the Great War.
9. Partha Chatterjee, *Nationalist Thought*. On his description of the East-West dichotomy and the Orientalist problematic, see pp. 73 and 38.
10. Certainly, the prisoners were not the first to employ the 'matter versus spirit' dichotomy in their arguments about the Ottoman Empire. Prominent intellectuals, such as Ahmet Midhat in the nineteenth century and Mehmet Akif and Ziya Gökalp in the twentieth, also employed this dichotomy. Although organising the debate about cultural change in this way seems to have gained currency after 1908 in both Islamist (Mehmet Akif) and nationalist (Ziya Gökalp) thought, in general it was not the prevalent method in the

Ottoman context. This makes the writings of the officer prisoners all the more meaningful as it seems to be common among them. On Ahmet Midhat and his view of Europe, see Carter V. Findley, 'An Ottoman Occidentalist', pp. 15–49. See also Uriel Heyd, *Foundations of Turkish*; Ziya Gökalp, *Turkish Nationalism*.

11. The second story is reported by Mehmet Arif Ölçen, *Vetluga Memoir*, p. 215. In fact, this paternalistic criticism of the peasant soldier was not by the officer himself, but by Yusuf Akçura, who was in Russia after the Treaty of Brest Litovsk arranging for repatriation of some Ottoman POWs. When Yusuf Akçura asked the peasant soldier where he had been a captive, the soldier said 'in the city of Gorod'. The soldier did not realise 'gorod' (or 'grad') meant city in Russian. Further questions from Akçura did not result in a more accurate answer. Another example is about a former prisoner of war who wanted to escape from his camp in Burma and walk to Anatolia, a distance of about 4,100 nautical miles: Şevket S. Aydemir, *Suyu Arayan Adam*, pp. 109, note 1; 398. As the case of İbrahim Çelebi shows, the men had a general idea that the homeland was toward the west. Being told to go west from Siberia, İbrahim Çelebi ended up first in Ukraine, then farther south in Romania among the Gagauz Turks, who assisted him: Private letter dated 23 February 1999 and conversations with Dr Zekeriya Türkmen of ATASE Archives regarding his grandfather İbrahim Çelebi, February 1999, Ankara.
12. Aydemir, *Suyu Arayan Adam*, p. 105. The author was never a POW, but his view of the peasant soldier is no different from that of those officers who were POWs.
13. Aydemir, *Suyu Arayan Adam*, p. 104. We can see similar attitudes in the early republican novel *Yaban* by Yakub Kadri. In the novel, Sergeant Bekir answers the nationalist protagonist and his former officer during the Great War, Ahmet Celal, with the following words: 'We are not Turks sir . . . Glory be to God, we are Muslims. Those that you talk of [Turks] live in Haymana'. Yakub Kadri Karaosmanoğlu, *Yaban*, p. 172.
14. Rahmi Apak, *Yetmişlik Bir Subayın Hatıraları*, pp. 99–100, 231–2.
15. Faik Tonguç, *Birinci Dünya Savaşında*, p. 106. Aydemir, the non-POW officer mentioned above, states that one of his men answered the same question, 'Our prophet is Enver Paşa'. Aydemir, *Suyu Arayan Adam*, p. 103.
16. Ibid. p. 106.
17. For example, see Tonguç for bravery, *Birinci Dünya Savaşında*, p. 137. For representations of those soldiers who shot off their trigger fingers to get out of fighting, see Ahmet Göze, *Rusya'a Üç Esaret Yılı*, pp. 51–2. For deserters see Tonguç, p. 162.
18. 'Hiss-i Şevkat ve Muavenet', *Vaveyla*, 18 Kanun-i evvel 1331/31 December 1915, number 4, p. 3.
19. Ibid. p. 3.
20. Ibid. p. 3.
21. Ibid. p. 3.
22. Mitchell, *Rule of Experts*, p. 191.
23. I suggest that this was not the product of some paranoiac fantasy. On Sevres Syndrome as such paranoia, see Fatma Müge Göçek's very informative chapter on 'Sevres Syndrome', in *The Transformation of Turkey*.
24. *İlm ile âlem bütün, nail bugün ulviyete / Biz se düşmüş, batmışız, saplanmışız sefalete / Karnımız aç, sırtımız çıplak, zebunuz, titreriz. . .* 'Biz', *Nilüfer*, 3 Şubat 1336/3 February 1920, number 2, p. 3. For similar expressions of despair see "C" Kampında hamiyet yarışı', *Yarın*, 13 Şubat 1336/13 February 1920, number 11, p. 5.

25. 'Gençliğin Vazifesi', *Nilüfer*, 6 Nisan 1336/6 April 1920, number 17, p. 3.
26. 'Yas Tutma', *Türk Varlığı*, 15 Kanun-i Sani/15 January 1920, number 24, p. 6.
27. 'Sanayi', Memleketin Fen ve San'at İhtiyacı', *Türk Varlığı*, 1 Mart 1336/1 March 1920, number 27, p. 10.
28. Ibid. p. 10.
29. 'Garb'dan Şark'a', *Türk Varlığı*, 1 Mart 1336/1 March 1920, number 27, p. 2.
30. Ibid. p. 2. Gökalp also explained how societies pass through four main stages of development (primitive/tribal society, society based on ethnic affinity, based on common religion, and finally those united common culture, nation). Heyd, *Foundations of Turkish Nationalism*, p. 60.
31. 'Bizde Hayalcilik', *Yarın*, 1 Nisan 1336/1 April 1920, number 20, p. 4. For another similar example see 'Temaşa', *Yarın*, 19 Mart 1336/19 March 1920, number 18.
32. 'Bizde Hayalcilik', *Yarın*, 1 Nisan 1336/1 April 1920, number 20, pp. 4–5.
33. Ibid. pp. 4–5.
34. Ibid. pp. 4–5.
35. This is reminiscent of Ziya Gökalp's critiques of the 'lethargy of the Turkish people'. Gökalp used his critique to motivate Turks to shake off that lethargy, much like the prisoner here was doing. Heyd, *Foundations of Turkish Nationalism*, p. 167.
36. 'Dün, Bugün, Yarın', *Yarın*, 9 Kanun-i Sani 1336/9 January 1920, number 3, p. 2. For similar expressions see Tonguç, *Birinci Dünya Savaşında*, pp. 82–9.
37. 'Hayat Yolunda', *Türk Varlığı*, 1 Mart 1336/1 March 1920, number 27, p. 7.
38. Ibid. p. 8. The author described the dilemma colourfully. In the 'depths of his soul', the peasant heard the 'merciless' voice of 'life', which told him 'I, too, exist. You have to take care of me because you have to live'. But the 'demons of hell' (*zebaniler*) gave another message about death and afterlife. 'One is positive (*müsbet*), the other negative (*menfi*)'. One talked of 'reality', asking to work and work hard to get through a 'great problem of existence', (*derd-i kebir-i mevcûdiyyet*) created by life. The other, 'filled with negative and superstitious thoughts', was an issue for the next world (*mes'ele-i uhreviyat*) connected to an 'imagined life' (*hayat-ı mevhum*) after death. Since the issue was about 'unknowing' Muslims' concern about 'flourishing in tomorrow's world without first flourishing in this world', the people's 'fear' about the next life became the obstacle to enjoying life and investing in this world. The result of such behaviour, according to the same writer, was that in the end one could keep neither one nor the other, and finally ended up completely 'empty-handed' (*sıfr'ül-yed*). For similar sentiments, see 'Dünya Sevgisi', *Yarın*, 30 Kanun-i Sani 1336/30 January 1920, number 8, p. 2; 'Silahlı Sosyalistler', *Türk Varlığı*, 15 Mart 1336/15 March 1920, number 28, p. 2.
39. 'Dünya Sevgisi', *Yarın*, 30 Kanun-i Sani 1336/30 January 1920, number 3, p. 2
40. 'Ruh-i Müşterek', *Yarın*, 6 Şubat 1336/6 February 1920, number 10, p. 4.
41. Ibid. p. 4.
42. Ibid. p. 4.
43. This call was not new in essence, the nineteenth-century Islamic modernist intellectuals would have wholeheartedly agreed with the need for religious transformation. Albert Hourani, *Arabic Thought in the Liberal Age, 1798–1939*.
44. 'Ruh-i Müşterek', *Yarın*, 6 Şubat 1336/6 February 1920, number 10, p. 4
45. 'İçtimaiyat', *Yarın*, 12 Nisan 1336/12 April 1920, number 21, p. 2.
46. 'Kamplarda Mesai', *Yarın*, 25 Kanun-i Sani 1336/25 January 1920, number 7, p. 2.
47. Şevket S. Aydemir noted that when he asked his company of soldiers how many had a

mosque in their village, only 'a few' stepped up, but when he asked how many had a village school, none came forward. Aydemir, *Suyu Arayan Adam*, pp. 103–4.

48. 'Garb'dan Şark'a', *Türk Varlığı*, 1 Mart 1336/1 March 1920, number 27, p. 2. Yet again bringing up the issue of self-sacrifice for others' benefit, one prisoner pointed to 'our' devotion to the subjects (*reaya*) of the empire; this devotion was 'determined by our inherited moral principles'. Literally meaning 'the flock', the term *reaya* has two meanings. More traditionally, it refers to all non-military (non-*askeri*) tax-paying groups in the empire, which would have included Muslims, Christians and Jews. However, in this particular context, it refers specifically to non-Muslim groups in the empire.
49. 'Kadın ve Kadınlık', *Türk Varlığı*, 1 Mart 1336/1 March 1920, number 27, p. 14. Some of the distance the prisoners put between themselves as Turks and the state can be blamed on the prisoners feeling abandoned, but there was much more to it than that.
50. Mehmet Ö. Alkan, 'Modernization from Empire to Republic', p. 50.
51. See Yücel Yanıkdağ, 'Educating the Peasants', pp. 91–107.
52. 'Türk Esir Efradına Mekteb', *Vaveyla*, 1 Haziran 1332/14 June 1916, number 28, p. 12.
53. 'Mesud Bir Gün', *Yarın*, 20 Kanun-i Sani 1336/20 January 1920, number 6, p. 6.
54. See Aydemir, *Suyu Arayan Adam*, on this issue.
55. 'Şiir', *Yarın*, 30 Kanun-i Sani 1336/30 January 1920, number 8, p. 8.
56. '"A" Kampında unutulmaz bir gece', *Yarın*, 9 Kanun-i Sani 1336/9 January 1920, number 3, p. 5.
57. 'İlan', and '"C" Kampında hamiyet yarışı', in *Yarın*, 13 Şubat 1336/13 February 1920, number 11, p. 5. It should be remembered that many POWs were still in captivity in 1922.
58. 'İkinci Kampta Mükâfat Merasimi', *Yarın*, 16 Kanun-i Sani 1336/16 January 1920, number 5, p. 7. See, also Yanıkdağ, 'Educating the Peasants', pp. 91–107.
59. 'Me'sud bir Gün', *Yarın*, 20 Kanun-i Sani 1336/20 January 1920, number 6, p. 6.
60. Ibid. p. 6.
61. 'İkinci Kampta Mükâfat Merasimi', *Yarın*, 16 Kanun-i Sani 1336/16 January 1920, number 5, p. 7; 'Kamplarda mesai', *Yarın*, 25 Kanun-i Sani 1336/25 January 1920, number 7, p.2. For a sample list of those who graduated, along with their grades and their graduation presents, see 'Şehadetnâme Alanlar', *Yarın*, 13 Kanun-i Sani 1336/13 January 1920, number 4, p. 5.
62. 'İkinci Kampta Mükâfat Merasimi', *Yarın*, 16 Kanun-i Sani 1336/16 January 1920, number 5, p.7.
63. 'Me'sud bir Gün', *Yarın*, 20 Kanun-i Sani 1336/20 January 1920, number 6, p. 6.
64. 'İçtimai Dertlerimizden – Bilgisizlik', *Yarın*, 1 Kanun-i Sani 1336/1 January 1920, number 1, p. 3.
65. Ibid. p. 3.
66. 'Yaşamak İçin Bilgi Gerekir', *Türk Varlığı*, 1 Nisan 1336/1 April 1920, number 29, p. 7.
67. 'İçtimai Dertlerimizden – Bilgisizlik', *Yarın*, 1 Kanun-i Sani 1336/1 January 1920, number 1, p. 4.
68. Ibid. p. 4.
69. 'A Kampında Unutulmaz bir Gece', *Yarın*, 9 Kanun-i Sani 1336/9 January 1920, number 3, pp. 3–4.
70. 'Halk Edebiyatı', *Vaveyla*, 31 Mart 1333/31 March 1917, number 67, p. 2. It should be remembered that the Ottomans had no national written language. Ottoman Turkish was a combination of Turkish, Arabic and Persian languages.

71. 'Halk Edebiyatı', *Vaveyla*, 31 Mart 1333/31 March 1917, number 67, p. 2.
72. Findley, 'The Advent of Ideology', p. 159; Carter V. Findley, *Ottoman Civil Officialdom*, p. 175.
73. I am not suggesting that there is a direct connection between the prisoners and the Village Institutes, but that it is a possibility. On the Village Institutes, see M. Asım Karaömerlioğlu, 'The Cult of the Peasant' and 'The Village Institutes Experience in Turkey', pp. 47–73; M. Rauf İnan, *Bir Ömrün Öyküsü*.
74. Some of the Ottoman prisoners even suggested the establishment of financial institutions in rural areas to help the peasants financially. The idea was to help the peasants directly so that they would not be indebted to or 'tricked' by greedy usurers and large landholders. 'İktisadiyat', *Yarın*, 30 Kanun-i Sani 1336/30 January 1920, number 8, p. 4.
75. T. B. M. M., 'Kırk Birinci Birleşim', 17 Nisan 1940, Pazartesi', in *Zabıt Ceridesi*, 6 Dönem, volume 10, pp. 74–5.
76. Again, the use of only the first names in the Ottoman Empire and republican Turkey until 1934 makes it impossible to find connections between the POWs and those who may have been involved in the Village Institutes project. It should also be mentioned that less than a decade after its initiation, Feridun Fikri Düşünsel turned against the Institiutes for a variety of reasons. Three among them were: (1) the Institutes were not used for the original purpose intended; (2) not enough of them existed; and (3) rather than creating unity and rapprochement between the rural and urban people, they seemed to reinforce the division.
77. For the Ottoman women's movement, see among others, Serpil Çakır, *Osmanlı Kadın Hareketi*. I acknowledge also the existence of the short-lived Köycüler Cemiyeti, which included among its founders Great War veterans who were also graduates of the Military Medical School.
78. It should be mentioned that the ideas of Ziya Gökalp were moving away from the elitism of the period at the start of the Great War. In his *Halka Doğru* ('To the People') movement and generally in his nationalist ideas, he suggested that the elite needed 'go to the people' and bring them 'civilization'. While this has more than a hint of elitism, it was part of an even exchange; in return, the elite needed to learn national culture from the peasants. Gökalp viewed the people as a 'living national cultural museum', among whom the elite would be 'nationalized'. In this, Gökalp was highlighting the importance of 'national culture', and the people as its repository. The camp newspapers and captivity diaries and memoirs, however, do not portray the peasant as the repository of national culture. In this, the ideas of the officer prisoners do not correlate with those of Ziya Gökalp, who is considered to be the ideological father of Turkish nationalism. He is credited with influencing the People's Houses movement of the 1930s, and ethnographic and folkloric research of the early republican years. François Georgeon, *Osmanlı Türk Modernleşmesi*, pp. 34, 100.
79. 'Gaye', *Türk Varlığı*, 15 Kanun-i Sani 1336/15 January 1920, number 24, p. 247.
80. 'Gençliğin Vazifesi', *Nilüfer*, 6 Nisan 1336/6 April 1920, number 17, p. 3.
81. Ibid. p. 3.
82. 'Yaşamak İçin Bilgi Gerekir', *Türk Varlığı*, 1 Nisan 1336/1 April 1920, number 29, p. 7.
83. Heyd, *Foundations of Turkish Nationalism*, pp. 48–9.
84. Ibid. pp. 50–1. As the prisoners were still writing about his ideas at the end of the war, Ziya Gökalp himself was arrested by the British occupation forces in Istanbul and sent to the island of Malta, where he would spend two years from 1919–21.

85. 'Gayesizlik', *Türk Varlığı*, 1 Şubat 1336/1 February 1920, number 25, p. 244. This particular issue is missing two pages from the original. Because of the similarity in issue discussed, I decided that a section for which I do not have a title belongs with the article titled 'Gayesizlik'.
86. 'Gayesizlik', *Türk Varlığı*, 1 Şubat 1336/1 February 1920, number 25, p. 1.
87. 'Ruh-i Müşterek', *Yarın*, 6 Şubat 1336/6 February 1920, number 10, p. 5. For other optimistic statements and mentality, see 'İçtimaiyat', *Işık*, 10 Haziran 1335/10 June 1919, number 29, p. 1.
88. 'Ruh-i Müşterek', *Yarın*, 6 Şubat 1336/6 February 1920, number 10, p. 5.
89. '"A" Kampında Unutulmaz bir Gece', *Yarın*, 9 Kanun-i Sani 1336/9 January 1920, number 3, p. 4.
90. 'İçtimaiyat', *Yarın*, 12 Nisan 1336/12 April 1920, number 21, p. 2.
91. Officer prisoners also disapproved of the idea of being a civil servant as a career choice. A number of them urged their comrades to avoid seeking government jobs. Others suggested that they should discourage their children as well. They suggested turning to something entrepreneurial or technical, such as engineering. One asked, why do 'we prefer a civil servant's job that pays 300 *kuruş* to making 800 to 1,000 *kuruş* earned with the sweat of our brow working in a job in industry'; avoiding civil servant employment would help both the individual and uplift the nation: 'Sanayi': Memleketin Fen ve San'at İhtiyacı', *Türk Varlığı*, 1 Mart 1336/1 March 1920, number 27, p. 9. See also 'Bugün, Yarın – 2', *Yarın*, 13 Kanun-i Sani 1336/13 January 1920, number 4, p. 2, where the author criticises the tendency among parents to encourage their children to aim for civil service jobs.
92. My earlier work, 'Savior Sons of the Nation' (Yanıkdağ, '"Ill-Fated Sons" of the Nation', chapter 2), suggested that both modernist and Westernist points of view among the prisoners were clearly evident, but since then I have discovered new and more comprehensive evidence. Some editorials that had seemed to suggest a Westernist line, eventually revealed themselves to be more along the lines of modernist thought. Arguably, with a smaller source base, I was getting only a partial picture of what they were arguing.
93. 'İçtimai Hastalıklarımız', *Nilüfer*, 30 Kanun-i Sâni 1336/30 January 1920, number 1, pp. 6–7.
94. Ibid. pp. 6–7. The word 'culture' is used in the Ottoman original.
95. Perhaps it was also problematic to define 'nation' in a multinational empire such as the Ottoman Empire. For the various meanings attached to *millet* and its evolution, see Bernard Lewis, *The Political Language of Islam*, pp. 38–42, 131–32, note 27.
96. 'Muhavere', *Ne Münasebet*, 15 Mart 1920/15 March 1920, number 10, p. 2. *Makam*, or *maqam* in Arabic, can be roughly translated as melodic mode or contour of classical Turkish or Middle Eastern music. Each *makam* has a complex set of rules of composition and performance. Intervallic structure and melodic development differ from one *makam* to another.
97. Ibid. p. 2. The copy of this newspaper was in such bad condition that it made the already not very legible writing more difficult to decipher. However, three colleagues confirmed one particularly illegible word as *hüseynî*.
98. If he became literate in captivity through the educating efforts of the officers, his poem may represent either a synthesis of his own identification prior to schooling or what was taught him by his officers.

99. *Bayram*: holiday. For a brief description of *bayram*s, see Donald, *The Ottoman Empire*, pp. 163–6.
100. 'Destan', *Vaveyla*, 1 Teşrin-i Sani 1331/14 November 1915, number 1, p.12.
101. 'Destan, [continued]', *Vaveyla*, 4 Kanun-i Evvel 1331/17 December 1915, number 2, p. 12.
102. It should be remembered that there were Jews and Christians in the Ottoman army if mostly in the rank of officers, although they may not have been among this man's captive compatriots in Krasnoyarsk.
103. 'İhmal edilen ihtiyaçlardan biri', *Vaveyla*, 4 Kanun-i Evvel 1331/17 December 1915, number 2, p.1.
104. 'Kurban Bayramı', *Işık*, 6 Eylül 1335/6 September 1919, number 70, p. 1. One of the most important ethnogenesis myths of the Turkic peoples. Ergenekon is an ancient epic story about the regeneration of the Gökturks after major setbacks. According to the epic, the word Ergenekon refers to the valley surrounded by high mountains on all sides where the defeated Turks had taken refuge. Finally, when they were numerous and powerful enough the Gökturks broke their way out and conquered the neighbouring peoples. The departure from Ergenekon, or *Nevruz*, is celebrated on 21 March. For more detailed information on Ergenekon, see Devin Deweese, *Islamization and Native Religion*.
105. Başkatipzade Ragıp Bey, *Tarih-i Hayatım*, p. 118.
106. 'Turân, Nedir ve Nerededir?' *Türk Varlığı*, 1 Nisan 1336/1 April 1920, number 29, p. 6. Büyük Orta is Central Asia in a larger sense, the region between the Urals and Hindu Kush.
107. See the Mughals of India referred to as a 'Turkish empire' and a 'Turkish dynasty' in 'Turan', *Niyet*, 31 Temmuz 1917/31 July 1917, reprinted in Tonguç, *Birinci Dünya Savaşında*, p. 270.
108. Alkan, 'Modernization from Empire to Republic', p. 53.
109. See, for example, 'İlk Türkler ve teşkil etdikleri saltanatlar', Moğolistan'dan Atilla'ya kadar Türkler', *Yarın*, 3 Şubat 1336/3 February 1920, number 9 and 'İlmi Sütunlar', 'Han', *İzmir*, 9 Şubat 1336/9 February 1920, number 7, p.3; see also 'Kültigin Kitabesi', *Yarın*, 1 Nisan 1336/1 April 1920, number 20, .
110. Hüsamettin Tuğaç, *Bir Neslin Dramı*, p. 122. It is possible that in captivity narratives written well after captivity, some of the Turkic knowledge might have been acquired after repatriation.
111. Halil Ataman, *Esaret Yılları*, pp. 133, 197. See also İnkilap Tarihi Arşivi, 97/33/33-8; Başkatipzade Ragıp Bey, *Tarih-i Hayatım*, p. 95 for references to *ırkdaş*' (co-racials) and 'our northern Turkish brothers' (*Şimal Türk kardeşlerimiz*).
112. 'Yas Tutma', *Türk Varlığı*, 15 Kanun-i Sani 1336/15 January 1920, number 24, p. 6.
113. 'İçtimaiyat', *Işık*, 10 Haziran 1335/10 June 1919, number 29, p. 1.
114. Ibid. p. 1.
115. 'Gayesizlik', *Türk Varlığı*, 1 Şubat 1336/1 February 1920, number 25, p. 244. (This particular issue is missing two pages from the original. Because of the similarity in issue discussed, I decided that a section for which I do not have a title belongs with the article titled 'Gayesizlik'.)
116. 'İçtimaiyat', *Işık*, 10 Haziran 1335/10 June 1919, number 29, p. 1. Another article in a different newspaper put it somewhat similarly: 'when we look at those nations who are secure in their existence, what we see first . . . is a glory of skill and current of knowledge

(*nur-ı marifet, bir seyyal-i irfan*)' in 'Gençlik ve Âti', *Badiye*, 1 Teşrin-i Sani 1335 /1 November 1920, number 3, p. 1.
117. 'İçtimaiyat', *Işık*, 22 Temmuz 1336/22 July 1920, number 46, p. 1.
118. 'Dün, Bugün, Yarın', *Yarın*, 9 Kanun-i Sani 1336/9 January 1920, number 3, p. 2.
119. Meltem Ahıska, 'Occidentalism', p. 353.
120. 'Gençlik ve Âti', *Badiye*, 1 Teşrin-i Sani 1335/1 November 1919, number 3, p. 1.
121. 'İçtimaiyat', *Işık*, 22 Temmuz 1336/22 July 1920, number 46, p. 1.
122. 'Gençlik ve Âti', *Badiye*, 1 Teşrin-i Sani 1335/1 November 1919, number 3, p. 1.
123. 'Gaye', *Türk Varlığı*, 15 Kanun-i Sani 1336/15 January 1920, number 24, p. 247.
124. 'İyi Alâmetler', *Esaret*, 4 Kânun-ı Evvel 1335/4 December 1919, number 36, p. 1.

CHAPTER

4

PRISONERS AS DISEASE CARRIERS: CASES OF PELLAGRA AND TRACHOMA

The report of the Committee of Enquiry regarding the prevalence of pellagra amongst Turkish prisoners of war will stand for years to come as a record of one of the best and most scientific enquiries ever accomplished by a nation at war.

Not only did the Committee clear up the problem of pellagra in Egypt, but it has put on record observations that will have to be remembered for everyone who has in future to draw up any diet scale.

The Lancet commenting on the 1918 pellagra investigation
The Lancet (8 May 1920), p. 1,027

From neuro-psychiatrists to generalists to epidemiologists, nearly all doctors viewed soldiers returning home – whether from far away provinces or nearby battlefronts – as disease carriers. In 1915, Dr Mazhar Osman, the leading neuro-psychiatrist of the time, wrote that military service and wars in distant regions of the empire had always been an avenue for new diseases into Anatolia.[1] As a result, he stated, Anatolia had become home for a number of diseases. Because of their numbers and the lengthy time they spent in contact with foreign populations in distant and strange places, prisoners of war were usually singled out as 'disease carriers', bringing back diseases – contagious or non-contagious – they acquired while in prison camps in Russia, Egypt, India and Burma. Neuro-psychiatrist Dr Nazım Şakir, by using a process of elimination, linked repatriated prisoners to the appearance of lethargic encephalitis (a brain disease character-ised by high fever, headache, sore throat, lethargy and double vision) in Istanbul, which killed a significant number of people in the capital city and beyond.[2] The prisoners also brought back malaria, dysentery, trachoma and pellagra. As mental health specialist Dr Şükrü Hazım wrote, the latter two were encountered in larger numbers among the prisoners being repatriated: 'A significant portion of our prisoners being repatriated are disabled with two important diseases: one is trachoma, the other is pellagra'.[3]

This chapter will examine the post-war politics and medical discourse surrounding pellagra, a non-contagious disease, and trachoma, a highly contagious one. After the war, a fierce debate developed between British camp doctors and officials and Ottoman (and later Turkish) doctors and officials over the medical mistreatment of Ottoman prisoners. In this medical debate, prisoners became contested objects. Turkish concern over pellagra was short-lived, partially because the disease was not contagious, but the struggle over trachoma lasted for decades. In the post-1925 period, what was officially called the 'Fight against Trachoma' allowed the republican state to extend its presence and authority into remote regions under the guise of bringing the nation back to health and, therefore, civilisation. Fighting diseases brought back by the prisoners provided the pretext for extending hygiene, civilisation, and modernity among the 'uncivilized' and 'unhygienic' peasants.[4]

PELLAGRA IN BRITISH CAMPS: QUESTION OF RESPONSIBILITY

About 150,000 Ottoman soldiers were taken captive by the British during the war, most in the final year of the war when fronts were quickly collapsing. In 1918, several thousand of the over 100,000 Ottoman prisoners interned in Egypt became sick and died at an alarming rate. Before dying as a result of this epidemic, each prisoner, as one British doctor put it, turned into a 'living skeleton'.[5] The cause of their death was a disease called pellagra, a semi-mysterious disease with an unknown aetiology at that time.

First identified in the eighteenth century, pellagra's aetiology was not discovered until the 1930s. At that time, doctors discovered that the cause of the disease was a lack of vitamin B3, or niacin. Niacin is needed by the body to efficiently process carbohydrates, proteins and fats, and for the normal functioning of the brain and the nervous system. In the absence of niacin, the body does not efficiently process the nutrients it needs from consumed foods and thus 'starves' or 'wastes' itself. Meanwhile, the nervous system also malfunctions.

Sometimes it was called the disease of the four Ds – dermatitis, diarrhoea, dementia and death. Patients with pellagra developed symmetric skin lesions especially in places where skin was exposed to the sun. This was the most easily identified sign of pellagra. The second D, standing for diarrhoea, was usually the initial symptom to appear, but, until the skin lesions developed it could not be directly connected to pellagra. Dementia, while showing itself initially in mild forms from irritability to loss of memory, could later develop into full-blown psychosis. If the body was unable to extract nutrients from food, death soon followed. Among the Ottoman prisoners in Egypt, there were many severe cases and therefore many deaths.

The first significant signs of pellagra in the Egyptian prison camps appeared in the winter of 1916–17, but early 1918 witnessed a dramatic increase in pellagra as the number of captured Ottomans swelled rapidly.[6] One British doctor professed that, with the capture of so many Ottomans, 'unexpectedly favourable opportunities became available in 1918 to British Army medical officers for investigating pellagra'.[7] Concerned that, if contagious, the disease might have an effect on British troops, General Edmund Allenby authorised two special investigations into pellagra in 1918 and in 1920.[8] Led by Colonel F. D. Boyd and Lieutenant Colonel P. S. Lelean, the First Committee worked from October to December 1918. It produced its *Report of a Committee of Enquiry Regarding the Prevalence of Pellagra among Turkish Prisoners of War*, in early 1919. While the work done by the First Committee might have been first rate, inventive and methodical, it could not discover the underlying causes of the disease. Some random measures were taken, which resulted in curbing the rate of increase of new cases. A Second Committee was appointed in the spring of 1920, eighteen months after the end of the war, because there were still some thousands of Ottoman prisoners in Egypt, and many of them continued to die. The second effort was headed by Major A. C. Hammond-Searle and Captain A. G. Stevenson. Their report, *Report on the Investigations of Pellagra among Turkish Prisoners of War in Egypt in 1920*, was published in Alexandria in September 1920.[9]

In addition to their overall failure, the two British inquiries also failed to accurately identify how many Ottoman prisoners suffered from pellagra and how many died from it. They were better at gathering statistics on how many were diagnosed and hospitalised. Despite their critical attitude regarding the 'incompetency' of their Ottoman counterparts, British doctors cannot be considered as competent as they assumed themselves to be. Although the statistics are grossly misleading, the Second Committee revealed that among 105,668 Ottoman prisoners of war, 9,257 (or 8.7 per cent) were hospitalised as pellagrous.[10] Since, as even the British doctors admitted, 'there were probably many other undiagnosed instances', the actual number of pellagrous prisoners was much higher than 9,257.[11] In compiling its statistics the Second Committee found it could not really trust the documentation supplied to it by other British institutions. For instance, the Second Committee discovered some irregularities in how the pellagra ward in the POW hospital reported numbers.[12]

Therefore, the Second Committee determined that it needed to test the accuracy of doctors' diagnoses and hospital record keeping by examining all prisoner patients in a sample hospital for signs of pellagra, not just those already diagnosed. Expecting to find that most hospitalised patients showing signs of pellagra had been properly diagnosed and properly placed in the pellagra wards, instead they discovered 525 additional Ottoman patients who presented with signs of pellagra. These patients had other diseases as well, but they had not been counted among those who had pellagra. Expanding their search to the rest of the prison camp, the committee identified 950 additional cases in a camp population of 17,488.[13] In short, while the camp hospital records showed that fewer than twenty prisoners had pellagra, the investigative committee actually identified 1,475 pellagra cases. Since the disease was not that difficult to identify, clearly the medical staff hospitalised only the most severely incapacitated. The First Committee did not provide exact numbers regarding admissions and deaths, but only rough graphs. However, reading the imprecise graphs, one can estimate that roughly 5,025 Ottomans were hospitalised in 1918 and of those approximately 1,245 (24 per cent) died. As the Second Committee readily admitted, the drop in the number of cases in 1920 was not because of the disease subsiding, but because prisoners were suddenly being repatriated in large numbers. Thus, a great number of pellagrous men were sent home to Turkey for Ottoman doctors to contend with. There is no indication at all that the British officials informed the Ottoman government of the condition of the pellagrous soldiers being repatriated.

Unfortunately, there are no British statistics for 1916 and 1917 even though the number of pellagra cases in these two years, as one RAMC (Royal Army Medical Corps) doctor admitted, 'was large enough to warrant the use of the term epidemic'.[14] After the war Ottoman and Turkish doctors developed their own estimates of the number of pellagrous soldiers. One Ottoman medical officer, Dr A. Rıza, who as a prisoner had assisted British doctors in his camp, estimated the total number of all pellagrous soldiers in all of the Egyptian camps to be approximately 20,000. Another medical officer, Dr Abdülkadir Noyan, who had not been a prisoner of war but who had interviewed Ottoman doctors who were prisoners in Egypt, concluded that 8,000 to 10,000 cases of pellagra occurred in Egyptian camps.[15] Whose statistics are closer to what actually took place is difficult to determine. However, since the Second Committee pointed to clear under-reporting or misdiagnosis by British officials, the reality might be closer to Dr A. Rıza's estimate.

When one casts a wider net, the likelihood of under-reporting becomes clearer. Working from camp records, the Second Committee reported that in August 1919, 164 pellagra patients were admitted to all POW hospitals and of these ninety-one individuals died.[16] However, August 1919 'Intelligence

Table 4.1 Ottoman pellagra hospital admissions and deaths: official British statistics

Year	Pellagra Admissions	Deaths	Death Rate
1918 (estimated from graph)	5,025	1,245	24.0%
1919	3,729	1,611	44.2%
Jan–July 1920	659	200	30.3%
Total Jan 1918–July 1920	9,340	3,056	32.71%

Sources: A. C. Hammond-Searle and A. G. Stevenson, *Report of Investigations, 1920*, pp. 3, 9; Francis D. Boyd and P. S. Lelean, *Report of a Committee of Enquiry Regarding the Prevalence of Pellagra among Turkish Prisoners of War*, Chart 2.[17]

Summaries' sent to London from the Egyptian prison camps listed a total of 1,510 patients in the hospitals and of this number 1,345 or 89 per cent were Ottomans. In the same month, 220 of the prisoner patients died.[18] The 'Summary' gave neither the exact number of Ottoman dead nor the cause of death. However, one might conjecture that since the Ottomans constituted 89 per cent of the patients, approximately 89 per cent of the dead were also Ottomans. That is, 196 out of 220; this number is more than twice the number of pellagra deaths reported by the Second Committee. It is possible that 105 additional Ottomans could have died from other causes, but it is also possible that the documents forwarded to the Second Committee deliberately under-reported the scourge of pellagra. If the deaths were not caused by pellagra, then the British camp hospitals might have had another health problem on their hands that they did not recognise.

Members of the First Pellagra Committee raised several questions that they sought to answer. What caused the disease? Could it be transmitted from one individual to another? Had the prisoners developed the disease before or after capture? And most perplexing, why did it seem to strike Ottomans but not Germans who served in the same Ottoman armies in Palestine and Syria, and were now housed in the same prison camps? At the POW camp at Maadi, there were several thousand German POWs. Although separated from the Ottomans by a simple barbed wire fence, no Germans were diagnosed with pellagra throughout 1918, while several thousand Ottomans contracted the disease. How could this be?[19]

Without getting into the minutiae of various tests, assumptions and theories, we can present some of the key assumptions and conclusions of the First Committee. First, pellagra was the result of dietary deficiencies; it was not contagious. Post mortem examinations revealed that all those who had and died with pellagra did not really die because of pellagra. That is, generally the cause of death was another opportunistic disease – dysentery, tuberculosis, etc – that existed at the same time as pellagra in the prisoners' bodies. The British doctors called these 'inter-current' diseases, which took advantage of the prisoners' extremely weakened immune system due to pellagra and usually became the cause of death. The First Committee implemented an extensive study of the domiciles of the prisoners and exactly when and where they first noticed even the slightest signs of skin lesions in an attempt to establish that the Ottoman soldiers had brought the disease with them into captivity. Accordingly, with three Ottoman prisoner doctors as translators, they interviewed 518 pellagrous prisoners of war in Kantara camp.[20] This was called an endemicity return. Of the 518 pellagrous prisoners, 474 were said to know where and when they first noticed the symptoms. Out of the 474 prisoners, 405 reported seeing the symptoms before capture and 69 after capture. The committee produced a map showing both the domiciles of the prisoners and where they first noticed the onset of symptoms (see Figure 4.1). The map showed that pellagrous soldiers came from all regions of the empire, so no clear pattern could be established to show that the disease was endemic to a specific part of the Ottoman Empire. However, the map also showed that the onset of symptoms had generally occurred in the regions of Lebanon, Palestine and Suez, which was not at all surprising because this was where almost all of the patients had been stationed or had fought. The committee decided these were the areas where 'Turks were most concentrated when suffering maximum privations'.[21]

Therefore, the committee convinced itself that it had uncovered the source of the problem. Since the symptoms appeared prior to capture, it had to be because the Ottoman army could not feed its soldiers properly, especially in the regions of Palestine and Sinai. The Committee estimated that 18 per cent of fresh captures had pellagra at the time of capture. Captured Ottoman documents, the Committee claimed, offered further evidence that Ottoman soldiers had not been fed properly by their own army due to significant food and transportation shortages.[22] In the Ottoman-Turkish memoirs and medical literature that appeared after the war, a number of officers and doctors confirmed serious food shortages on the Ottoman side, particularly towards the end of the war.[23] However, these same people pointed out that the shortages were sporadic and happened mostly when troops changed locations frequently. Furthermore, Ottoman officials, especially the Ottoman-Turkish military doctors (non-prisoners), insisted that while they encountered scurvy and occasionally war (or hunger) oedema among the Ottoman soldiers in the field, they never encountered pellagra, even after extended periods of food shortages.[24]

The First Committee claimed that three captive Ottoman doctors had interrogated the prisoners about the first appearances of their skin lesions. However, the claim about prisoners being largely pellagrous when captured was challenged by Dr A. Rıza, who had been in another camp. He asserted that he and six other

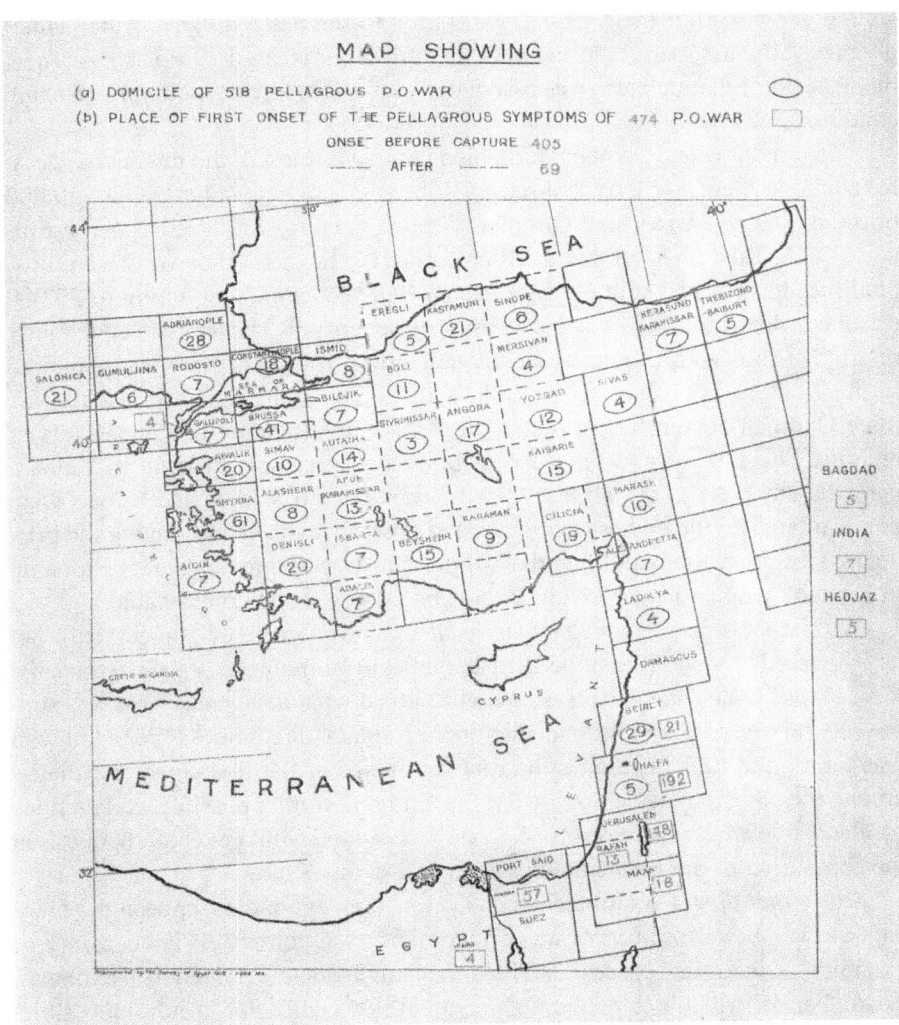

Figure 4.1 Pellagra map: 'endemicity return'
Source: From Boyd and Lelean, *Report of a Committee of Enquiry Regarding the Prevalence of Pellagra among Turkish Prisoners of War*, appendix

captured Ottoman doctors were asked to examine 14,000 Ottoman prisoners who arrived fresh from the front at the Salhieh camp. 'We examined these new[ly captured] prisoners one by one', he reported, 'and could not find even the smallest of pellagra symptoms'. When a second large contingent of new prisoners arrived from the Hejaz after months of being besieged, the Ottoman doctors, he insisted, found a significant number of scurvy cases, but again no pellagra.

'A few months after their arrival, we started to see pellagra among the [same] prisoners', he asserted, 'and the numbers rapidly increased'.[25] For Dr A. Rıza, this was proof that pellagra was associated almost exclusively with prison camp conditions.

Then, months later, when the Salhieh camp was closed, the prisoners, Dr A. Rıza among them, were transferred to Bilbeis, a camp containing about 40,000 prisoners, about twenty-five Ottoman-Turkish doctors, and a 3,000-bed hospital.[26] Dr A. Rıza claimed that at Bilbeis only the most serious cases were hospitalised. In fact, according to him, nearly half the camp, amounting to 20,000 prisoners, had pellagra to some degree of severity.[27] The British endemicity return that showed prisoners as mostly pellagrous prior to capture was compiled in the Kantara camp, not at the Bilbeis or Salhieh camps. Unfortunately, the three Ottoman doctors who assisted the British investigation in Kantara left no records. There is, of course, the possibility that prisoners brought to Kantara were already pellagrous, while those who were sent to Salhieh and Bilbeis were not. Kantara had the highest outbreaks and possibly even deaths among the prisoners. However, the likelihood that all previously pellagrous soldiers ended up in Kantara, while none arrived in Bilbeis or Salhieh, seems improbable.

Was it that A. Rıza, moved by nationalistic pride, denied or exaggerated what he witnessed? Or was it that the British medical committee, so eager to trace the disease to pre-internment causes, misrepresented what it saw and what was supposedly reported by the Ottoman doctors in Kantara? It is impossible to tell who was telling the truth regarding the time and place of the first signs of pellagra among the captured men. Admittedly, there might be other possible explanations for the discrepancy. But even the Second Committee would eventually question the conclusion of the First Committee regarding this issue.

Since the First Committee's conclusion that symptoms appeared before capture was based on interviews of Ottomans by Ottomans, it is necessary to examine the interview process and how the British doctors judged its usefulness. A number of British doctors complained that it was difficult, if not impossible, to get reliable information from the Ottoman prisoners about their health history. Dr Douglas Bigland of the RAMC, who was in the prison camps during the first investigation and who worked closely with the Second Committee, observed the following:

> In attempting to get a true history of his case from a Turk one feels almost sympathetic towards the gentlemen whose life-work it is to discover, if possible, the truth concerning our incomes. At best, in either case a good guess is the most that can be hoped for. In our country, too, a man's ignorance acts as a check upon his gift for telling lies, but with a Turk it is otherwise. Nevertheless, the statements

of prisoners, in my opinion, are of some value when repeated cross-examinations are made at different times, and if when any discrepancies in the story arise the whole history is dismissed.[28]

Unable or unwilling to make sense of the prisoners' accounts of their medical histories, the doctor concluded that the prisoners were inveterate liars. Bigland's views were likely shared by his colleagues. The invented image of the 'ignorant Turk' influenced both their dealings with the prisoners and their unwillingness to trust the prisoners' accounts. We do not know the exact content of the lies, but clearly they had to do with the patients' medical history. So, the prisoners must have given accounts of their history, which the doctor believed were lies. Here was something where the 'ignorant Turk' surpassed the 'ignorant British', but it would have made no Ottoman officer proud.

Articles published by the British doctors contain a number of other similarly Orientalist and racialist commentaries. This Orientalist point of view blinded the doctors mentally, and therefore medically, to the truth and allowed them to pick and choose what 'facts' they would find useful in diagnosing and treating pellagra.[29] In this way, an account that a prisoner may have noticed some blemish on his skin prior to capture could be taken as fact, but other answers could be dismissed because the prisoners were notoriously untrustworthy liars. For example, one significant sign of pellagra was loss of appetite, but some British doctors could easily dismiss it as a real symptom among the prisoners: 'The appetite was, as a rule, poor, but how much of this symptom was due to pellagra and how much to the extraordinary outlook of the Turk upon questions of disease and death it is impossible to say'.[30] The same RAMC doctor who listed depression, hysteria, psychasthenia and other mental disorders as symptoms of pellagra asked his readers to believe that the sick prisoners gave up eating not due to an actual loss of appetite, but because of their fatalism. His Orientalist perspective caused him to interpret actual loss of appetite as the prisoners' conscious act of giving up on life and hastening their own death. The loss of appetite became yet another 'lie', rather than a real symptom of the disease from which the prisoners were suffering.[31] In this way, all other possibilities – from real loss of appetite, difficulty in digestion, extreme diarrhoea, depression, lack of energy (to even difficulty in sitting up in bed) – became secondary to the diagnosis of 'fatalism' and passive suicide.[32]

Interestingly, the patients' otherworldly 'fatalism' and therefore death-wishes did not keep them from asking 'this worldly' question about the doctors' incomes. Scholars have pointed out the contradictory nature of colonial (Orientalist) discourse. Now the 'Turk' was both 'simple-minded and yet the most worldly and accomplished liar'.[33] He was 'fatalistic' enough to give up on eating, but also full of this worldly materialistic envy as evidenced in his attempts at discovering the salary of the enemy doctors. Perhaps these prisoner patients had been through the camp schools where they learned to love the material world as well, but had not quite given up on the other world. Alternatively, the Ottoman officers had partially misjudged their peasant soldiers' disregard for this world.

Pellagra, and its accompanying ailments, was what the doctors called a 'wasting' disease. The lack of appetite and other causes resulted in the extreme emaciation of the prisoners. In comparison to an average healthy Ottoman prisoner, the afflicted prisoners lost 30 per cent of their body weight at the mid-stage of the disease. Those who were at the advanced stage of the disease were truly no more than skin and bones, as British doctors readily admitted.[34] For some British doctors 'the great emaciation presented by some of the patients resembl[ed] nothing so much as the appalling pictures indelibly associated in one's mind with Indian famines'.[35] Externally, the sick men lost incredible amounts of weight. Some of the advanced cases could not even be weighed. The weight of *mildly* sick prisoners ranged between 100 and 110 pounds (45–50 kg).[36] Given that the average weight of a healthy Ottoman prisoner was about 144 pounds (65 kg), this was already more than a 30 per cent drop. One British doctor, W. Burridge, admitted that when he was put in charge of the South Labour Camp at Kantara, and inspected 3,500 Ottoman prisoners, he found 318 of them to be no longer fit for labour. In his words, they were 'living skeletons'. 'Never before', he said, 'had I seen such an advanced grade of emaciation, nor have I since'.[37]

As the first 'living skeletons' died, the British doctors autopsied, or in the words of one former prisoner who worked in the hospital, 'opened up many corpses'.[38] In these several hundred autopsies, various 'outstanding features' presented themselves. What did they find as the doctors extended their gaze beneath the wrinkled skin and into the depths of the body? As Dr Bigland expressed it:

> Certain cases died apparently from dysentery, which when examined post mortem revealed very slight intestinal lesions; cases which, in the vivid language of the fifth year medical student, should not have died. So marked was this that one had recourse to a metaphysical explanation based upon Mahomedan ideals and the fatalism of the East.[39]

As the 'mystery' persisted, the doctors methodically continued with their investigations of the corpses: they measured, heated, diluted, examined, weighed and compared everything from bile to faeces to intestines to hearts in their search

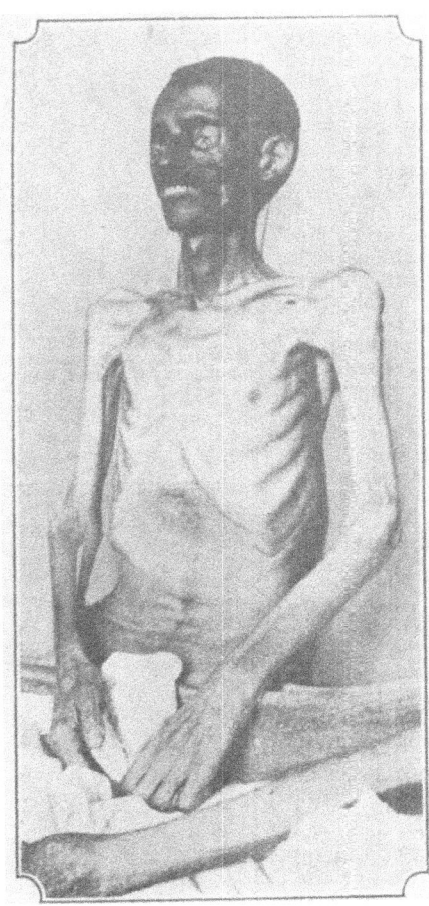
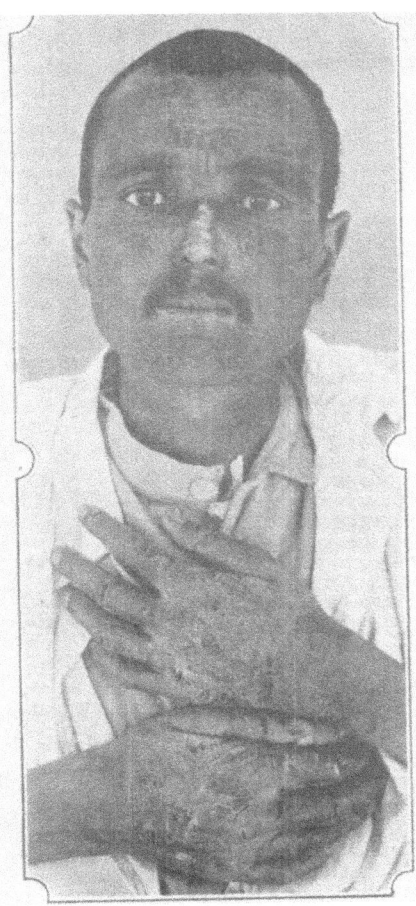

Figure 4.2 Pellagra victim, post mortem
Source: Reprinted from A. Douglas Bigland, 'The Pellagra Outbreak in Egypt – I: Pellagra Among Ottoman Prisoners of War', *The Lancet* 195 (1 May 1920), pp. 947–53, with permission from Elsevier.

Figure 4.3 Pellagra victim: classic skin marks of pellagra on hands and face
Source: Reprinted from A. Douglas Bigland, 'The Pellagra Outbreak in Egypt – I: Pellagra Among Ottoman Prisoners of War', *The Lancet* 195 (1 May 1920), pp. 947–53, with permission from Elsevier.

for a cause. They found that hearts and livers in the sick men had shrunk to nearly one-half the size of healthy organs. The average heart of a prisoner who died from pellagra or one of the other diseases ranged from 5.96 to 7.5 ounces, whereas the normal average was eleven ounces. In one fifty-cases sample, the doctors concluded that the heart was wasted by 45.8 per cent, the liver by 26.4 per cent and the pancreas by 48.2 per cent.[40]

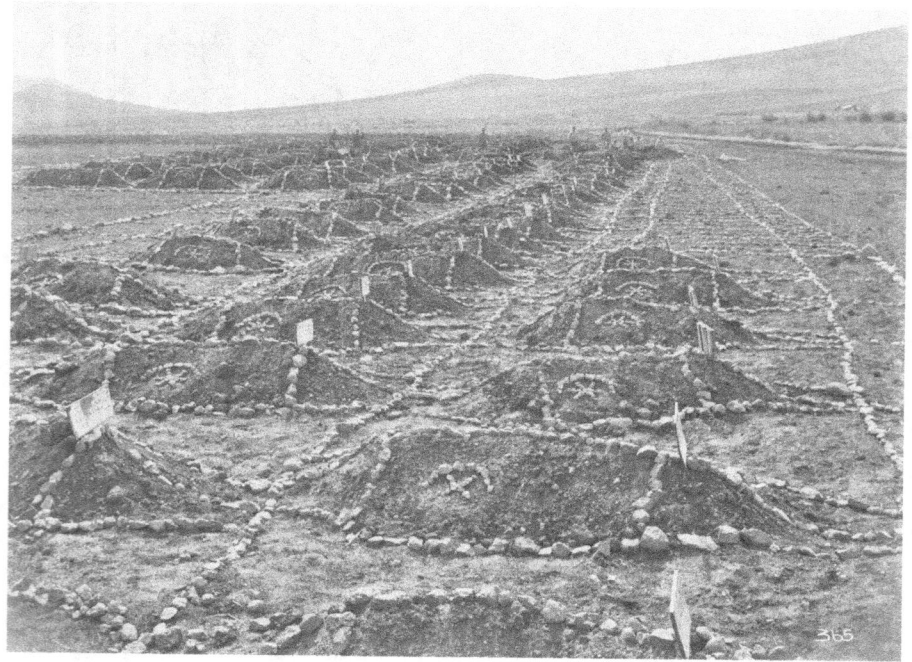

Figure 4.4 Mounds at the cemetery at the Turkish prisoner of war camp, Kaukab [Iraq]
Source: Courtesy of Australian War Memorial, B00365

Other diseases ailing the pellagrous prisoners

The autopsies conducted by the Second Committee sought to identify the cause of death for each prisoner identified as pellagrous. In all cases pellagra was present, but the autopsies revealed that in almost all of them the cause of death was another disease that existed concurrently with pellagra. They theorised that pellagra rendered the body weak and thus allowed other opportunistic diseases to advance rapidly and kill the patient. In a fifty-person sample, autopsies conducted to identify the direct cause of death concluded that twenty-eight (56 per cent) deaths could be attributed to bronchopneumonia. Twelve (24 per cent) were classified as death from dysentery and eight (16 per cent) were found to have died from pulmonary tuberculosis. Only in two cases (4 per cent) was pellagra credited as being the direct cause of death.[41]

As the Table 4.2 reveals, these prisoners had several morbid diseases, although only one or a combination might have eventually killed them. Other autopsies revealed further diseases: nephritis, syphilis, scurvy, Banti's disease,

Table 4.2 Morbid conditions present in autopsied POWs

Condition	Number	Percentage
Pellagra	50	100
Pneumonia	29	58
Dysentery, bacillary	25	50
Dysentery, amoebic	5	10
Tuberculosis (various forms)	15	30
Malaria (old)	8	16
Pleural effusion	4	8
Intestinal worms	4	8

Source: *Report of Investigations, 1920*, p. 28.

hepatic cirrhosis (alcoholic type), lepto-meningitis and pyemia.[42] Certainly, the prisoners' bodies reflected the 'hardships' encountered during war. The First Committee continuously referred to these 'hardships' to explain pellagra and to minimise British responsibility for the disease. During and after the war, Ottoman-Turkish doctors never denied the presence of other diseases among the soldiers, but they always adamantly denied that the soldiers were already pellagrous when captured. Therefore, there is no doubt that British autopsies discovered other diseases among the pellagrous dead. However, attributing the cause of death to another disease that the prisoners might have actually brought into the camps would certainly reduce the responsibility of pellagra as the real culprit. Was there a plan to downplay the lethal effects of a condition which clearly was being exacerbated by the camp diet?

The British medical officers who conducted the investigations had several agendas. Some saw medical 'opportunities' to advance science and their careers. Others saw likely failure in the obstacles created by what they felt to be uncooperative patients bent on sabotaging the investigation. And some surely were motivated by the Hippocratic oath even if their medical perspectives were tainted and dulled by their Orientalist attitudes. The doctors knew that dementia and other mental problems were signs of pellagra, and they had observed many such signs of 'dullness of mentality', among the pellagrous prisoners.[43] Yet, they never considered the 'discrepancies' in the prisoners' statements as resulting from mental problems caused by the disease. Additionally, even if some of the patients were uncooperative, was it really unreasonable for these patients to refuse to collaborate with the captor doctor? As Frantz Fanon showed, prison camps change the doctor-patient relationship. If the German prisoner did not trust the French doctor and begged the doctor to spare his life before treatment, why would an Ottoman trust a British doctor when so many of them were dying in the camp hospitals under those very doctors' supposed 'care'?[44]

Camp diet

Among significant confusion as expressed by the investigating doctors, a few things seemed to be certain. Foremost, pellagra was nutrition related. Not all prisoners in captivity in Egypt ate the same diet. Since German, Austrian and Bulgarian prisoners in British captivity did not become pellagrous, and since, with one exception, Ottoman officers did not succumb to the disease, the culprit had to be embedded in the enlisted men's diets. Accordingly, the next step was taken to compare the diets of Ottoman prisoners before and after capture and to compare both to the diet furnished for European prisoners in Egypt. This the British did.

The 1917 Kress von Kressenstein report listed the following food items Ottoman authorities supplied to its troops in Sinai: 680 grams of bread (wheat, barley, maize), net 40 grams of meat, 150 grams of bulgur (cracked wheat), 10 grams of oil, 30 grams of vegetable (mostly onions), 15 grams of dates, 70 grams of rice. This amounted to 2,603 calories. Reportedly, the troops in Palestine had only 2,372 calories.[45] What the British authorities did not take into account was that lower calories and lower protein of their pre-capture diet did not prove the

Table 4.3 Pre-capture and prison camp diets compared

Date	Diet description	Protein value		Fats	Carbs	Cals
		Biological	Gross			
Sep 1917	Pre-capture diet-1: information from captured report by General Officer commanding Sinai Front, General von Kressenstein	30.4	82.4	27.52	490	2,603
Autumn 1918	Pre-capture diet-2: information from supply personnel and other reliable first line prisoners of war (average of 9 estimates)	3.4	85.6	30.34	430	2,396
Nov 1917	POW rations scale: non-labour	39.1	92.0	27.55	515	2,744
Nov 1918	POW rations scale: non-labour (after committee intervention)	39.9	97.0	42.50	524	2,941
3/1918 to 11/1918	POW rations scale: labour	48.7	109.3	47.30	610	3,390
6/1918 to 10/1918	POW rations actual issue: labour[46]	45.6	102.4	33.33	560	3,026

Source: Committee of Enquiry, 1918, p. 17.

existence of pellagra among the Ottoman soldiers before they were captured. They did not consider, for example, a lower calorie diet could possibly contain the element niacin, the absence of which caused pellagra. In fact, bulgur wheat, which Ottomans received as soldiers, but not as prisoners, is rich in niacin. Furthermore, the Ottoman soldiers were also given dates as part of their daily diet; however, in the prison camps they may have been given more olives than dates as the dietary list gives 'dates or olives'. Dates are rich in the vitamin B-complex (including niacin), C and niacin, and they are a very good source of antioxidants such as carotenoids and phenolics. Carotenoids are especially useful in maintaining eye health. Although British doctors dismissed Ottoman rations as low in calories, they did not take into account that wheat bread, especially if it was whole grain, bulgur, and dates together may have contained significant amount of that ingredient – niacin. All this might have staved off pellagra and the nutritional eye diseases the prisoners developed in the camps.[47] This accounts for the fact that Ottoman soldiers could get scurvy or other nutrition-related diseases, but be free of pellagra as the Ottoman doctors claimed.

According to Dr A. Rıza, he and nineteen other Ottoman doctors in his prison camp were approached by the Second Pellagra Committee and asked to draft an opinion on pellagra cases among the prisoners. The original report of the Ottoman doctors cannot be found. All that remains is an account of it written by Dr A. Rıza in 1932. Citing the absence of pellagra among the European prisoners, the Ottoman officers and even among Ottoman soldiers who worked in the officer camp, Dr A. Rıza attributed the European's health to their access to a 'variety' of 'fresher' foods with higher 'calories', which he identified as 'nutritional value of foods', such as protein, biological protein (he calls this *biyos*), nuclein and others.[48]

Unfortunately, there are no adequate records with calorie values of the pre-1918 camp diet. In order to compare Ottoman and European prisoner diet, the researcher must look to the post-pellagra outbreak period when the diet was the improved version of the pre-1918 diet.

Believing that increased calorie intake might help with pellagra, and actually seeking to stop the outbreak, the British augmented the diet given to Ottomans by the latter half of 1918. The new and improved calorie value of the 'Non-European Prisoners of War' diet was higher by a thousand calories than that of the European prisoners, but most of the calories for the Ottomans came from thirty-two ounces of 'native' bread versus the nine ounces of 'English bread' given to Europeans. The problem, which the doctors did not yet understand, was that the native bread was nearly worthless in terms of the critical ingredient niacin or vitamin B-3. The European prisoners received at least three important foods high in niacin that the Ottomans did not receive: herring, potatoes and

Table 4.4 *European and non-European POW rations in Egypt*

Rations For European (German, Austrian and Bulgarian) POWs			Rations For 'Non-European' (Ottoman) POWs		
Item	Amount	Frequency	Item	Amount	Frequency
bread	9 oz	daily	bread	32 oz	daily
broken biscuits	4 oz	daily	meat (including bone)	4 oz	daily
meat OR	4 oz	twice a week	OR preserved meat	3 oz	daily
preserved meat	3 oz	twice a week	vegetables	4 oz	daily
bacon	1¾ oz	5 days a week	rice	3 oz	daily
salted, smoked, or pickled herring	10 oz	once a week	oil or margarine	¾ oz	daily
			salt	½ oz	daily
tea	¼ oz	daily	onions	½ oz	daily
sugar	1 oz	daily	tea	¼ oz	daily
salt	¼ oz	daily	sugar	1 oz	daily
potatoes	20 oz	daily	dates or olives	2 oz	daily
fresh vegetables	4 oz	daily	lentils or beans (extra issue, added especially to increase protein)	4 oz	4 days a week
split peas or beans	2 oz	daily			
rice	1.3 oz	daily			
oatmeal	1 oz	daily			
cheese	4/7 oz	daily			
margarine	3/7 oz	daily			
pepper	1/100 oz	daily			
maize meal	½ oz	daily			
Total calories	2,613.5		Total calories	3,680.5	

Source: *Report of Investigations, 1920*, pp. 10, 14–15.

bacon. As the prisoners were overwhelmingly Muslim in religion, they would not have eaten the bacon because of religious restrictions on swine flesh. Since the British asked the prisoners about their diet back at home, they knew that both potatoes and fish had been regularly consumed by the Ottomans in civilian life. If they had been inclined to accommodate the prisoners, the doctors could have easily recommended that such items be added to the prisoners' rations, but they were not. Given how the doctors felt about the prisoners' assumed inclination to lie, perhaps they felt these men were not being truthful about the diet they consumed at home.[49]

The First Pellagra Committee determined that 'biological value of protein' (B.P.V.) was a key factor in the development of pellagra. As a result, in the revised diet, Ottomans received approximately a thousand calories more than the European prisoners, due largely to the addition of lentils and beans. This increased the diet's gross protein value, but it did not solve the pellagra problem.[50]

Table 4.5 *Further comparison of rations: nutritional values*

Rations	Protein		Gross fat	Gross carbs	Calories
	Gross	B.P.V.			
European ration	102.6	62.6	43.6	429	2,613.5
Non-European ration (without extra lentils/beans)	108.4	49.8	40.4	628.1	3,510.8
Non-European with extra issues	121.6	54.9	41.4	653.8	3,680.5

Source: Report of Investigations, 1920, pp. 11, 13, 15.

For Ottoman soldiers, the captivity diet was seemingly better and clearly more consistent than army food in Palestine and Sinai in the last two years of the war. Nonetheless, the Ottoman prisoners still complained of its quality. One educated soldier, Sergeant İbrahimoğlu Bekir from Ankara, who worked in the pellagra ward in Egypt, left a graphic account of his experiences with food while in captivity:

> When we became prisoners, they sent us to Sidi Bishr. We stayed there 10 months; what we ate and drank was in good order. They gave us wheat bread, vegetables, and meat. We then came to Bilbeis [camp]. There, they gave us bread made from maize and rice; we could [actually] see the corn kernels and rice pieces in the loaf. This bread usually smelled of mold and it was very light, and did not have much substance to it. No vegetable at all; meat was only two–three times a week and that only being horse meat in one tiny piece.[51]

With the move to Bilbeis and the change in diet, numerous health problems developed. Upon repatriation, he reported the below to an Ottoman doctor who noticed the signs of pellagra among the repatriated prisoners:

> In one camp with 2,000 men, 1,500 of us could not see at night . . . After that was this thing called pellagra. [Our] hands and feet were burning like fire. Later they became red, irritated, runny with mucous, and then covered in scabs. Diarrhoea was particularly bad, sir. Those who were sick were melting away [*eriyip gidiyordular*]. Only 5 per cent [of the sick] could be saved. Bismuths, shots were no good; they used needles on some of us. Even these did not help. They opened up many corpses. They [the British doctors] were astonished too, sir. They could not find a virus or the like. Those who could be saved were sent to the convalescent homes (likely means hospital here). [There] they gave us wheat bread, chicken, meat and other items. But it was too late, sir.[52]

The words of Sergeant İbrahimoğlu Bekir convey the problems of pellagra rather well. His comment that only 5 per cent were saved most likely refers to the worst cases that were hospitalised. The First Committee report confirms his account of inedible bread. The Committee found that some breads at various camps were 'defectively aerated', 'rancid' and infested with weevils ('weevily'). Along with improperly cooked beans, which made digestion difficult, the Committee argued that insufficient aeration of the bread and other problems led to 'defective or insufficient absorption' of nutrients from the food eaten by the prisoners. The First Committee even argued that up to one-third of protein from food eaten might be lost in the intestines because of such seemingly minor issues as 'defective aeration' of bread or 'improperly soaked beans prior to boiling'.[53] In short, what seemed like a sufficient diet on paper may not have been as good in reality.

A significant part of the post-war controversy was the attempt to assign blame for the cause of pellagra. The British, while refusing to concede that the diet they fed the prisoners caused pellagra, would only grant that the diet had been insufficient to counteract pellagra, apparent or latent, in the prisoners. Dr Douglass Bigland deflected responsibility from the British on to the prisoners when he asserted:

> Turks before capture were suffering from food deficiency and that for some time after capture they were subject to a diet not very much better. This may account for the fact that some were pellagrous when captured and others developed the disease after capture. Even if it be asserted that all the prisoners were really chronic pellagrins, it appears that the diets supplied in our camps were not sufficient to inhibit recurrences.[54]

However, from late 1918 to mid-1919, some 7,000 Germans were held as prisoners in Egypt, but they remained pellagra free. These prisoners were from the German units fighting along the Ottoman fronts, most of whom were captured between September and November 1918. The First Committee used this fact to argue that the Ottomans had gone through dietary 'hardships' which the Germans had not, which explained why the Ottomans had pellagra when captured and the Germans did not. However, soon after the First Committee concluded its report and disbanded, pellagra began appearing among the German prisoners. In mid-1919, seventy-nine Germans became pellagrous. The Second Committee had to confront this unsettling new reality. They believed that, since pellagra developed over a period of three to six months, the Germans had to have developed the disease while in captivity. Therefore, the First Committee's most fundamental conclusion was simply wrong. Accordingly, there was no clear evidence as to which patients were pellagrous before capture and which 'developed the disease during and as a result of deprivations during captivity'.[55] The Second Committee accepted as fact that pellagra could, and at least partially did, originate during imprisonment.

The Second Committee had to take into account two other developments. First, two Germans captured in East Africa developed pellagra thirteen months after being interned in Egypt.[56] Second, in August 1920, just as the Second Committee was concluding its investigation, 400 Ottoman prisoners arrived in Egypt from prison camps in India, Burma, and Mesopotamia. Inspected by the Second Committee doctors upon arrival, they showed no signs of pellagra. Additionally, they assured the doctors that they had not experienced symptoms in the past. The British camps from which they had come had not reported any pellagra cases.[57] However, within six to ten weeks after arrival in Egypt, three of these men showed clear signs of pellagra. The newly sick men had been in captivity as long as five years in other locations without any signs of pellagra. Therefore, it is reasonable to conclude that the diet in the Egyptian camps was the critical factor in causing pellagra.[58] But mindsets and preconceptions die hard.

What was particularly disturbing was the speed at which the disease manifested itself in the Egyptian camps. The experiences of the Ottomans arriving from South Asia shattered the theory that clinical pellagra needed a minimum of three to six months to develop, as it had developed in as little as six weeks after arrival in the Egyptian camps. The German cases were perplexing to the British doctors because most German prisoners supplemented their camp diet with 'liberal purchases from the camp canteen', financed not only by the small salaries they earned, but also through the financial help provided by the German Embassy after 1918.[59] The availability of 'canteen' provisions very likely was a factor in keeping the Germans largely free of pellagra. But if, right after the end of the war, even some Germans were getting pellagra, then the camp diet for both Ottomans and Europeans was inadequate to stave off pellagra. Germans developed pellagra belatedly because their diet was significantly richer in niacin than that of the 'Non-European diet'. If the Ottoman government could have afforded to help its imprisoned soldiers to purchase additional food from the canteens, perhaps fewer of its soldiers would have developed pellagra.[60]

Additional factors, downplayed or completely ignored by the First Committee, did point to an important pattern in the development of pellagra. Because Ottoman prisoners could earn small wages in exchange for their labour while imprisoned, some enlisted men (the very ones whose diet put them most at risk, and who did not see any connection between sickness and labour) were 'happy' to work for pay, according to the British.[61] In 1920, Lieutenant Colonel P. S.

Lelean, a member of the First Committee, engaged in an exchange in *The Lancet* with Drs D. Bigland and J. I. Enright. He acknowledged that 'apparently healthy prisoners, selected (by pellagra experts) from volunteers in non-labour camps where many of them had been confined for long periods, became definitely pellagrous remarkably quickly (within three weeks in some instances) after transfer to labour camps'.[62] The First Committee had hinted at, but then dismissed, this evidence that implicated British prison camp conditions for the development of pellagra, while admitting that of the 500 healthy ('very fit') 'non-labour' men sent to Kantara labour camp, forty-two showed pellagra symptoms 'within 8 days'.[63] The doctors explained this away by suggesting that these selected men had not been healthy after all. Rather, they now suggested that they must have had 'latent' pellagra with 'deranged digestion and deficient power of assimilation, who while remaining healthy when at rest, rapidly developed into clinical pellagrins when put to work'.[64] Therefore, the authorities ordered that this group cease all labour. Dr Woodcock, a protozoologist and low ranking member of the First Committee, had witnessed this in the Kantara labour camp where most cases of pellagra appeared, but decided not to argue with his First Committee colleagues' contrary conclusions. In 1920, in response to Lieutenant Colonel Lelean's *Lancet* article, he spoke out saying: 'had not the labour been knocked off, one would hesitate to say how many of the 'apparently healthy' Turks would not have gone on to show a manifestly pellagrous condition'.[65]

Pellagra, even when it did not result in death by internal starvation, produced numerous painful side effects. Dr Douglas Bigland confessed that 'surgical cases with wounds show great difficulty in healing and fractured bones complicated with pellagra would not unite'. This became so clear to the British medical personnel that they eventually decided 'severe limb injuries with pellagra were treated by immediate amputation'.[66] In the final analysis, the death rates from pellagra provided by the British should have included not only those whose bodies starved, but also those many more who were operated on, or suffered wounds that did not heal, because their nutritionally deprived bodies could not fight infections.

British doctors, especially those of the First Committee, and Ottoman-Turkish doctors certainly disagreed over the timing and cause of pellagra. Another issue of contention was how many Ottomans had died needlessly of pellagra. Even now, an estimate would be difficult to produce. The doctors of the Second Committee discovered important evidence that there had been cases of significant under-reporting of pellagra cases. If pellagra cases were not identified and reported properly and the actual numbers were always higher than what was incorrectly reported, is it not possible that pellagra deaths were not always identified as such? Undoubtedly, we can attribute some of this under-reporting to pellagra frequently masking its role as killer and remaining hidden in the background in innumerable cases. Ultimately, pellagra's path of destruction was significantly larger than what the British reported at the time.

Night blindness

A second nutrition-related health issue that affected a large number of prisoners was night blindness, or nyctalopia. One Ottoman sergeant reported that 'in a prison camp with 2,000 enlisted men, 1,500 could not see anything at night'.[67] Here again, British officials acknowledged the condition but significantly downplayed the numbers affected by it. Although the sergeant called the condition *tavuk karası* – the popular term for retinitis pigmentosa, a condition whose symptoms are similar to nyctalopia – *tavuk karası* was an incorrect label. Nyctalopia is nutrition-related, while retinitis pigmentosa is genetic and not caused by nutrition.[68]

That significant numbers of prisoners experienced 'night blindness', or nyctalopia, was attested to by both British and Ottoman doctors. Dr W. Burridge noted that 5 to 10 per cent of all prisoners suffered from eye problems, and drew attention to the presence of night-blindness as yet another indicator of inadequate nutrition.[69] Dr James W. Barrett, attached to the First Australian General Hospital at Heliopolis in Egypt, observed that some of the eye problems among the Ottoman prisoners were due to nutritional amblyopia, 'occur[ing] in Turkish prisoners of war' due to pellagra.[70] The problem with a statement like this was that Barrett did not acknowledge what could have caused pellagra – camp diet or pre-captivity diet. Stated as such, it only said that pellagra caused some of the eye problems. Yet, we know what caused pellagra. Ottoman doctors employed in the camp hospitals also reported about night-blindness seen among the men.

The medical profession attributed night-blindness to a lack of fats in the diet, but in truth the cause was almost always a vitamin A deficiency.[71] Ironically enough, not too far from the prison camps was an ancient Egyptian papyri describing 'night blindness' as a disease encountered in ancient Egypt; the same papyri also provided a correct prescription for its cure – eating liver.[72] Liver would have helped the prisoners both with night blindness and pellagra, as it also contains niacin. Night blindness was associated with several symptoms from corneal clouding, to xerophthalmia (dryness due to eye's inability to produce tears), to keratomalacia (further severe dryness), and at the same time secretion of a sticky red substance around the eyes.[73] Experiments conducted on animals around the same time period showed that a diet that was not well-balanced was sufficient to produce, relatively quickly, keratomalacia, a severe dryness of the eyes that is a sign of oncoming night blindness. Vitamin A deprivations of eight to ten weeks caused rapid weight loss, unsteady gait and difficulty in breathing.[74] If the diet improved quickly enough, and included vitamin A, the night blindness would be cured, but the longer the deficiency, the more damage the retinas suffered. Continual deficiency eventually caused permanent blindness.

The prisoners' diets were woefully lacking in vitamin A. Consider the 1918 diet of the prisoners – bread, canned meat, 'vegetables', rice, onion, dates or olives, daily lentils or beans. None of these items are considered to be a good source of vitamin A.[75] As luck would have it, the 'European diet' fed to German, Austrian and Bulgarian prisoners, contained enough vitamin A to keep their eyes healthy.[76] But the lack of vitamin A created additional health problems for the Ottomans, since this vitamin also helped prevent or fight off infections by producing the white blood cells that destroy harmful bacteria and viruses. Here, one cannot help but think of Dr Bigland's comment above that certain prisoners died from diseases that should not have killed them. Pellagra and night blindness fall into that category, not only because they are both caused by nutritional deficiency, but also because that deficiency made the body vulnerable to a host of opportunistic diseases.

EYE DISEASES: TRACHOMA AND OPHTHALMIA

Sometime in mid-1919, a group of newly released Ottoman prisoners from Egypt arrived in the city of Izmir. Their condition greatly alarmed the Ottoman authorities. An alarming number of the group was blind in one or both eyes. The Ottoman government, which had surrendered unconditionally and was under foreign occupation, dispatched a formal protest to the British government charging that the British had shown unacceptable medical neglect toward Ottoman prisoners in captivity.[77]

In forging a response, British authorities consulted Lieutenant Colonel H. L. Eason, an eye specialist in an Egyptian hospital. His thesis was a familiar one. The reason for high incidence of blindness was that 'both ophthalmia and trachoma have occurred among Turkish Prisoners of War owing to the fact that these diseases were common in Palestine and Turkey before and during the War, were rife in the Turkish Army, and that prisoners arrived already infected'.[78] According to Eason, Ottoman military doctors in captivity had acknowledged severe outbreaks of ophthalmia among the troops prior to capture. Moreover, he continued, after the capture of Jerusalem by the British in 1917, the military patients in the Ottoman hospital there were sent to the POW hospital in Cairo. Seventy-eight of an unstated number, whom he had personally examined, were suffering from eye diseases. He explained that he encountered:

29 cases of purulent ophthalmia with ulcer of the cornea; of them, 15 had perforated cornea which caused blindness; an additional 30 out of the 78 were blind in one or both eyes as a result of recent ophthalmia ... The ophthalmia epidemics [in the prison camps] were due to the continual infection of camps by fresh arrivals of prisoners already suffering from the disease ... and their [the prisoners'] personal habits ... The complaints [of the Ottoman government] with reference to Trachoma are even more unjustifiable. The Ottoman Government must be aware that in common with Egyptians and all other Eastern people who live in hot climates under insanitary conditions, the Turks suffer extensively from trachoma ... [I]t has been my experience that a very high percentage of Turkish Prisoners have had active trachoma when captured.[79]

Although his response was dismissive, claiming that the Turkish prisoners tended to be infected upon capture, Eason fully accepted that trachoma was a very serious problem. He eventually published a lengthy article on trachoma in Egypt during the war. Eason used both ophthalmia and trachoma as separate conditions but some doctors used the terms interchangeably, referring to all eye diseases as ophthalmia. Trachoma, also called Egyptian ophthalmia, is a chronic inflammation caused by a parasitic organism similar to a bacterium (*Chlamydia trachomatis*). Untreated, it damages the corneas of the eye and causes blindness. It is transmitted by insects and is highly contagious in early stages through hand-to-eye contact or by the sharing of towels or handkerchiefs. If identified early, trachoma can be treated with heavy and extended antibiotic treatment. Ophthalmia is severe inflammation of the eye especially, but not exclusively, involving the conjunctiva. It may be indicative of a number of conditions including sympathetic ophthalmia (inflammation of both eyes following trauma to one eye), trachoma and actinic conjunctivitis (inflammation resulting from extended exposure to ultraviolet rays), among others.[80]

Allied occupation of Istanbul cut short the Ottoman protest on the matter. However, the subject of blind prisoners resurfaced in Ankara, the seat of the nationalist uprising against the Allied occupation. Likely taking their cue from a story published in *Öğüt*, a nationalist newspaper in Konya, two members of the Nationalist Assembly in Ankara – Faik [Kaltakkıran] Bey and Mehmet Şeref [Aykut] Bey – brought up the subject in the chamber in May 1921. The two introduced a motion to declare as guilty 'the British doctors, prison camp commandant, and officers' for causing 15,000 prisoners to go blind. The motion and Mehmet Şeref Bey's speech afterwards declared that thousands of Ottoman prisoners had been forced to submerge completely in creosol solutions ostensibly for delousing. This concoction, he argued, was intentionally mixed in such a way as to damage the prisoners' eyes and blind them. Going a step further, Mehmet Şeref Bey declared that 'in this way the British extracted (*çıkarmışlardır*) the eyes of 15,000 Turks'. A few days later, a resolution easily passed the National Assembly. Signed by the nationalist ministers and Mustafa Kemal, it both called for further investigation and declared that the prisoners had been purposefully blinded. This was, the resolution stated, a crime against humanity.[81]

Nothing seems to have come of the resolution and there are no records of 'further investigations'. Yet for many Turks, the issue was not forgotten. A 1922 captivity narrative of a former Ottoman civil official, Eyüb Sabri Bey, who had also been imprisoned in Egypt, charged that any of the prisoners who made the mistake of complaining of eye problems was sent to the camp hospital against his will. In about a week or two later, the same prisoner returned blind, having had one or both eyes surgically removed (enucleated). Differing from the Assembly, he charged that the prisoners' eyes were removed by British and Armenian camp doctors. The Armenian camp doctors he referred to were presumably those Armenian-Ottomans who, like other Ottoman doctors, served in the camps. Although the book did not make much of an impact at its first printing, and not much more when it was reprinted decades later in 1973, we need to note for future reference his inclusion of Armenians with the British.[82]

The camps: creosol and trachoma

While the early 1920s controversy over the blind prisoners seems to have quickly dissipated, it is still worth asking whether there might have been any credibility to the charges. Several prisoners described the general experience of the delousing as beginning with stripping down, then going through the creosol solution, followed by showers to wash away the remnant of the solution. Finally, they were given clean clothes to wear.

One prisoner, Nureddin, remembered that the solution created a slight sensation of burning and discomfort over his whole body. In a memoir serialised in the daily *Vakit*, under the title of 'Turkish Youths in Egyptian Deserts', he recollected the experience of delousing. That day's subtitle of the memoir was 'Prisoners in the outfit of Adam' (Hz. Adem):

> Let me narrate how we were forced to shower in this location; perhaps the readers will find the story remarkable. [There was a very large barrel and] now completely naked, we had to get inside this barrel . . . Right by the large barrel was a soldier, who emptied a bucket of liquid over our heads once we entered the large barrel; the barrel itself was only half full. This experience was different than a typical shower or a bath; while in a typical shower one pours water over

Pellagra and Trachoma 143

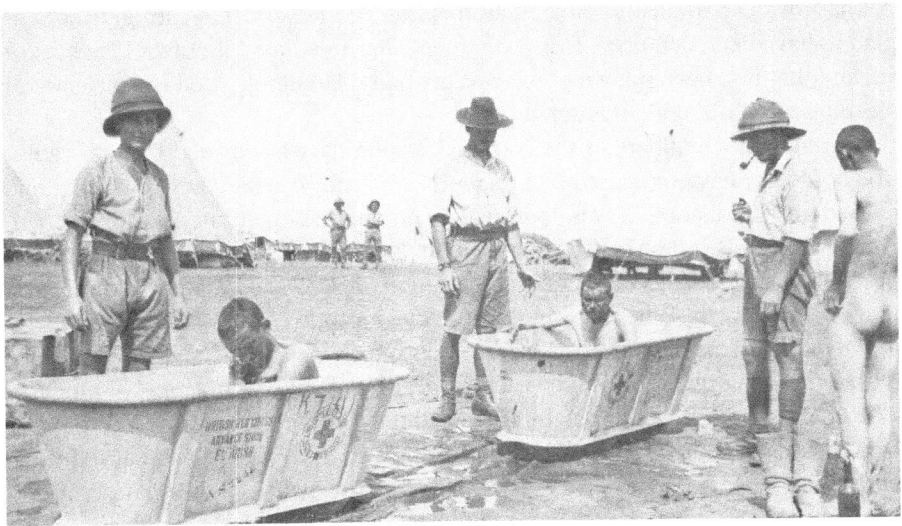

Figure 4.5 Turkish prisoners of war being disinfected under supervision at the Standing Hospital field ambulance
Source: Courtesy of Australian War Memorial, H00847

one's head, ours was different. The liquid poured over our head was called . . . lin [partially illegible], which was a type of antiseptic liquid. It was meant to kill the microbes [germs] on our bodies. Right after the bath in this [liquid] which badly irritated our bodies, we showered and cleaned ourselves with regular water. [The spectacle of] this hygienic measure is probably still alive in the memories of those prisoner friends.[83]

Although methods for delousing prisoners may have differed from one camp to another, the narrator here describes only that a bucket of creosol solution was poured over his head. This was not a full head-to-toe submersion in the liquid. The passage instead suggests that the prisoner was less upset with the disinfection process and skin irritation than he was with having to be naked in front of friends and foreign soldiers.

Another prisoner, Ahmet Altınay, related that

after we were captured, they lined us up. There was a barrel as tall as us. There was some medicated chemical inside. They got everyone as naked as the time we were given birth; [and told us] to get in the barrel and submerge until our heads got wet. Meanwhile our clothes were sterilized . . . [Afterwards], I slept well that day. There were no lice left, or anything else.[84]

Altınay did experience complete submersion in creosol. Interestingly, he was glad to have been deloused, from which he felt immediate relief from the host of vermin that had been gnawing away at his body. He highlighted the pleasure of sleeping well following the delousing.

Perhaps the members of the National Assembly who pushed for the resolution could not have imagined that trachoma, vitamin A deficiency or ophthalmia caused the blindness that was so prevalent among the repatriated prisoners. Yet, since there had to be a reason for so many blind men, the most logical cause, given the prisoners' accounts of their common experiences, was their immersion in a chemical bath. When nothing else seemed to make sense that did. But why was that experience mentioned so prominently? As Chapters 1 and 2 showed, for Ottomans, avoiding public nudity was a question of cultural practice, of modesty and of religious proscription. In forcing the Ottomans to undress not only in front of their captors, but also in front of their friends, the British caused them embarrassment. Arguably, the reason in some cases why the story of delousing is told by the prisoners as an 'important' event worthy of mention is based on the experience of nakedness, not the chemical solution or the fact that it might have irritated the bodies of some. Another possibility is that, for those who had suffered from lice for months or years, the organised, efficient way of delousing was an impressive novelty. This procedure also marked their entry into the permanent prison camps, a memorable event in itself. Eye disease or blindness for another reason was not what marked the experience for Altınay. He did not contract trachoma or did not go blind because of creosol, but he slept well because he was no longer bothered by filth and lice.

Treating eye problems in camps

In a lengthy post-war article on the problem of trachoma and ophthalmia, Dr H. L. Eason referred to his experiences with Ottoman prisoners in Egypt:

> Before the war ophthalmia was, next to malaria, the most prevalent disease in Palestine. From conversations I have had with Turkish and Syrian doctors who were attached to the Turkish army, it appears that ophthalmia did not occur until the troops reached the neighbourhood of Jerusalem and Gaza, where the climatic conditions and the habits and customs of the natives more nearly approach those of Egypt than do those of the populations of the more mountainous country further north. I am told that there were numerous outbreaks of purulent ophthalmia among the Turkish troops in these districts, and they were severe in character.[85]

Prior to August 1918, he insisted, there were only limited incidents of ophthalmia in the Ottoman camps. However, from August to the end of December 1918, in Kantara camp alone, some 3,600 prisoners were admitted to hospitals specifically for eye-related problems. The camp hospital in Heliopolis kept monthly figures on eye patients admitted: 100 in July, 400 in August, 500 in September, 1,000 in October, 1,200 in November, and down to 500 in December.[86] In two camps within the space of four to five months, 7,300 Ottoman POWs were seen or operated on for ophthalmic problems alone. He did not provide statistics on the specific nature of the treatment the patients received.

Not always sure of what treatment method to follow, British and Ottoman doctors under their control in the camps experimented with several options. Some treatments seemed to work, while others made things worse by destroying the conjunctiva (the thin membrane that covers the inner surface of the eyelid and the white part of the eyeball) thus leading to further infection. 'Cauterization with pure carbolic acid for corneal ulcers was equally useless in many cases' and did not stop epidemics. Regular daily prophylactic treatment of every prisoner, with or without an eye disease, was, according to Eason, more successful.[87] Nonetheless, some men became completely blind in one or both eyes; panophthalmitis (inflammation of all layers of the eye) and staphyloma (abnormal protrusion of the uveal tissue through a weak point in the eyeball) caused 'the total destruction of a great many eyes'. Eason confirmed that at the Heliopolis camp, where most of the 'patients eventually arrived', 418 eyes were surgically removed (enucleation) in 1918.[88] Here, undoubtedly, was the origin of the Eyüb Sabri Bey's story about operations to remove eyes even though he was in a different camp.

Of course, what Eason revealed in terms of statistics pertained only to 1918. He complained that it was nearly impossible to keep accurate statistics because they sometimes saw the same patient more than once, and because prisoners were continually transferred from one prison camp or hospital to another. Ottoman statistics were incomplete as well; an Ottoman pamphlet revealed that in two large repatriations, one in August 1919 and one 'some time afterwards', a total of 2,609 cases out of 54,734 enlisted men were found to be suffering from severe scaring due to trachoma and ophthalmia. The statistics provided in Table 4.6, collected by the Ottoman and Turkish authorities, revealed the prevalence of trachoma among the prisoners, and the work of the British camp authorities. The Ottoman doctors, in examining the men, classified them into ten categories.[89]

During the same time, 4,245 officers were repatriated from Egypt as well, but not a single one was listed as having, or was hospitalised due to, symptoms of trachoma. However, 128 officers were hospitalised for other

Table 4.6 Study of 2,609 trachoma patients repatriated in August 1919 and at a later unlisted date

General nature of treatment	Category (where and how treated)	Numbers
Operations conducted in Egypt [or later transferred there]	Both eyes removed (*istisâl edilen*)[90] while in Egypt	64
	Both eyes operated on in [the island of] Limni [Lemnos][91]	1
	One eye removed (*istisâl*) while in Egypt	27
	Left eye removed (*ihraç*) in Limni	1
	Left eye removed (*ihraç*) on the Iraq front	1
	One eye removed in Egypt, but still have one healthy eye	80
	One eye removed in Limni, but still have one healthy eye	1
Received treatment in Egypt	Blind in both eyes	448
	Fully blind in one eye and have partial sight in the other	333
No treatment received	Repatriated from Egypt but still have trachoma	1,653
Grand total		2,609

Source: adapted from Sıhhat ve İçtimai Muavenet Vekaleti, *Trahom Hakkında Halka Nasayih*, p. 4.

reasons, along with 8,392 enlisted men who had other unlisted illnesses, but no trachoma.[92]

The trachoma epidemic comes home to Turkey

Trachoma was prevalent enough in parts of the Ottoman Empire that prior to the war the government had inaugurated a short-lived and possibly half-hearted campaign to combat it. Writing in 1919, one Ottoman-Turkish doctor recalled that the Ottoman state had made a commitment to fight trachoma before the war, but the war cut the effort short. Disappointed in the outcome, Dr Muhtar considered the state's decision to be short sighted. 'I don't know why the war became an obstacle to this [effort]', he opined.

> As long as the war continued there was more of a need for this struggle [against trachoma]. Even if we do not have completely reliable statistics, it can be said that during the war the army could not make use of many (*pek çok*) enlisted men because of their trachoma; an enlisted man with trachoma always stayed like an invalid and a crippled limb of the army.[93]

A post-war official publication described the geography of trachoma in Anatolia. Prior to 1914 trachoma could be found only in certain southern and south-eastern *vilayet*s (provinces), but after the war it spread to various other parts of the Anatolian peninsula.[94]

Trachoma was only one of several diseases that swept over Anatolia, both during and after the war. Even a quick survey of medical journals and official government publications in the 1920s reveals that the Anatolia of this time period was facing major health crises. Though neither the only one nor the most dangerous by any means, trachoma was one of the major diseases threatening the population. Dr Muhtar insisted that trachoma was almost as ruinous to Anatolia and Turks as the *masâ'ib-i selâse*, or the three calamities facing the empire: syphilis, malaria and tuberculosis.[95]

In 1920, even before the founding of the republic in 1923, it was estimated that perhaps 3 million people were infected with trachoma.[96] This would amount to more than one-fifth of the estimated 1923 population. Certain areas of Anatolia had more than their share of trachoma cases. For example, the province of Adıyaman, in the south east, was known as 'the province of blind people' (*körler memleketi*) during the early republic.[97] The prevalence of various diseases, especially trachoma, in post-war Turkey was such a dramatic and disturbing sight that it filtered into the popular poetry of Fazıl Hüsnü Dağlarca as late as 1965. In a fit of anger he questioned officials about not only diseases but also other social ills and shortcomings in a poem called 'An Ode from Outside'.

> You! Ali Bey, you Veli Bey are this:
> Guilty in front of future generations.
> You will somehow govern your nation
> And it will reach modern civilization?
> Ahead is dark, behind is dark, right is dark, and left is dark.
> Are we getting buried in the black earth?
>
> A country, half of it dirt poor,
> Half eats only bread and salt.
> Its dogs, cows, bears are asleep
> All of its intellectuals are sleepless.
> About a million of the community are stricken with trachoma, a million with malaria,
> Another million with tuberculosis, don't we know all this?[98]

Of course, Dağlarca's numbers are only meant to be poetic approximates, as in 'millions', and are not to be taken as actual statistics. These diseases became all the more significant because the officials, doctors and civilians were still reeling from the nation's death toll in the Great War and War of Independence. During the years between the end of the Great War in 1918 and the founding of the republic in 1923, both the government in Istanbul and nationalist leaders attempted in various and modest ways to deal with the problem of diseases, though some of the latter would accuse the former of not doing anything.

How did trachoma become such a big problem in Anatolia? One publication laid out the history of trachoma as a series of waves of introduction. The work identified four different time periods and ways in which this disease entered Anatolia. Initially, it was introduced by the returning veterans of the Ottoman-Mamluk war in 1517. Three hundred years later, it was reintroduced by the Egyptian fellahin soldiers of Ibrahim Pasha, who invaded south-eastern and central Anatolia by way of Syria in the 1830s. The disease existed at Mediterranean port cities such as Antalya, Alanya, Mersin, Iskenderun and Adana. Egyptian merchants, who carried the disease, passed it onto the 'Turks' who traded with them. In the estimation of the Ottoman-Turkish doctors of the 1920s, the connection to Egypt was quite clear. Many such doctors called trachoma 'the Egyptian disease' (*Mısır hastalığı*).[99]

The final reintroduction, the one that was critical for the new Turkish republic, was by the repatriated prisoners who had succumbed to trachoma while in Egyptian prison camps or while fighting in Palestine, Syria or Yemen. They then spread the disease widely among the Anatolian population.[100] Another pamphlet, published in 1921 while the last of the prisoners were still returning, directed its readers' attention to the connection between the repatriated prisoners and their relatives who were by then showing signs of trachoma. Warning that it would soon get worse because 'those hundreds or [even] thousands of enlisted men and officers who returned from captivity are traveling to various parts of the country [to their hometowns]', it urged the imperial government to take precautions to stop the disease from spreading further among the populace. The author, Dr Mehmed Emin, added that even the American medical mission working in Turkey linked the spread of the disease to 'not examining the eyes of the prisoners upon repatriation and failing to cure them' before they were allowed to go to Anatolia.[101] Surely, a 'cure' would be impossible for those whose condition was advanced, but doctors probably meant treatment or operation until the men were no longer contagious.

Strangely enough, both for the British captors and for the Ottoman and nationalist authorities, the prisoners became 'porters' carrying diseases from one place to another. Both the British and Ottoman-Turkish sides insisted that there had been no or very little disease until the prisoners introduced it from the outside. For the British the homeland of the prisoners was already a source of the

Pellagra and Trachoma 149

disease, but for the imperial and nationalist authorities, the source became the camps in Egypt.

National mobilisation against trachoma

With his 1919 article, Dr Muhtar, an eye disease specialist in Kilis in south-eastern Anatolia, advised that instead of copying or importing European procedure and knowledge 'randomly', the state should bring in its 'seasoned specialists', and involve the Imperial Medical School in educating and training all medical professionals on the dangers and treatment of trachoma. 'Because', he argued, 'trachoma is found only infrequently in its typical [classic] form in our country', non-specialists do not, and will not, know how to deal with the epidemic that would spread even further.[102]

The political, military and demographic disruption of the 1918–23 period stifled both Istanbul's and Ankara's efforts to deal with national health issues. In 1925, two years after the founding of the Turkish republic, the state finally declared a 'mobilisation' (*seferberlik*) to deal with trachoma and other communicable diseases. The state's use of military terminology – as in 'call to arms' or *seferberlik* – was not by chance. Behind this effort was Dr Refik Saydam, the former Ottoman military doctor now turned Minister of Health, who would later serve as Minister of the Interior and Prime Minister. While various pamphlets or informative booklets on the topic of trachoma had been appearing for a number of years, something comprehensive was needed to give direction to what was now officially called the 'struggle against trachoma'.

Before they could act, the state and health professionals needed, as a foundation, an accurate portrayal of present health conditions in the country. The first step toward meeting this need was pioneered by Dr Vefik Hüsnü (Bulat), a military or former military doctor, who delivered a report called 'Turkey's Trachoma Geography' at the meeting of the Second National Medical Congress in Ankara in 1927. At the request of the Minister of Health Refik Saydam, Dr Vefik Hüsnü had travelled and researched throughout eastern and south-eastern Anatolia in order to compile the report.[103] Vefik Hüsnü's study divided Turkey into four trachoma zones. For each, he estimated the percentage of those affected with trachoma, the possible rate of increase and local issues related to the geography of each province within those zones.[104] The author insisted that irrespective of zones, an almost universal contributor to the spread of the disease was what he called 'living without consideration for hygiene' (*hıfzısıhhaya riayetsiz yaşamak*). Vefik Hüsnü did not neglect to provide a summary of the worldwide diffusion of the disease, making sure to cover all continents.[105]

Dr Vefik Hüsnü's 'Turkey's Trachoma Geography' became a model for the later, much larger efforts through the 1920s and 1930s, which were sponsored by the state to study the health and social geography of the nation's provinces for each of the nation's major health issues. Eventually, nineteen detailed studies were produced.[106] They helped the state to determine which diseases existed in which regions, and how best to deal with them. The process of compiling the studies brought representatives of the state into direct contact with local communities, some of which had been at least partially isolated. The agents and officials of the state appeared in the provinces to measure, study, examine the geography, diseases and the people, for the purpose of what some have called 'national territorialisation of space', or the projecting of national meaning onto a specific area in order to construct a national homeland.[107] 'National territorialisation of space', in this way, provided rational justification for the state and its efforts. Faced with a sobering picture, national leaders had to admit that the homeland was in medical crisis. As bad as the situation was, it gave the same leaders a reason to justify the state's presence in formerly isolated areas, while at the same time passing the blame onto the former Ottoman state. The republic would now cure the same people that the sultanate could not or did not.

This national territorialisation of space is necessary at all times for the nation-state to establish its legitimacy. Scholar Arjun Appadurai argues that 'the nation-state creates vast networks of formal and informal techniques for the nationalization of all space considered to be under its sovereign authority'. It does this through such diverse apparatuses as court houses, museums, hospitals, village dispensaries, post offices, and so on.[108] Village dispensaries and province hospitals to deal with trachoma (and other diseases) were exactly what the republican elite had in mind to keep the nation healthy. These people were needed not only as witnesses to the state's concern for their health, but also as healthy individuals who would be more productive.

The first two dispensaries, one with ten beds and the other with twenty, were opened in Adıyaman and Malatya in 1925.[109] Others followed slowly in provinces in the south, east and southeast. One doctor estimated, based on some months of service in Adana, that nearly 90 per cent of the population was afflicted with trachoma. In his estimate, Maraş, Urfa, Gaziantep and Kilis in the southeast and Antalya in the south were not too far behind.[110] Other official or non-official sources estimated that the rate of infection in the south and the southeast averaged 70 per cent.[111] Other provinces with a lesser, but still significant, rate of infection included Erzurum, Bitlis, Van, Muş, Aydın and Manisa.[112]

For the leading health professionals and nationalist leaders of the early republican period, the prevalence of curable diseases signalled a lack of civilisation and modernity. Eliminating such diseases would bring the nation closer to the level of civilised modernity. The aim itself was not that different to what the prisoner officers had in mind; they too wanted to attain contemporary civilisation as represented by the West. However, there were also some differences. For the prisoner officers, it was the peasants' ignorance, 'wild' behaviour and even otherworldly concerns that kept the nation back. For the health professionals, it was the peasants' diseased bodies and unhygienic lifestyles that frustrated the efforts to reach the level of modern civilisation. If the health professionals and others as the agents of the state could teach the people about rules of hygiene and cure them of their most dangerous ills, then the aim would be a few steps closer. A number of doctors made significant efforts in order to make this happen, either as part of some national commission or as individual doctors who were nevertheless concerned about the same issues.

Dr Nuri Fehmi, who would soon be appointed as the man in charge of the campaign against trachoma, was one such person. He looked to evidence from Switzerland to try to understand how to deal with trachoma. There were relatively few cases of trachoma in Switzerland, and he insisted that it was partially due to that country's geography and topography. However, he claimed that the low rate of infection was based mostly 'on the [Swiss] people's perfect attention to cleanliness and hygiene'.[113] This would have been no surprise to other doctors working on trachoma or other related eye diseases. In fact, in 1927, Dr S. Şükrü had asserted something very similar: 'trachoma is more generally found among those groups of people exposed to physiological poverty, those who do not pay attention to general hygiene, [those who live with] destituteness, poverty, [and] misery'.[114] He was seconded by Dr Muhtar: 'Trachoma is friend (*arkadaş*) to those poor people who ordinarily live in poverty and in [a state of] filth'. He added that it is nearly impossible to find a person without trachoma in those families who live a life of privation (*ma'işet*) and have common use of various ('personal') belongings.[115] Similarly, the 1924 version of *Trahom Hakkında Halka Nasayih* indicated: 'trachoma's spread from one to another can happen very quickly among those who live in tribal groups and in bad conditions [such as] Arab and Kurdish peoples, Circassians and Jews'.[115] Certainly, the disease was just as likely to spread quickly among poor Turks and other ethnic groups who were forced to share personal items or lived in very close quarters out of economic necessity. However, the *Nasayih*, while pointing to poverty and communal lifestyle as the crucial factors, only identified these groups by name. In later versions of the booklet, the ethno-religious connection was edited out completely.

Given the conditions and the lack of knowledge about hygiene and cleanliness among peasants, the state had to take the lead in eradicating the disease. The state's efforts to combat trachoma included the establishment of stationary dispensaries, mobile units and a few hospitals. Its doctors also launched a public relations campaign of sorts professing the republic's concern for its citizens, with the effort to combat blindness and trachoma as projects in progress. The aim was to demonstrate that the republic could accomplish what the Ottoman state could not. *Sıhhıye Mecmuası*, the official journal of the Ministry of Health, argued that the 'struggle against trachoma is the [unique] work of the republic'.[117] Dr Nuri Fehmi [Ayberk] went so far as to declare that one could not even find the word 'trachoma' in Ottoman government publications. According to him, it only appeared in state publications in 1924, a year after the founding of the republic.[118] This was an overstatement of great magnitude. However, it was true that there was a dramatic change in the state's attitude toward, and assuming responsibility for, the nation's health during the republican period.[119]

Once the 'mobilisation' was declared in 1925, state officials started to appear in the provinces where trachoma was prevalent. An official publication of the Ministry of Health, *Sıhhıye Mecmuası Fevkalade Nüshası: Vekaletin 10 Yıllık Mesaisi*, reported in 1933 that from 1925 to 1932 some 2 million patients were 'treated' for trachoma. While more than 1.9 million received outpatient treatment, at least 38,000 – more than twice the number of repatriated blind prisoners – required eye operations by Turkish doctors to preserve their lives and health.[120] These were impressive numbers given that the population of Turkey was only 16 million in 1935 and that the 'struggle against trachoma' had begun in 1925 with just two small dispensaries.

Nonetheless, the doctors who would come to lead the fight against trachoma after 1934 downplayed the accomplishments of the pre-1934 period. Dr Nuri Fehmi Ayberk, who took charge in 1934, insisted that the so called 'war against trachoma' had not only failed to provide services to a large enough population, but had greatly exaggerated its accomplishments.[121] Rather than counting the number of patients treated, the previous administration publicised the total number of 'treatments' administered to all patients, whose numbers were not that large. Similarly, to increase the programme's numbers, even the simplest of procedures were sometimes listed as full-fledged 'operations'.[122]

A propaganda piece, *Onbeşinci Yıl Kitabı*, published by the Republican Peoples Party in 1938 at least partially corrected these 'mistakes' and exaggerations to which Dr Nuri Fehmi Ayberk referred. This book distinguished between 'treatment' and 'examination'. Whereas the earlier and official *Sıhhıye Mecmuası Fevkalade Nüshası* had reported 2 million patients by 1933, the new publication exposed the fact that while there had been 2 million *treatments*, there had been only 70,000 patients in hospitals and dispensaries. The numbers for the mobile treatment and examination units were relatively close or even higher than those of the stationary hospital.[123]

Ayberk studied the methods of nine countries: Syria, Palestine, Egypt, Tunisia, Italy, Greece, Yugoslavia, Hungary and Poland. Finding the anti-trachoma efforts in Egypt, Hungary, Poland and the Jewish settlements in Palestine to be the most effective, he formed a plan to attack trachoma in Turkey. Ayberk eliminated the mobile units and increased the number of dispensaries and available beds.[124] Since there were thousands of children who were blind or partially blind due to eye diseases, the state opened special primary schools for them.[125]

Ayberk was aided in his efforts by recent regulations and laws relating to health and hygiene in the republic. Although there had been a number of regulations for dealing with trachoma and those who suffered from it, the state decided to legislate for hygiene even more strictly in 1930. The 1930 law, which covered a wide range of social and medical issues, expanded the powers of the state and its officials, and made its civilising mission easier and legal, through the fact that it was also made mandatory.

The second section of the law (items 29 through 128) regulated the 'fight against contagious and epidemic diseases'. The fourth chapter of that section dealt specifically with the 'fight against trachoma', while others addressed malaria, tuberculosis and venereal diseases.[126] With the introduction of the law, it became mandatory to report cases of trachoma to the state. In areas where the number of patients with trachoma reached a certain threshold, the Ministry of Health would appoint a committee to improve care and build new medical facilities. These committees had the state's authority to summon the people to medical institutions they established. Dr Mazhar Osman summarised the policy, noting that the state 'started to treat those who came forward with pleasure and those who did not come forward by force'.[127] The committees also had the authority to ban any patient deemed to be contagious from places where they might infect others. The laws and regulations applied to the whole nation, but the 'fight against trachoma regions' (*trahom mücadele mıntıkası*) were mostly in the south-eastern part of Anatolia.[128]

The 1930 hygiene law gave the state, its doctors and officials the authority to investigate, treat and summon people afflicted with trachoma and a number of other diseases. The state, guided and goaded by socio-medical 'experts', wanted to eradicate social and real diseases to reach modernity and the level of civilisation they desired. Of course, this could be done by expanding its control and surveillance of citizens and their daily lives in capillary forms. This does not mean that the republican state achieved that power, but it certainly had more of it than the Ottoman state did only a decade earlier.

PRISONERS AS CONTESTED OBJECTS

Health conditions of the repatriated prisoners of war shocked the authorities and inaugurated both a political and a medical controversy in which prisoners became contested political and medical objects. In its resolution relating to the repatriated blind prisoners, the nationalist government in Ankara was openly accusatory in levelling the charge that 'English doctors, commandants, and officers [in the Egyptian POW camps] had purposefully invalided [*malul etmek*] 15,000 prisoners . . .'.[129] The resolution was introduced by two members of the assembly – Faik and Mehmet Şeref Beys – and who they were and their recent experiences were important. After occupying Istanbul, the British arrested and sent to exile in Malta (March 1919–October 1920) a number of Ottoman civil and military officials, as well as intellectuals. Before becoming members of the National Assembly in Ankara, both Faik and Mehmet Şeref Beys had been prisoners in Malta.[130] In 1921, they introduced a resolution about the British mistreatment of prisoners in Egypt. A closer reading of the discussions in the Assembly reveals that while the resolution was about Egypt, their speeches were more about those imprisoned in Malta. It is possible that what they read about the repatriated blind prisoners from Egypt made sense in the context of how they were treated in Malta. Because nothing revealing came of the resolution to further investigate, we might surmise that the members of the Assembly were informed by Ottoman-Turkish doctors, who were already writing on this issue, that the cause of the soldiers' blindness was trachoma.

Into the later 1920s and 1930s, the issue of the prisoners frequently came up when physicians wrote about various diseases plaguing Turkey. In these publications, Turkish doctors challenged their British counterparts on the grounds of prisoner health, but they also wrote more generally about the health of the nation in order to reflect its march towards modern civilisation. Accordingly, the issue became significantly larger than the individual harm done to the health of the Ottoman, now Turkish, prisoners. The British had surveyed, enumerated, measured and discoursed upon the demographic and epidemiological properties of the bodies of sick Ottoman prisoners. From this, they had drawn conclusions about the nation and homeland, conclusions with which Ottoman-Turkish doctors did not agree. Starting during the last few years of the Ottoman Empire, but especially during the early republican years, these 'medico-Orientalist' interpretations and diagnoses of 'Turkish' prisoners, the Turkish homeland and the Turkish nation did not go uncontested by nationalist doctors.

This contestation took place in several stages. Ottoman-Turkish health professionals declared that, despite their all-knowing attitude, the British diagnoses of Ottoman prisoners and their postulations about diseases of Turks were distorted by their misinformed 'Orientalist' assumptions. Many of the diseases that the British attributed to the prisoners and their homeland were not endemic to Turkey. Additionally, the nationalist doctors argued, the epidemics of pellagra, trachoma or dysentery that had swept Anatolia after the war had come into

Turkey from foreign regions with the returning prisoners and veterans. Even if something like trachoma was acquired in Palestine or Syria, these places were now 'enemy' territory. Even pellagra, widely accepted by the Ottoman-Turkish doctors to be a disease produced by food deficiency and therefore not contagious, was regularly mentioned in the context of Ottoman prisoners 'bringing' it home from out there somewhere.[131]

A significant charge the Ottoman-Turkish doctors levelled against the British was that their medical opinions were discredited because of their prejudiced assumptions about the Ottomans and Turks. These assumptions, the argument ran, clouded the Europeans' judgment and thus their diagnoses. Dr A. Rıza, who became involved in the investigations regarding pellagra in the Egyptian camps, charged that the British doctors were stubbornly determined to establish a causal connection between the disease and the Ottoman soldiers' pre-war residences as evidenced by their 'pellagra map' project.[132] A. Rıza was more than a sceptic. In a 1932 article, he charged that because of their bias, the British doctors focused on non-essential issues and had therefore failed to understand the nature of pellagra and other diseases among the prisoners. He stood by the report he and his Ottoman colleagues had prepared for the Second Committee. Nothing that had happened since the prison camps changed his mind. In fact, new evidence provided by an American researcher in 1926 would have proven him to be correct, though niacin deficiency as the causative factor would not be discovered until 1937.[133] According to him, his report had asserted that pellagra was not bacteriological and had nothing to do with physical stature, age, race, climate, gender or status, but was simply a matter of better nutrition provided by fresher foods.[134] Dr A. Rıza was not alone in this regard. Other doctors in Turkey continued to argue well into the 1930s that British failure to provide wholesome food to the captured men caused disease, most notably pellagra. Dr Abdulkadir Noyan insisted: 'the general diet of the prisoners consisted of bread made of adulterated flour which became stale very quickly, mostly maggot-ridden and hollowed out [*çoğu kurtlanmış ve içi kısmen boşalmış*] Egyptian broad-beans, very small amount of meat, and low-quality date marmalade'.[135]

When it came to diseases such as trachoma and dysentery, the connection between the appearance of the diseases in Turkey proper and the repatriated POWs became even more pronounced. Dr Osman Şerafeddin argued that 'many of the enlisted men, prisoners of war in Egypt and India fell victim to this disease [dysentery] and brought it to the motherland'.[136] Abdulkadir Noyan seconded this finding, declaring: 'these [amoebic dysentery] seeds [*tohumları*] could not survive in some of our cold and moderate climate [regions]. But, they continue to exist as isolated incidents in some other moderate and warmer provinces'.[137]

For Noyan, the motherland's climate alone was enough to partially reduce the danger of dysentery introduced by the repatriated prisoners.

Ottoman-Turkish doctors believed that many European doctors were biased against them and their empire and nation. Although a number of them had fought against this kind of bias, in 1921 as the prisoners were still being repatriated, a European publication triggered an important response in the form of a critical article from Mazhar Osman. In challenging European science and men of science, he was speaking for those doctors who dealt with trachoma and pellagra. The content of his critique reached all the way back to the late nineteenth century.

At an International Medical Congress in 1897, German psychiatrist Baron Richard von Krafft-Ebing had given a talk on syphilis. He had earlier demonstrated the connection between syphilis and general paresis – a form of neuro-syphilis resulting from damage caused to the brain by untreated syphilis – prior to serological tests, such as the Wasserman test (which is still in use today).[138] In this address, he suggested that the 'syphilization and civilization' combination was the cause of general paresis of the insane (hereafter G.P.). He and other European scientists argued that G.P. was more common among 'brain workers' than those who earned their living by physical labour. Since the nervous system of white men was thought to be more highly organised than that of other 'races', and 'brain workers' could only exist among the civilised, Caucasians were judged to be more vulnerable to G.P.[139] By this definition, G.P. became a measure of civilisation, defined by the 'lack' of G.P. in a given location. Therefore, the 'lack' of G.P. in a given location proved 'lack' of civilisation and therefore indicated savagery. Krafft-Ebing's observation was soon confirmed by other European men of medicine. Two such names were Ernst Rudin, Swiss psychiatrist and racial hygienist, and renowned German psychiatrist Emil Kraepelin, with whom Mazhar Osman studied while in Germany.[140]

European scientists' equation of G.P. with civilisation and its absence with barbarity attracted the attention of Ottoman and, later, Turkish doctors. A number of them rejected the assertions out of hand. Among others, this medical theory was most vociferously attacked by Mazhar Osman. In his 1921 article titled 'Sendemi Brutus?' or 'Even You, Brutus?' Mazhar Osman wrote:

> Westerners come to the East with various legendary burdens on their minds that resemble the tales in One-Thousand and One Nights. And in every corner they look for things that will satisfy [and confirm] their imaginations [of the East]. They become entranced by this illusion and therefore see and interpret everything they encounter according to this illusion; in this way they make

judgments about us. This is true ... even of those who are most learned and erudite.[141]

With these comments, Mazhar Osman suggested that even men of science took the Orient-Occident dichotomy as a starting point for nearly everything pertaining to the East. Understandably, he was more offended and surprised by what he called the unscientific findings of those German doctors who had served in Turkey. He first took on Dr Ernst von During, Professor of dermatology in Istanbul from 1889 to 1902, then a certain Professor Müller. Both had maintained that G.P. and *tabes dorsalis*, another form of neuro-syphilis, were non-existent among Ottomans, thereby implying that Ottomans lacked civilisation.[142] Mazhar Osman went on the offensive:

> During the Great War Professor Müller, even though he had served in Turkey for two years and conducted [many] medical examinations during this period, told us at a meeting of the Imperial Medical Academy that he had never encountered G.P. and tabes, and consequently he had arrived at the conclusion that the syphilis virus in Turkey did not cause neurological disorders. And as he told us this, he firmly believed that he was actually teaching us something. We invited this expert to Şişli LaPaix hospital. We showed him that eleven percent of those hospitalized had either G.P. or tabes. Because his silly tales were corrected, he [suddenly] ceased to be merry.[143]

According to Mazhar Osman, Müller still did not amend his theories, despite having been presented with irrefutable evidence. He even went on to write a work called 'Psychology of Turks', in which he said 'many other things about our nature'. Mazhar Osman continued: 'whatever the professor heard about Turks since he was a child, he wrote in this work ... and in this way he introduced his misinformed thesis about the psychology of Easterners to other [European] men of science'. It is interesting to note that Mazhar Osman seamlessly switched between Turks and Easterners (*Şarklılar*), as the prisoners of war did in some of their writings we encountered in Chapter 3. He claimed to have encountered many misinformed interpretations about Turkey or about diseases in Turkey. Some of these European works gave statistics without stating where these numbers came from, he added. Yet, they always arrived at similar conclusions. According to these people, he said, 'if there were not enough factories in Turkey or if no small industry existed', the reason for this disappointing state of affairs could only be one thing: 'the laziness of the people'.[144]

These charges against the European doctors continued well into the 1930s, and Mazhar Osman was not the only critic. A number of other Ottoman and

Turkish doctors, ranging from generalists to epidemiologists to dermatologists, shared his point of view. Abdulkadir Noyan charged that European doctors' 'exaggerations and overgeneralizations [about us] ... resulted from baseless opinions'.[145] European men of science had failed to move beyond the Orient-Occident dichotomy – when they were writing about, diagnosing and even treating diseases found, or presumed to be found, among Orientals. Europeans' assumptions about Turks undermined their scientific judgment, which was supposed to be objective. Science itself might be value neutral, but scientists were not without prejudices and biases, which then influenced the science they practiced. As Mazhar Osman suggested, if they went looking for lazy and syphilitic Turks, they were going to find them in great numbers.

In addition to exposing the cultural biases of European doctors, Mazhar Osman continued to challenge the notion that neuro-syphilis could not exist in Turkey or among non-Westerners. He argued that the number of cases of G.P. was not really much lower in Turkey than in Europe. The problem, he contended, was not the absence of the G.P., but the absence of diagnoses –especially in remote parts of the empire (or, later on, the nation-state).[146] In other words, there were many cases of G.P. but not enough doctors to diagnose them all. He estimated that between 6 to 12 percent of all those entering the mental asylums in Turkey had G.P. Although he did not believe in their theory, he still played along, trying to disprove their reasoning. Finally, he took on the whole concept of 'syphilization and civilization'. He claimed that, in his experience of treating soldiers during the occupation of Istanbul, he had occasion to treat non-Europeans from an array of places, which included colonial troops fighting for France and England. During this time, he encountered something interesting: 'general paresis among the French Senegalese and Madagascan soldiers during the occupation years'.[147]

He had one last thing to tackle. In his 1928 publication he referred to some recent medical statistics from two Istanbul hospitals, which had shown that Greek (Rum) Istanbulites were slightly more likely to have G.P. than Turks. He argued that 'the difference in the percentage did not result from a larger educated class' among Greeks in Istanbul, as the European scientists might assume. Rather, what accounted for the higher rate of G.P. among the Istanbulite Greeks was 'prostitutes, pubs and nightclubs'. Mazhar Osman was firm: 'In whatever location syphilis and prostitution are found, general paresis is likely to be found in larger numbers there'.[148]

In mounting an offensive against European doctors, the likes of Mazhar Osman were not only correcting the Other's erroneous knowledge about Turkey or negotiating an acceptable place for Turkey in some imagined hierarchy of nations. By pointing out the biases of many of the European doctors, they were attacking the discourse of inherent difference upheld by European doctors. Motivated by a sense of patriotism and nationalism, they were doing nothing short of confronting the premise of an East–West dichotomy as the starting point of medical diagnoses. Their arguments in publications, intended for European eyes and ears, were nothing short of aiming to establish equality with other peoples who considered themselves more civilised. By studying or training in Europe, Ottoman and Turkish doctors had already accepted the scientific advancements of the West. However, Western science was not uncritically adopted by these doctors. As the foregoing demonstrates, they were using the tools of Western science to produce evidence intended to debunk Western, 'Orientalist' medical and scientific discourses. Consequently, one might conclude that Western science, located in the material sphere by scholar Partha Chatterjee, was not accepted without further questioning and challenge by the peoples of the colonised or semi-colonised world.

FINDING A HYGIENIC AND HEALTHY PLACE FOR THE NATION

It was clearly important to Mazhar Osman and other doctors, as citizens of the Turkish republic, to establish their nation's equality with peoples and nations who were presumed to be advanced and civilised. The propelling factor was a sense of nationalism and patriotism among the doctors. They were torn between their professional responsibilities, realistically to face the nation's health problems, and their patriotic duty to protect the nation's image. On the one hand, it was their patriotic duty to expose the dire health situation the nation faced regarding diseases ranging from mental to physical, and from intestinal to visual. On the other hand, they were determined that Turkey be respected by the world as a civilised nation equal to those in Europe. Since they were not armed with sufficient statistics or health surveys of the population of Turkey, especially from the early decades, they instead attempted to show that the diseases plaguing Turkey existed in various other places around the world, especially in advanced nations, which they imagined proved Turkey's level of civilisation

In their medical writings, trachoma and pellagra were cited as appearing both in Europe and in the less developed world. They pointed out that trachoma could be found not only in 'North Africa, Egypt, Arabia, Syria, Palestine', but also in 'Austria, Hungary, eastern Prussia, Poland, Italy, and Ireland, and even in London'.[149] If the rate of trachoma infection was not as high in London as in parts of Anatolia, the prisoners as disease carriers from British-run Egyptian camps were to blame. The story was the same for pellagra: the Turkish diet was sufficient and fresh enough to ward off the disease. However, pellagra was found in Portugal, Spain, France, Romania, Italy, Mexico, and occasionally in

England. To deliver the final blow to the belief that certain diseases were signs of backwardness, Dr Şükrü Yusuf cited the case of a country he considered more advanced than European countries: '10,663 people', he related, 'had died of pellagra in 1915 in the United States'.[150]

Nuri Ayberk, who later became the director of the 'struggle against trachoma', said 'there is no race exempt from trachoma', in a publication in which he listed fourteen countries where significant numbers of trachoma cases could be found. Leading the list was Egypt. Turkey ranked fifth in the list, certainly above countries like England and Switzerland, but also below four others, including Greece. The fight was not hopeless. The more advanced nations had overcome the disease, thus giving hope to Turkey.[151]

CONCLUSION

Without question, towards the end of the Great War, the Ottoman military found it increasingly difficult to properly feed the fighting troops in Syria, Palestine and the Hijaz. Ottoman military doctors in the field readily admitted to encountering trachoma, malaria, scurvy, dysentery and other diseases among the troops, but they denied witnessing pellagra. Even if we allow for some pellagra prior to capture, what is undeniable is that many cases of pellagra developed in the camps due to a calorie-rich but niacin-poor prison camp diet. The 'non-European' diet was simply not rich enough in niacin to keep the prisoners free from pellagra. Consequently, so many of those confirmed healthy as they entered the camps soon developed pellagra.

As to the blind prisoners of war, there is absolutely no evidence of any intentional wrongdoing, especially in terms of prisoners becoming blind after delousing with creosol. It was pure and simple: trachoma and other contagious eye diseases were the main, but not the only, causes of blindness among the prisoners. Trachoma in particular spread among the men quickly both before and after capture. A number of Ottoman-Turkish doctors – prisoners and non-prisoners – acknowledged that trachoma existed among the troops before capture. It continued to spread in the camps among the soldiers because the men did not carefully follow doctors' instructions to avoid sharing personal items such as towels and pillows. However, the prisoners also suffered from nutrition-related eye diseases, which were caused by lack of adequate vitamin A in their diet. This much was admitted by a number of British doctors in the camps. What we do not know is the severity of vitamin A deficiency and the number of prisoners involved. However, given that many thousands of Ottomans were still in British prison camps by 1920 and vitamin A deficiency lasted for so many years, it would not be unreasonable to suggest that many prisoners also suffered from nutrition-related eye problems. As the foregoing has suggested, prolonged deficiency can cause permanent damage to eyes or even blindness.

True, all this was unintentional in the sense the captors did not knowingly and purposefully withhold niacin and vitamin A from the Ottoman prisoners of war. They did not even know niacin was the cause of pellagra. But, they did know pellagra was caused by lack of proper nutrition, just as they knew that some eye diseases were nutrition-related. The camp doctors and officials intended no direct and intentional harm to the prisoners; however, their Orientalist, racialist and even racist attitudes were so ingrained, so beyond question in their minds, that when what 'Turks' said as patients or what they reported about their diets at home contradicted these mind-sets, Turks could only be lying 'non-Europeans' who knew less about themselves than the European doctors did. Therefore, a 'non-European' diet was concocted for the Ottoman prisoners of war, which lacked the variety and significantly better nutritional quality of the 'European diet'. The end result was the unintentional but still grave harm done to the prisoners of war by the thousands. Admittedly, the Second Pellagra Committee was more sensitive and attuned to the mistakes made by people on their side. Yet, they also could not divorce themselves from the similarly racialist attitudes and 'wilful ignorance' of the other men of science.

POSTSCRIPT: OLD BLIND SOLDIERS NEVER DIE

On 9 October 1998, almost exactly ninety years after the official end of the Great War, an article appeared about the 'Turkish' prisoners of World War I in *Aksiyon*, the weekend magazine of the Turkish daily *Zaman*. Just like many other magazines, newspapers, journalists and amateur 'historians' regularly do in Turkey, this article also equated Turks with Ottomans as if there were no other ethnic or religious groups among the Ottoman soldiers and prisoners of war. The provocative title, featured in full page on the front cover was, 'Turks as Test Animals: [How] the British Blinded 15,000 Turks under Scientific Pretext'.[152] The article was the result of the reporter's accidental discovery of the aforementioned discussions and the resolution passed in the Nationalist Assembly in 1921. They were in no way a 'new discovery', as such, but they allowed a seventy-plus-years-old charge to be thrust back into the public arena. As the title of the article indicated, the Nationalist Assembly of 1921 was said to have determined that the prisoners were blinded by means of submerging them in creosol solution, purposefully mixed so as to be caustic to the eyes. The charge was levelled against the 'British doctors, camp commandants and officers'. Having found the scant records, the author requested help from various government agencies, but received no further enlightenment, for no one had systematically worked on this topic. Unfortunately, that meant that the discussion in the 1921 Assembly would, by default, be accepted as fact in the sensationalised newspaper article. The fact that the resolution itself had called for further investigation into the matter was completely ignored.[153]

Although the original public excitement over the *Aksiyon* article slowly subsided, the image of the blind prisoners was too emotionally graphic to completely die. In fact, as time would show, in this brief apparent disappearance, the story metamorphosed into something to fit into a different agenda. Several academics and journalist-turned 'historian-writers' claimed to have 'new findings' pointing to the 'real culprits' behind the war crimes inflicted on 'Turkish' prisoners of long ago. The new thesis maintained that the British were complicit in allowing it to happen, but the crime of intentionally blinding the 'Turkish' prisoners was now put squarely on the shoulders of traitorous (Ottoman-)Armenian doctors or translators working in the Egyptian prison camps. Newspaper stories reported on these 'new findings', giving them credibility. The 'new findings' were turned into cleverly constructed 2–3 minute PowerPoint files emailed as attachments from one end of the world to the other. When played, the file showed images of 'Turkish' prisoners and played the Turkish national anthem, or Janissary military music. PowerPoint files turned into websites, and websites into documentary films. Books of questionable scholarly quality, written only to proffer a politically driven thesis, were celebrated.[154]

In 2004, a captivity memoir was published titled *Katran Kazanında Sterilize* or *Sterilization in a Tar Cauldron*. Two-thirds of the work is the transliteration of a diary kept by Ahmet Altınay, a former prisoner of war in Egypt. The rest consists of an extended introductory essay by two transliterators. In this essay, they briefly state that 'it is clear that some Armenian doctors especially played a role in [medical] operations that blinded the Turkish prisoners who came to them for treatment'.[155] Aside from the 1921 resolution, which called for further investigation into the alleged plot, the only evidence the authors cite for the intentional medical mistreatment by the Armenian doctors came from the aforementioned memoir of Eyüb Sabri Bey, the Ottoman civil official imprisoned in Egypt. Then, they note two pieces of information from a Red Cross report on the prisoners in Egypt. First, 20 per cent of prisoners in Heliopolis had conjunctivitis. Second, the Red Cross report listed one British and two Armenians among the medical officials in that particular camp. Therefore, while ignoring the conjunctivitis issue, they note: 'the information that the British doctor Colonel E. G. Garnen was accompanied by two on duty Armenian doctors named Arsen Khoren and Leon Samuel confirms Eyüb Sabri Bey's assertions'[156] Therefore, the mere presence of the two Armenian doctors in the camp becomes confirmation of Eyüb Sabri Bey's allegations, while the problem of conjuctivitis is dismissed.

The proponents of this theory are not even aware of it, but this line of reasoning also assumes that the Turkish prisoner doctors in the camps looked the other way while Armenian and British doctors supposedly blinded Turkish prisoners of war by the thousands. Were they part of the 'conspiracy' too? As the foregoing showed, Turkish doctors in the camps and those who cursorily inspected them when they were repatriated noted only the prevelance of trachoma and conjunctivitis. The problem with the 'British or Armenians blinded them' thesis in this particular book is that the diary offers absolutely no evidence that either the British or Armenians actually did anything to intentionally blind the prisoners – either during delousing, or afterwards with operations. In fact, it was Ahmet Altınay who claimed that after the disinfection he was completely free of lice for the first time in a long time and, as a result, slept well thereafter.[157] However, the transliterators' introduction creates the context of intentional blinding of the prisoners and allows the diary to be read within that setting – even if Ahmet Efendi found relief in his sterilisation in a tar cauldron.

In terms of influencing public perception, the journalistic myth-making has been appallingly successful in advancing the 'purposeful blinding of prisoners' narrative. Perhaps this success also required that in the victims' narrative the identity of the alleged perpetrators change from British to Armenian in order to gain more traction. Does it matter if a 'public' historical narrative does not correspond to the records and standards of professional historical research? Apparently, in some cases it matters very little. The process of historical production, one historian has argued, 'does not stop with the last sentence of a professional historian since the public is quite likely to contribute to history if only by adding its own readings to – and about – the scholarly productions'. And sometimes the narrative about an event might be constructed well before the historian reaches the scene.[158]

NOTES

1. Mazhar Osman [Uzman], 'Türkler Mütereddimi', pp. 58–61.
2. Nazım Şakir [Şakar], *Emraz-ı Asabiye Dersleri*, p. 41. What caused lethargic encephalitis is still not known for certain. Ottoman-Turkish doctors usually called it '*uyku hastalığı*' ('sleepy sickness') but knew it was different from 'sleeping sickness' transmitted by the tsetse fly. The disease attacked the brain, leaving the victim in a statue-like condition – motionless and speechless. Between 1915 and 1926, there was an epidemic of lethargic encephalitis around the world.
3. Şükrü Hazım [Tiner], 'Pellagra', p. 249.
4. Substantial historical evidence for diseases among prisoners exists only for those held by the British. Because there is only a scattering of mentions of diseases among prisoners in Russia, it is not possible to study epidemics in Russian prison camps, even though we discovered in Chapter 1 that Ottoman doctors and officers predicted that many died

because of disease and ill-treatment even before reaching the camps. While in camps, there were major outbreaks of typhus among all prisoners in Russia, which likely killed tens of thousands of people.

5. W. Burridge, 'Pellagra among the Prisoners in Egypt', p. 764.
6. J. I. Enright, 'The Pellagra Outbreak in Egypt', p. 998.
7. Anon., 'Recent Researches on Pellagra in Egypt', p. 189.
8. Eran Dolev, 'The Story of the Pellagra Outbreak', p. 228. Dolev believes that General Allenby had two other reasons for the investigations: (1) he saw an 'opportunity' in which the disease might be investigated closely; and (2) because he thought 'a future serious political attack at home was inevitable, in view of the devastation caused among the prisoners of war'. Eran Dolev, *Allenby's Military Medicine*, p. 173. Dolev unquestionably accepts the conclusions of the First Committee.
9. Anon., 'Recent Researches on Pellagra in Egypt', p. 189.
10. It should be noted that the 1918 committee reported the number of captured Ottoman soldiers as roughly over 109,000, not the 105,668 the Second Committee reported. Secondly, the Second Committee's statistics clearly came from the 'working papers' of the First when it provided the number of the hospitalised, but the First never thought this as an important thing to mention.
11. Anon., 'Recent Researches on Pellagra in Egypt', p. 189.
12. A. C. Hammond-Searle and A. G. Stevenson, *Report of Investigations on Pellagra among Turkish Prisoners of War, in Egypt, 1920*, p. 5. (Hereafter, *Report of Investigations, 1920*.)
13. *Report of Investigations, 1920*, pp. 5–6.
14. Douglas Bigland, 'The Pellagra Outbreak in Egypt', p. 947. Yet, the numbers may be less than one hundred according to the imprecise graph.
15. A. Rıza, 'Pellagra ve Vitaminler', p. 131. Unfortunately, Dr A. Rıza is not very precise with his information, but neither were the British. Dr Abdülkadir Noyan's statistics, gathered from others, might reflect the hospitalised cases only, rather than actual occurance. Noyan, 'Vitaminsizlik Hastalıkları Ordu ve Memleketimizdeki Durumu', p. 49.
16. *Report of Investigations, 1920*, p. 3.
17. Francis D. Boyd and P. S. Lelean, *Report of a Committee of Enquiry Regarding the Prevalence of Pellagra among Turkish Prisoners of War*, Chart 2. (Hereafter, *Committee of Enquiry, 1918*.)
18. Public Record Office, WO 95/ 4750, Intelligence Summary for August, 1918.
19. Almost as soon as the work of the First Committee ended about 79 German POWs were diagnosed with pellagra. See Enright, 'The Pellagra Outbreak in Egypt', pp. 998–1003. See also Anon., 'Pellagra in Egypt in 1918', p. 1,027.
20. The report gives these names as Drs Hakimian, Kalfayan and Anastassiades, but I could not find anything published by them. *Committee of Enquiry, 1918*, p. 52.
21. *Committee of Enquiry, 1918*, map and pp. 179–80.
22. The documents cited by the committee belonged to German General Friedrich Kress von Kressenstein who was serving in the Ottoman army during the Great War. *Committee of Enquiry, 1918*, pp. 60–1, 17–19.
23. Abdülkadir Noyan, *Son Harplerde*, pp. 94–107.
24. A. Rıza, 'Pellagra ve Vitaminler', pp. 129–30; Noyan, 'Vitaminsizlik Hastalıkları', p. 49.

25. A. Rıza, 'Pellagra ve Vitaminler', pp. 129–30. A. Rıza and other non-POW Ottoman doctors claimed that even though they had occasionally encountered scurvy among the Ottoman soldiers in the field, they almost never encountered pellagra even during times of food shortage. A. Rıza's observation that while the Ottoman soldiers suffered from scurvy and even beri beri during hard times, pellagra did not make an appearance is seconded by other doctors who served during the Great War. Noyan, 'Vitaminsizlik Hastalıkları', pp. 48–9; Osman Şerafeddin Çelik, 'Bir Pellagra Vak'ası', p. 17; Dr Bedreddin, 'Pollagra bir Avitaminose Hastalığımıdır?', pp. 104–5.
26. A. Rıza, 'Pellagra ve Vitaminler', pp. 129–30.
27. Ibid. pp. 129–30.
28. Bigland, 'Pellagra Outbreak in Egypt', p. 948.
29. This has been part of the argument in my 'Mısır'daki Osmanlı Esirlerinde', pp. 26–33.
30. Bigland, 'Pellagra Outbreak in Egypt', p. 948.
31. Ibid. pp. 947, 949.
32. J. I. Enright, 'War Oedema in Turkish Prisoners of War', p. 314.
33. Homi Bhabha, *Location of Culture*, p. 82.
34. *Report of Investigations, 1920*, p. 36. It is relatively clear that these average weights were not for the most seriously ill, but of those who were moderate to serious.
35. Douglas Bigland, 'Oedema as a Symptom', p. 243.
36. *Report of Investigations, 1920*, p. 36. It is relatively clear that these average weights were not for the most seriously ill, but of those who were moderate to serious.
37. Burridge, 'Pellagra among the Prisoners in Egypt', pp. 764–5.
38. 'Çok cenaze açtılar . . .' is how the former prisoner, Sergeant İbrahimoğlu Bekir of Ankara, put it in his statement to an Ottoman doctor. Said Cemil, 'Pellagra', p. 1,087.
39. Bigland, 'Oedema as a Symptom', p. 243. When pellagra rendered the patient's body weak, the patient contracted another ailment such as dysentery, pneumonia and others. In the end it was not pellagra that killed, but one of the concurrent diseases that appeared as a result of pellagra.
40. *Report of Investigations, 1920*, p. 29.
41. Ibid. pp. 27–8.
42. *Committee of Enquiry, 1918*, pp. 42–3.
43. Ibid. pp. 29–33.
44. Frantz Fanon, 'Medicine and Colonialism', p. 231. For instance, in one POW hospital (Abbasia), the death rate averaged about 12–14.5 per cent in January 1918 and August 1919. Public Record Office WO 95/4750/ Intelligence summary for January 1918 and August 1919.
45. *Committee of Enquiry, 1918*, pp. 17, 60–1.
46. If I have read the chart and explanation correctly, there was considerable difference in what the ration looked like on paper (3,390 calories) and what was actually distributed as ration (3,026 calories). While some variance could be understood, when a few mg of this or that vitamin was crucially important, a 300 calorie difference could mean significantly more.
47. See http://transition.usaid.gov/our_work/humanitarian_assistance/ffp/crg/downloads/fsbulgur.pdf and http://www.ars.usda.gov/SP2UserFiles/Place/12354500/Data/SR25/reports/sr25fg20.pdf (accessed in December 2012). NIH now recommends 16mg of niacin per day. On dates, see M. A. al-Farsi, 'Nutritional and Functional Properties of Dates', pp. 877–8.

48. A. Rıza, 'Pellagra ve Vitaminler', p. 130. Nuclein is any of the substances found in the nucleus of a cell consisting chiefly of proteins, phosphoric acid and nucleic acids.
49. Yücel Yanıkdağ, 'Mısır'daki Osmanlı Esirlerinde', pp. 26–33.
50. *Committee of Enquiry, 1918*, p. 20.
51. Said Cemil, 'Pellagra', p. 1,087.
52. Ibid. p. 1,087.
53. *Committee of Enquiry, 1918*, pp. 57–8. Sergeant İbrahimoğlu Bekir's comment about 'rice' in the bread also does not add up. However, he might have confused millet grains for rice, or it is possible in his camp there was further (or a different kind of) adulteration of the bread that the committee did not examine.
54. Bigland, 'The Pellagra Outbreak in Egypt', p. 953.
55. *Report of Investigations, 1920*, p. 48; Bigland, 'The Pellagra Outbreak in Egypt', p. 953.
56. *Report of Investigations, 1920*, p. 48.
57. Here was the source of the problem. The British medical committees still concerned themselves with calories and protein count. It was true that the ration of the POW in India was lower in calories and possibly even in protein, but they also received items in India and Burma that they did not receive in Egypt. Here's a quick look at the daily diet at Sumerpur (Rajputana). Wheat meal (atta), 453.6 grams; rice, 226.8 grams; lentils (dall), 85 grams; ghee, 28.35 grams; vegetables 226.8 grams; potatoes (instead of vegetables), 113.4 grams; onions, 56.70 grams; meat (goat), 186.18 grams. Red Cross, *Reports on British Prison-Camps in India and Burma*, p. 19.
58. *Report of Investigations, 1920*, p. 64–5.
59. Anon., 'Pellagra in Egypt in 1918', p. 1,027.
60. Prisoners probably did not feel 'hungry', as they were getting enough calories, but the food was not nutritious enough. Even if they received aid from the Ottoman state, there was no guarantee that they would have purchased additional food items to supplement their diets. We should also remember that in some cases the intestinal diseases such as dysentery among the Ottomans might have also slowed down the absorption of nutrients from the already faulty diet. Dr Woodcock, the protozoologist attached to the First Committee, noted helminthic infections in the intestines of Ottoman prisoners. These are basically parasitic worms living inside the intestines of the patients; they disrupt nutrient absorption. H. M. Woodcock, 'Helminthic Infections and Pellagra', p. 320.
61. *Report of Investigations, 1920*, p.
62. P. S. Lelean, 'Pellagra', p. 157.
63. *Committee of Enquiry, 1918*, pp. 18–19.
64. Ibid. pp. 18–19.
65. Woodcock, 'Helminthic Infections and Pellagra', p. 320.
66. Bigland, 'Pellagra Outbreak in Egypt', p. 950. One might ask a question here, which Bigland did not address: if wounds showed 'great difficulty' in healing, how would an amputation heal?
67. Said Cemil, 'Pellagra', p. 1087.
68. Nyctalopia is a condition that lies somewhere between pellagra and trachoma in the sense that it was nutrition-related like pellagra, on the one hand, and an eye problem that could lead to permanent blindness, like trachoma, on the other.
69. Burridge, 'Pellagra among the Prisoners in Egypt', pp. 764–5.
70. Alan S. Walker, *Australia in the War of 1939–1945*, p. 661.
71. Burridge, 'Pellagra among the Prisoners in Egypt', p. 765. Night-blindness is only one

of the medical problems vitamin A-deficiency might cause. Vitamin A helps form and maintains healthy teeth, skeletal and soft tissue, mucous membranes and skin.
72. John E. Dowling, 'Vitamin A Deficiency and Night Blindness', p. 648.
73. Ibid p. 657.
74. Ibid. p. 657. See also James W. Barrett, 'Trachoma and Visual Standards during the War', p. 303.
75. Although it is not listed among 'good sources' of vitamin A, meat, as such, contains an amount of vitamin A. I was not able to determine whether that applies to 'canned meat' as well.
76. Among the food items they received are cheese, oatmeal, fish and polenta, which are good sources of vitamin A. Fish oil, which the fish the European POWs were given presumably contained some of, is also a very good source of vitamin A.
77. Public Record Office, F.O. 383/535236-38.
78. PRO, F.O. 383/535236-38. For trachoma in Palestine see also Royal Commission, *Palestine Royal Commission Report, 1936* (London: HMSO, 1937), p. 310.
79. PRO, F.O. 383/535236-38.
80. So as not to be too technical for the reader and to avoid fruitless arguments about whether a doctor meant trachoma or ophthalmic, I will mostly ignore the distinction except where it is crucially important.
81. T. B. M. M., 'Otuz Yedinci İçtima, 28. 5. 1337, Cumartesi', in *Zabıt Ceridesi*, Devre 1, Volume 10, pp. 328–9; Mehmet Ali Eren, 'İngilizler 15 bin Türk'ü kör etti', pp. 26–30.
82. Eyüb Sabri, *Bir Esirin Hatıraları*, originally published in 1922, but later reprinted as *Esaret Hatıraları*, 1978.
83. Nureddin, 'Mısır Çöllerinde Türk Gençleri, 12', *Vakit* (1924). Without too much speculation, we might suggest that the burning sensation was the result of chapped and cracked skin resulting from years of fighting in dry desert conditions being irritated by the chemical solution.
84. Ahmet Altınay, *Katran Kazanında*, p. 58. I should add that this episode is mentioned not in the diary section of the book, but in a four-page section called 'Retired teacher Ahmet Altınay's [cassette]-taped remembrances about the Canal War and his captivity', inserted between the lengthy introduction and the actual diary itself.
85. H. L. Eason, 'Ophthalmic Practice', p. 99.
86. Ibid. p. 99.
87. Ibid. p. 104.
88. Ibid. pp. 101–3.
89. Sıhhat ve İçtimai Muavenet Vekaleti, *Trahom Hakkında Halka Nasayih*, p. 3.
90. I have translated *istisâl* (exterminate, uproot, excise) as removal per *Osmanlıca Tıp Terimleri Sözlüğü* and *Redhouse Sözlüğü*. In the same table, sometimes the word *ihraç* (removal, extraction, exportation) is used though presumably only to refer to the same action.
91. Presumably, the Island of Lemnos (Limni in Turkish) was used as a staging ground for prisoners captured during the war in Gallipoli; prisoners were later transferred to Egypt.
92. Sıhhat ve İçtimai Muavenet Vekaleti, *Trahom Hakkında Halka Nasayih*, p. 9. It is possible that some of these 8,392 men had pellagra as well as other medical conditions.
93. Muhtar, 'Memleketimizde Trahom', p. 160.
94. Sağlık ve Sosyal Yardım Bakanlığı, *Sağlık Hizmetlerinde 50 Yıl*, p. 130. Dr Rükneddin Fethi mentions encountering trachoma in Erzurum, Erzincan and Ağrı, among other

places. *Doğu Köylerinde*, pp. 61–2. See also the account of Arthur S. Tenner on trachoma work in Turkey and Syria at the end of the war, 'Experiences of an Eye Surgeon', pp. 203–7.
95. Muhtar, 'Memleketimizde Trahom', p. 159. The same 'three calamities' idea is also expressed in S. Şükrü, 'Trahom: Trachome', p. 1,358.
96. Meliha Özpekcan, 'Büyük Millet Meclisi Tutanaklarına Göre', p. 125. Sağlık ve Sosyal Yardım Bakanlığı, *Sağlık Hizmetlerinde 50 Yıl*, p. 130. It is possible that not all of these were exactly cases of trachoma, but other dangerous ophthalmological problems were probably thrown into the same category.
97. Sağlık ve Sosyal Yardım Bakanlığı, *Sağlık Hizmetlerinde 50 Yıl*, p. 130.
98. Fazıl Hüsnü Dağlarca, 'Dışardan Gazel', in Talât Sait Halman (trans.), *Fazıl Hüsnü Dağlarca*, p. 152.
99. At least one author objected to this terminology on the grounds that it implied the disease was found only in Egypt whereas it could also be found, in smaller numbers, in Europe as well. Sıhhat ve İçtimai Muavenet Vekalati, *Trahom Mücadele Talimatnamesi*; Niyazi İsmet, *Küçük Sıhhat Memurlarına*; Muhtar, 'Memleketimizde Trahom', p. 160.
100. Türkiye Cumhuriyeti, Sıhhat ve İçtimai Muavenet Vekaleti, *Trahom Hakkında Halka Nasayih*, p. 3.
101. Mehmed Emin, *Memleketimizde İntişar Etmekte*, pp. 2–3, 11–12.
102. Muhtar, 'Memleketimizde Trahom', p. 160.
103. Gürkan Sert, 'İkinci Milli Tıp Kongresinde', pp. 1517–19; İnci Hot, 'Ülkemizde Trahom ile Mücadele', p. 23.
104. Sert, 'İkinci Milli Tıp Kongresinde', pp. 1517–20.
105. Ibid. pp. 1517–20; Hot, 'Ülkemizde Trahom ile Mücadele', p. 23.
106. Feridun Frik, *Türkiye Cumhuriyetinde Tıb*, p. 19.
107. On this idea see R. J. Kaiser, 'Geography', pp. 315–33. A brief summary is in Umut Özkırımlı, *Contemporary Debates on Nationalism*, pp. 180–1.
108. Özkırımlı, *Contemporary Debates on Nationalism*, p. 174; Arjun Appadurai, *Modernity at Large*, p. 189.
109. Frik, *Türkiye Cumhuriyetinde Tıb*, p. 10; Sağlık ve Sosyal Yardım Bakanlığı, *Sağlık Hizmetlerinde 50 Yıl*, p. 130.
110. S. Şükrü, 'Trahom: Trachome', p. 1,357. Moving to the north, the author added that in his estimate 12.3 per cent of all eye diseases in Samsun were trachoma.
111. Sağlık ve Sosyal Yardım Bakanlığı, *Sağlık Hizmetlerinde 50 Yıl*, p. 131. Hot gives an 80 per cent rate of infection in Kilis: 'Ülkemizde Trahom ile Mücadele', p. 27.
112. Sıhhat ve İçtimai Muavenet Vekaleti, *Trahom Hakkında Halka Nasayih*, p. 5.
113. Nuri Fehmi [Ayberk], *Trahom*, p. 23. See also his 'Trahom' in Mazhar Osman [Uzman], *Sıhhat Almanakı*, pp. 760–1.
114. S. Şükrü, 'Trahom: Trachome', p. 1, 360.
115. Muhtar, 'Memleketimizde Trahom [II[', p. 382.
116. Sıhhat ve İçtimai Muavenet Vekaleti, *Trahom Hakkında Halka Nasayih*, p. 5.
117. Sıhhat ve İçtimai Muavenet Vekaleti, *Sıhhıye Mecmuası Fevkalade Nüshası*, p. 65.
118. Nuri Fehmi Ayberk, 'Türkiye Trahom Mücadelesi', pp. 127–8.
119. *Emraz-ı Sâriye ve İstilâiye Nizamnamesi* (Regulation of Contagious and Epidemic Diseases) of 1915 mentions trachoma as one of the diseases covered by the regulation. Filiz Koçak, 'Türkiye'de Sağlık Politikası'nın', pp. 155–7; Sert, 'İkinci Milli Türk Tıp Kongresinde', p. 1518.

120. Sıhhat ve İçtimai Muavenet Vekaleti, *Sıhhıye Mecmuası Fevkalade Nüshası*, p. 68.
121. Ayberk, 'Türkiye Trahom Mücadelesi Tarihçesine ait Hatıralarım', p. 134.
122. Ibid. p. 134.
123. Cumhuriyet Halk Partisi (Republican Peoples Party), *Onbeşinci Yıl Kitabı*, no page numbers, tables on trachoma. Feridun Frik adds that up to 1938, 16 million patients had been given medication; *Türkiye Cumhuriyetinde Tıb*, p. 10. This number is either exaggerated or he misstates what he means: 16 million doses of medication had been distributed to fewer patients is slightly more realistic.
124. This study is not specifically concerned with the success or failure of the struggle against trachoma.
125. Sağlık ve Sosyal Yardım Bakanlığı, *Sağlık Hizmetlerinde 50 Yıl*, p. 130; Frik, *Türkiye Cumhuriyetinde Tıb*, p. 10.
126. Dördüncü Fasıl: Trahom ile Mücadele, Umumi Hıfzısıhha Kanunu, 1593, 24 April 1930. Published in the *Resmi Gazete*, number 1489. Also available at http://www.mevzuat.adalet.gov.tr/html/487.html (accessed on 22 June 2010).
127. '*Müracaat edenleri memnuniyetle, etmeyenleri zorla tedaviye baslamıştır*'. Mazhar Osman [Uzman], 'Cumhuriyetin Sıhhat Siyaseti', p. 42.
128. Dördüncü Fasıl: Trahom ile Mücadele, Umumi Hıfzısıhha Kanunu, 1593, 24 April 1930. Published in the *Resmi Gazete*, number 1489. Also available at http://www.mevzuat.adalet.gov.tr/html/487.html (accessed on 22 June 2010).
129. Eren, 'İngilizler 15 bin Türk'ü kör etti', p. 28; T. B. M. M., 'Otuz Yedinci İçtima, 28. 5. 1337, Cumartesi', in *Zabıt Ceridesi*, Devre 1, Volume 10, pp. 328–9.
130. They were among the ranks of political, military and intellectual leadership, including Ziya Gökalp, arrested by the British in Istanbul when the capital city was invaded.
131. Mazhar Osman Uzman, 'Pellagra ve Sinir Sistemi Hastalıkları', p. 3.
132. A. Rıza, 'Pellagra ve Vitaminler', p. 130.
133. See Alan Kraut, *Goldberger's War*.
134. A. Rıza, 'Pellagra ve Vitaminler', p. 130.
135. Noyan, 'Vitaminsizlik Hastalıkları', p. 49.
136. Osman Şereffedin Çelik, 'Harp ve Sari Hastalıklar', p. 10.
137. Abdülkadir Noyan, 'Harp Salgınları=Epidemies de guerre', pp. 6–7.
138. It is also known as general paralysis of the insane.
139. Joseph Collins, 'The Etiology, Prognosis, and Treatment of General Paresis', p. 125, and 'Medical Profession and the Social Evil', p. 426. Burton Thom, 'Strain in Spirochetes', p. 11.
140. Mazhar Osman [Uzman], *Akıl Hastalıkları*, pp. 295–6 (this version mentions 'skin' only); Mazhar Osman Uzman, *Tababeti Ruhiye*, pp. 257, 261. We could add Fahrettin Kerim [Gökay] to this as well, *Ruh Hastalıkları*, p. 31; also Mazhar Osman [Uzman], *Psychiatria*, pp. 187–8.
141. Mazhar Osman [Uzman], 'Serdemi Brütüs?', p. 89.
142. Mazhar Osman Uzman, *Tababeti Ruhiye*, p. 336.
143. Mazhar Osman [Uzman], 'Serdemi Brütüs?', p. 89.
144. Ibid. p. 90.
145. Noyan, 'Harp Salgınları= Epidemies de guerre', p. 3.
146. Mazhar Osman [Uzman], *Psychiatria*, p. 188.
147. Mazhar Osman [Uzman], *Akıl Hastalıkları*, p. 296.
148. In Mazhar Osman [Uzman], *Akıl Hastalıkları*, p. 296, he says: 'prostitutes, pub and

nightclub *garçons*'. But in a later publication, this changes to: 'fahişeler, meyhane ve gazinolar'. Mazhar Osman [Uzman], *Psychiatria*, p. 187.
149. Mehmed Emin, *Memleketimizde İntişar Etmekte*, p. 6. See also Said Cemil, 'Pellagra', p. 1,085.
150. Şükrü Yusuf, 'Pellagra Hakkında', pp. 39–40; and Said Cemil, 'Pellagra', pp. 1,085–6.
151. Nuri Fehmi [Ayberk], *Trahom*, pp. 23, 25–6.
152. Eren, 'İngilizler 15 bin Türk'ü kör etti', pp. 26–30.
153. Ibid. pp. 26–30.
154. See, especially, Cezmi Yurtsever, *Gözlerim Eyvah*. See also the same person's personal website: http://cezmiyurtsever.com/index.php?option=com_content&task=view&id=199&Itemid=3 (accessed on 14 August 2010). There are hundreds of similar websites most simply copying and pasting each other.
155. Altınay, *Katran Kazanında Sterilize*, p. 17.
156. Ibid. pp. 17–18. Eyüb Sabri, *Bir Esirin Hatıraları*, originally published in 1922 but reprinted in 1978 as *Esaret Hatıraları*.
157. Altınay, *Katran Kazanında Sterilize*, p. 58.
158. Michel-Rolph Trouillot, *Silencing the Past*, pp. 25–6.

CHAPTER

5

WAR NEUROSES AND PRISONERS OF WAR: WARTIME NERVOUS BREAKDOWN AND THE POLITICS OF MEDICAL INTERPRETATION

A generation that had gone to school on a horse-drawn streetcar now stood under the open sky in a country side in which nothing remained unchanged but the clouds, and beneath those clouds, in a force-field of destructive currents and explosions, was the tiny, fragile human body.

Walter Benjamin, 'The Storyteller', p. 84

They said war is like a bath of steel, those who enter it would be steel-like. In reality, the opposite is the truth.

Dr Şükrü Hazım Tiner, *Eugenik Bahsine Umumi Bir Bakış*, p. 30

While primarily concerned with prisoners of war, this study must also examine the medical discourse concerning Ottoman soldiers who suffered nervous breakdowns at the front, or those who military-medical authorities accused of malingering. During the war, when medical professionals examined and diagnosed Ottoman soldiers who claimed to have suffered a nervous breakdown, or war neurosis, they frequently used prisoners of war as a point of comparison. Neuro-psychiatrists initially insisted that since they did not see war neurosis and related disorders among prisoners of war, that non-prisoners' claims to be suffering from war-related disorders were false. Therefore, the doctors perceived them as malingering or feigning illness. This chapter argues that the connection between prisoners and non-prisoners was already evident in the socio-medical discourse of neuro-psychiatrists both in the Ottoman Empire and Europe. However, about a decade after the end of the war, the neuro-psychiatrists retroactively diagnosed the former prisoners with some of the same mental disorders as those non-prisoners they had diagnosed during the war. At that point, whatever prior diagnostic distinction may have existed between the prisoners and non-prisoners in the way the doctors viewed their specific conditions disappeared altogether. By that point, the issues that mattered to the neuro-psychiatrists, social scientists and state officials, was how the mental and physical health of individuals impacted the nation (the subject of Chapter 6).

EUROPEAN DEBATES ON WAR NEUROSES: FROM SHELL SHOCK TO NERVOUS FRIGHT AND HYSTERIA

Medically and scientifically, the best minds in the Ottoman Empire followed the advances being made in the fields of psychiatry and the newly established field of neurology. Leading figures in European universities and hospitals such as Jean-Martin Charcot (1825–1893, Paris), Hermann Oppenheim (1858–1919, Berlin), Emil Kraepelin (1856–1926, Munich) and Joseph Babinski (1857–1932, Paris) were researching, teaching, practicing and writing about the latest developments.[1] Looking at it from the point of transfer of knowledge, the distance between Istanbul and Berlin or Munich were not as great as they might seem. A number of Ottoman and later Turkish neuro-psychiatrists had direct and indirect connections to these men. Some studied with them, others served as their assistants and interns, and still more attended their seminars and conferences on a regular basis. Ottoman men of medicine, rather than being passive importers of scientific knowledge, were an active part of this international medical community. Most of the Ottoman-Turkish neuro-psychiatrists considered herein – Mazhar Osman [Uzman], İhsan Şükrü [Aksel], Fahrettin Kerim [Gökay] and Nazım Şakir [Şakar] – trained in Germany.[2] Well-respected throughout the world, German neuropsychiatry remained influential in Turkey until the mid-1940s.[3] As intelligent professionals, Ottoman neuro-psychiatrists, while closely tied to the German school of psychiatry, also monitored international medical scholarship from England to the United States to Italy.[4]

World War I was the first event in which medical professionals examined and treated large numbers of soldiers who seemed to be suffering debilitating war-related nervous symptoms. Just a few months into the war, soldiers from all belligerent nations began to exhibit functional disorders of sight, hearing, speech and gait as well as insomnia, tremors and uncontrollable emotionality. But these symptoms were arising in soldiers who had not been necessarily physically injured in battle. In the absence of visible physical trauma, such as head and spinal injuries, some doctors surmised that the shock of the exploding shells transferred through air pressure or sound waves and caused micro lesions in the soldiers' brains, producing the symptoms displayed.[5] In fact, some early evidence involving Ottomans seemed to support this 'shell shock' theory, as it was originally termed in England.[6] After an intense naval bombardment in Gallipoli, allied soldiers captured an Ottoman trench in which they discovered a group of seven dead Ottomans, sitting together with their rifles across their knees. 'One man has his arm across the neck of his friend and a smile on his face as if the had been cracking a joke when death overwhelmed them. All now have the appearance of being merely asleep; for of the several I can only see one who shows any outward injury', recorded someone on the British side.[7] That the shock of exploding shells would violently tear soldiers' bodies apart was expected, but that they also seemed to maim men's nerves without leaving an external physical trace was simply puzzling.

The theory of invisible micro lesions in the brain was short-lived because the brains of autopsied soldiers revealed no such lesions. Other kinds of evidence also worked against the theory of 'shell shock'. For example, by mid-1915, European doctors noted that a large majority of men diagnosed with shell shock had not been in close enough proximity to exploding shells to have suffered commotional disorder or damage resulting from falling or exploding shells.[8] The absence of somatic (physical) signs and the discovery of hysterical symptoms, even among soldiers who were in rear areas, strengthened the arguments of those doctors who had believed all along that these conditions were psychogenic (originating in the psyche or emotions). For many doctors, two already well-establish diagnoses, previously used for private patients in peace time, seemed to fit the soldiers' symptoms: hysteria and neurasthenia. Hysteria presented as paralysis, catatonia, blindness, stuttering or mutism, and trembling or twitching. Neurasthenia, a form of nervous exhaustion, was characterised by exhaustion, anxiety, melancholia and sleeplessness.[9]

Neurasthenia was a mid-to-late nineteenth-century American invention, termed by neurologist Charles Beard. Seen as a 'disease of modern civilization, especially among higher classes of the most modern nations', neurasthenia was characterised by nervous exhaustion brought about by overwork. American doctors typically reserved the diagnosis of neurasthenia for upper-class people, whereas Germans stripped it of class specificity. British doctors preferred the American approach. In England, during the war, only officers suffering from war neuroses (shell shock) were diagnosed with neurasthenia, whereas the enlisted men exhibiting similar conditions were deemed to be hysterics.[10] Clearly, it was more the socio-economic background of the British neuro-psychiatrists, rather than the actual differences in symptoms, that determined the diagnosis.[11]

Until the late nineteenth century, only female patients were diagnosed with hysteria. Subsequently, the work of Charcot became influential in the 1880s. Since many of his 'hysterical' patients were not women but burly male labourers, he legitimated the diagnosis of male hysteria.[12] Yet, the belief in male hysteria was not accepted universally and it did not always lose its association with effeteness and hypochondria. Among the men Charcot diagnosed with male hysteria were victims of traumatic experiences, including railroad and factory accidents. The men displayed motor and sensory disturbances. Diagnosing them specifically with traumatic hysteria, Charcot believed that a provoking agent, a traumatic stimulus, could easily trigger these conditions in people with an inherited or constitutional disposition, or *diathèse*.[13] In terms of the causes of the disease (aetiology), he gave primacy to the pathogenic (or disease-producing) effects of emotions unleashed by trauma, in particular, fear. For him, both organic and psychological factors played a role in hysteria. Previously, hysteria was seen as a malady which did not submit to laws, but imitated other illnesses. Charcot argued that hysteria had its laws, phases and objective symptoms, while still imitating other illnesses. At the end of the century, Charcot's male hysteria diagnosis reached Germany, though a number of German doctors at the time regarded hysteria as a symptom of the shortcomings of French masculinity, and therefore unlikely to be found among German men.[14] The Great War forced the German doctors to reassess this view.

A leading German neurologist, Hermann Oppenheim, in response to Charcot's notion of traumatic hysteria, argued that patients showing the same symptoms suffered from traumatic neurosis. For Oppenheim, symptoms shared by victims of railway and factory accidents were the direct result of a physical jolt that caused microscopic alterations in the nervous system of the patient. Both diagnoses overlapped to some extent, but the difference was one of emphasis. Oppenheim stressed the primary pathogenic effect of traumatic events, rather than the wishes, fears or other mental processes associated with hysteria which Charcot emphasised. Although he did not completely reject the psychological factor, Oppenheim believed that the hysteria diagnosis placed too great an emphasis on the patient's morbid wishes, ideas and thoughts and thus blurred the distinction between real sickness and simulation (or malingering).[15]

Oppenheim's traumatic neurosis diagnosis triggered years of intense debate and controversy in German medical circles before, during and after the Great War. Originally, this debate revolved around the issue of awarding financial compensation to victims of industrial and railroad accidents in Germany. Many other German doctors rejected traumatic neurosis because, if made official, it could create an epidemic of 'pension neurosis' among the German working class. Believing that the working class would find the temptation of financial reward too great to resist, they diagnosed the same symptoms as hysterical reactions by lazy individuals seeking state disability pensions.[16]

After the war broke out, the debate over war neurosis picked up where the earlier debate over accident neurosis had left off, but now the stakes were higher.

Oppenheim continued to diagnose soldiers who broke down at or near the front with traumatic neurosis. However, his opponents, drawing on the international literature on male hysteria and motivated by patriotic feelings, viewed war neurotics in the same way as they did peacetime pension seekers – as lazy people trying to shirk their duties. Although these doctors did not deny the unique character of the Great War, they drew a distinction between the front soldiers' physical wounds and the more baffling nervous and psychological maladies that seemed to afflict both those at the front and those behind the lines in equal measure.[17]

Joseph Babinski, a disciple of Charcot, played an important role by 'dismembering' hysteria, which served to support the more militarist and patriotic assessment of the disorder now found among soldiers. In the early 1900s, Babinski proposed a much narrower definition of hysteria, calling it 'pithiatism', roughly meaning curable by persuasion. He argued that all but one of the areas covered by Charcot's definition could be explained in neurological terms as belonging to other disease categories. The remaining area encompassed only phenomena that were, or could be, provoked by suggestion. During the war, Babinski argued that the symptoms displayed by soldiers were not brought about by the trauma of war itself, but either by unintentional suggestion from doctors or by the patient's auto-suggestion and imitation. Defining suggestion as a pathological influence, he argued that hysteria was a disease with false symptoms; in this way, there was very little difference between suggested illness and simulated, or malingered, illness. Here, his theory of pithiatism became useful. He argued that the soldiers' symptoms could be removed by isolation and simple techniques of persuasion, or the *traitement brusque*. The idea that negative suggestions must be countered with positive suggestions opened the doors for a variety of therapeutic approaches. All of these approaches viewed hysteria as a curable condition; after the doctors worked their magic, the soldiers could be sent back to the front. Pressures of war and prevailing patriotism at the time brought Babinski's approach into favour first in France and later across Europe and the Ottoman Empire.[18]

In Germany, the question of the causes of war neurosis was decided by a professional debate in September 1916. Faced with an unprecedented crisis of shattered nerves among soldiers, which impacted the war effort, German neuropsychiatrists convened at a celebrated congress in Munich, where Oppenheim's traumatic neurosis theory was finally dismantled by his opponents. Leaving the 'unpatriotic' and 'uneconomical' nature of traumatic neurosis aside, Oppenheim was called to task for not being able to explain the striking absence of war neurosis among prisoners of war, who, prior to being captured, presumably experienced the same battle conditions as those afflicted with nervous disorders.

As Dr Robert Gaupp, an attendee at the same congress and one of Oppenheim's opponents, put it, a prisoner would not be served by hysteria because a hysterical condition would not guarantee a trip home from captivity. Additionally, the anti-Oppenheimian faction argued that neurotic symptoms among soldiers with serious wounds were rare. In addition, they pointed to the surprisingly high incidence of neurotic symptoms among soldiers who were behind the front lines, which supported the medical point that men's conditions did not directly result from war. Some neuro-psychiatrists at the congress debunked Oppenheim's tenet that traumatic neurosis was incurable with claims to have successfully cured a number of soldiers, using suggestive and psychic therapies. In short, the Munich congress resulted in the dethronement of traumatic neurosis as a somatic or physical disorder, and reinterpreted it as a psychogenic condition, originating in the soldiers' psyche.[19]

For many doctors, evidence that some soldiers recovered was proof that the condition was nothing more than hysteria, or even worse – malingering. In Munich, the emphasis shifted from the battlefield experience to the soldier's inner world: his 'will', 'attitude' and 'hereditary disposition'. Since the hysterical soldier was simply lacking the willpower to fight, the doctors' task was to use suggestive therapy to remove the symptoms and create willpower. But since hypnosis or the talking cure took special training (and was time consuming), many doctors preferred simpler, faster methods: isolation, extended cold baths (or showers), work therapy and finally electro-shock therapy to cure patients. The main proponent of the electrotherapeutic option was Dr Fritz Kaufmann of Mannheim, who referred to it as the 'method of violent suggestion'.[20]

Among the attendees at the Munich conference in 1916 was Dr Mazhar Osman, the leading psychiatrist in the Ottoman Empire. On his return, Mazhar Osman delivered a talk at the *Emraz-ı Akliye ve Asabiye Müsamereleri* (Mental and Nervous Diseases Meetings), which he had organised to periodically meet at the LaPaix French Hospital in Şişli, Istanbul.[21] He subsequently published, in Ottoman, a summary of the traumatic neurosis versus hysteria debate. Dr Mazhar Osman emphasised the overwhelming medical consensus reached at the Munich congress: that broken soldiers suffered from nothing more than hysteria. He found his German colleagues' evidence of very few cases of war neuroses among French prisoners of war compelling, concluding that it confirmed the somatic illegitimacy of the condition.[22]

At the same meetings (*müsamereler*) where Mazhar Osman delivered his lecture, his French-trained colleague Mustafa Hayrullah reported on both the French and German sides of the newest developments regarding war neurosis with his '*Harb-i Hazırın Emraz-ı Asabiye-i Akliyeye Öğrettikleri*' (Psychological and Neurological Lessons Learned in the Current War). Among other things, this demonstrated that the Ottoman neuro-psychiatrists were following their European colleagues' work relatively closely.[23] However, 'pension neurosis', a major issue in the German context, did not directly apply in the Ottoman case.[24] Yet, because the German doctors' interpretation of war neurosis was at least partially influenced by the pension issue, what the Ottoman neuro-psychiatrists learned from them carried that indirect influence of pension neurosis. Ottoman neuro-psychiatrists were just as influenced in their diagnostic practices by current medical and social thought, as well as by their patriotic and nationalistic sensibilities, as were military doctors.

The remainder of this chapter will look at the degree to which war neurosis existed in the Ottoman army. Then, it will tackle the question of whether it was true that no similar conditions existed among the prisoners of war. The intention here is not to attempt a retroactive diagnosis, but to examine how war-related mental disorders (hysteria and neurasthenia, hereafter referred to as 'war neuroses') were seen and interpreted by neuro-psychiatrists in the context of a masculinist war and their own concerns relating to national health.[25]

WAR NEUROSIS IN THE OTTOMAN EMPIRE

Before attending the 1916 Munich conference, Mazhar Osman had written an article entitled 'Are Turks Degenerate?' (*Türkler Mütereddimi*). But what did he mean by degenerate or degeneration? Whether using *dejenerans* or the more traditional *mütereddi*, what the neuro-psychiatrists meant was connected closely to the idea of 'racial degeneration', as initially advanced by Benedict-Augustin Morel, and enlarged upon by others.[26] This was the idea that major psychiatric illnesses were the result of the process of degeneration, or the increasing corruption of the 'germ plasm' (or, roughly, genes) from generation to generation. In explaining degeneration, Morel proposed two fundamental laws: the law of double fertilisation (or the impact of heredity) and the law of progressivity. The former stressed the risk of psychological inheritance from both parents, where each could contain 'the seeds of destruction'.[27] The latter concept, progressivity, as explained in 1860, had a profound impact on psychiatry and later on anthropology. This theory assigned blame to the passing of the 'bad seed' from one generation to another, and suggested that each new generation received a heavier and more destructive dose of that negative influence. That is to say, individuals, diseases or, as will be covered later, even nations and civilisations degenerated from bad to worse.[28] Thus, in asking and answering the question 'are Turks degenerate?', Mazhar Osman had a number of factors to consider. One of those was the question of war neurosis among the Ottoman troops, and what it indicated about national health and fitness.

Mazhar Osman directed his readers' attention to the dramatic prevalence of 'hysterical symptoms' among European troops. Similar conditions, he proclaimed, 'showed up only in incomparably small numbers among Turks ... barely approaching one percent' of the European numbers.[29] Despite certain signs of gloom about Turks' decline toward degeneration, this was, for the neuro-psychiatrists, a positive indication about the nation's mental health. Dr His, a German military doctor serving in the Ottoman Empire during the war, who was probably getting his information from the likes of Mazhar Osman, confirmed: 'The army of neurotics with shakers and people suffering from nervous heart and stomach diseases do not exist in Turkey [as it does in Germany]'. Dr His then offered the well-worn German excuse for the lack of Ottoman war neurotics: the absence of generous disability pension benefits in the Ottoman Empire that would guarantee a pension for each soldier.[30]

While not nearly as many as in Europe, there were nonetheless cases of war hysterics in the Ottoman Empire. Reportedly, Armenian-Ottoman physician Dr Yahoub Garabetyan was the first to notice a connection between exploding shells and symptoms of war neurosis which some soldiers exhibited. Noticing an artillery soldier in Gallipoli whose upper body leaned forward with arms drooped loosely by his sides and head plunged down between his shoulders, Dr Yahoub concluded in an unpublished conference paper that the soldier's *camptocormie* (*bel bükülmesi*) was caused by shells being fired and exploding around him. The awkward posture, much like that of a hunchback, was, he suggested, caused by the contracted and tightened stomach muscles. It mirrored the defensive position one might take when something is about to fall on them, except that it was now a permanent disfigurement.[31]

Several European historians have associated the prevalence of war neurosis with trench warfare, a kind of warfare not typical on the various Ottoman fronts. Eric Leed has argued that static trench warfare, rather than the above-ground war of movement more common in the Ottoman territories, was the crucial factor in the appearance of war neurosis. According to Leed, the immobility of trench warfare reduced soldiers to passivity in the face of industrialised slaughter. Such passivity in the midst of slaughter resulted in mental breakdowns.[32] If trench warfare was crucial to the appearance of symptoms, then examples of 'war neurotic' Ottoman troops should be found among those who fought in Gallipoli. Could Mazhar Osman have been correct in his estimation of the small number of war neurotics? Or was it something else? Was the Ottoman neuropsychiatric profession unable or unwilling to identify war neurotics when they indeed existed? Or was it, as Leed would have it, the nature of combat experienced by Ottoman soldiers?

Trying to answer whether war neurosis was prevalent in the Ottoman Empire

War Neuroses and Prisoners of War   179

or how many such people existed with any certainty is a difficult task, but some rough numbers can be estimated.³³ Considering the chaos created by the war, the post-war invasion and the War of Independence, even if the neuro-psychiatrists had kept careful records, they certainly do not exist now. As Chapter 1 made clear, there are too many unknowns in terms of the statistics relating to the Ottoman Great War: we do not even know with any degree of certainty how many soldiers died of wounds or disease. However, one can still attempt to extrapolate some numbers from the statistics of other belligerent countries. In Italy, 20,000 men broke down in the first three months of the war. However, the more permanently disabled were fewer in numbers. In Germany, more than 600,000 men were treated for neurological disorders during the war.³⁴ However, the permanently disabled were far fewer in numbers. For permanent cases, German and British sources give 200,000 and 80,000 respectively. Scholars have calculated that the number of war neurotics is roughly 4 per cent of all casualties. Applying this formula for purposes of getting a rough estimate, predicts the existence of 39,000 permanent and 117,000 temporary war neurotics among Ottoman combatants.³⁵ Several years after the war, a discourse emerged in Turkey among mental health professionals concerning the 'large numbers of men' failing consciously or unconsciously to perform their duties for the nation. It was only at that point that the neuro-psychiatrists openly acknowledged the larger number of war neurotics.

A problem remains. Is it accurate to attempt an estimate of Ottoman war neurotics based on European statistics if the Ottomans did not engage in prolonged trench warfare? The short answer is yes. Simply because Europeans happened mostly to be fighting in trench warfare, just when so many men started to suffer from war neurosis does not prove that this kind of warfare was the absolute crucial causative factor in the development of the disorder.³⁶ Trench warfare might have increased the number of war neurotics, but it does not mean that other forms of combat in an industrialised war did not produce war neuroses. Warfare on the Eastern Front was not characterised by trenches either, but judging from the volume of Russian medical literature on war neurosis, mental breakdown was a common problem among Russian soldiers as well.³⁷

Writing about Gallipoli, one British doctor claimed that every man leaving the battle zone was in a condition of profound neurasthenia.³⁸ Since Allied soldiers in Gallipoli were in such a state, were not Ottomans affected to a similar degree? What is the likelihood that the ordeal in the following account was only experienced by the soldiers on the Allied side?

[J]umping to what he took for solid ground, [he] found himself – as he put it with a gesture of infinite disgust – squelching thigh-deep in decomposed Turkish dead. For weeks this experience recurred to his consciousness both by night in dreams and by day in dreaded interruptions to his normal train of thought.[39]

Since Ottoman soldiers must also have had breakdowns in Gallipoli, there should be records and case studies on them. But there are none.

Should one, against all reason, assume that Ottoman troops were immune to such incidents? How could this 'immunity' possibly be explained? Could cultural differences alone have prevented mental breakdowns? What is more likely is that medical personnel did not recognise – or did not bother to treat and record – such cases. Ottoman soldiers, being mostly illiterate, left no record of their ordeals, thus adding to the incomplete impression of Ottoman 'immunity'. The kinds of experiences that pushed the Allied soldiers over the edge had to be experienced by the Ottomans in the opposing trenches. Moreover, the Ottomans – whether in Gallipoli or Palestine or Sarıkamış – faced more powerful guns and prolonged bombardments than did their enemies. The industrialised slaughter that rained on the ill-prepared and ill-equipped Ottoman troops was heavier and deadlier than anything the Ottomans could return.

As it was the case in the international medical community, even well after the war, Ottoman-Turkish neuro-psychiatrists continued to deny a direct connection between war and mental breakdown. Just as World War II began, Mazhar Osman set down his conclusions on the Great War's impact on fighting men. No doubt, he said, war affects the psyche in a number of ways. 'The psyche is always tense', because 'death is always in plain view'. A comrade who was alive 'only a few minutes ago might now be dead or missing a limb, or his head blown to pieces'. He continued, 'as if the exploding shells that churn up the earth and throw it in the air along with [severed] arms and legs were not enough, of course, a human being can become confused by the thunder-like loud noise and shock [that follows]'.[40] He was repeating in 1941 what he had also pronounced in 1928. 'Those incredible artillery sounds, a single artillery shell tearing to pieces hundreds of bodies, tense nerves in trenches, expectation of an enemy attack any moment, cold, hunger, losing those you love ... [all these] should have increased the number of cases of insanity caused by the war'. 'But', he quickly followed, 'it did not'. Moreover, he added, 'no specifically war-related insanity was encountered' in noticeable numbers among the troops, and specialists diagnosed only 'hysteria, neurasthenia, tics [twitching] ... melancholy, manias, schizophrenia'.[41] For twenty-five years, despite mounting evidence to the contrary, Mazhar Osman and many others like him in Turkey or elsewhere stubbornly held to a view that they had adopted in 1916.

Writing several months after the end of the Great War, in a piece titled the 'Psychopaths', Dr Hüseyin Kenan took a similar line, insisting: 'like the commotional issues resulting from war, what was known as war neurosis was confirmed to be nothing more than public demonstration [*tezahürat*] of hysteria and neurasthenia'.[42] Both Mazhar Osman and Hüseyin Kenan believed that intense fear could result in hysterical reactions, but these would be short in duration and easily treated. Furthermore, the symptoms had not been specifically caused by the war. Thus, they managed to divorce the experience of war from the conditions exhibited by the soldiers. While doctors – both in the Ottoman Empire and Europe – acknowledged that this was a different kind of industrialised war, their separation of the war experience from the symptoms or diseases that resulted from war served to shift the emphasis from the battlefield experience to individual 'determinants'. In short, war revealed, but did not cause, these psycho-neurological conditions.

For the doctors, the question remained: why did some men develop hysteria and related disorders, while others did not? In 'Hysteria According to Babinski', Dr Şükrü Hazım, a former student of Mazhar Osman, highlighted yet another complicating factor that undermined the legitimacy of war neurosis. Following his European colleagues, he argued that 'in this war, hysterical symptoms were never observed in the front trenches [*avcı siperleri*]'. Rather, the symptoms appeared [*tezahür*] in public view only when the person in question 'was out of the danger [zone] and was in the rear lines'.[43] He was using this evidence to suggest a few things. First, war neurosis was not caused by combat but possibly by the fear of having to return to the combat zone, which could result from a lack of willpower. Of course, this raised the possibility of the condition being nothing more than malingering.

In his same 1919 'Hysteria According to Babinski', article, Dr Şükrü Hazım acknowledged the hitherto largely hidden explanation for the alleged lack of hysteria and neurasthenia among Ottoman soldiers. He declared, 'it is true that hysteria did not seem to show a great increase in numbers among the enlisted men of our country', but, he confessed, 'the real reason for this must be found in the fact that our doctors tended to deem hysteria [and hysterical symptoms] as malingering and opted for punishment', rather than treatment, of soldiers they suspected of malingering.[44] Dr Nazım Şakir, possibly the only neuro-psychiatrist to serve in the field during the war, seconded Şükrü Hazım's point. In the Ottoman Empire, Nazım Şakir argued, 'no one took responsibility for these sick men [hysterics]. Wherever they were they were generally treated like malingerers and cowards, spent their lives in transfer stations and prisons'.[45] With these revelations, an important issue surfaced: the assumed relationship between hysterical symptoms and malingering.

A few words about malingering are in order. Although one was simulation of illness and the other an illness, medical professionals assumed a direct connection between malingering and hysteria. From the neuro-psychiatrists' perspective, malingering was always potentially present in the cases of functional neuroses like hysteria. Even Sigmund Freud, who tended not to see malingerers everywhere, said 'all neurotics are simulators, they simulate without knowing it'.[46] Many neuro-psychiatrists found the line between malingering and hysteria to be a blurry one. Following Babinski's teachings, Şükrü Hazım, for example, argued that 'hysteria is a compulsion of malingering'. What gave him this certainty was that he found 'persuasion and counter suggestion' (*ikna ve mukabil telkin*) in curing soldiers to be effective.[47] Dr Nazım Şakir, who was usually much more measured in what he said, wrote as late as 1946: 'a hysteric is a malingerer, who does not consciously simulate' illness. He meant that hysteria was unconscious malingering.[48] Mazhar Osman was more direct: hysteria 'is, in fact, malingering' [*adeta*].[49] Şükrü Hazım defined the hysteric as someone 'who wants to get everyone's attention, often a cheater, a thoughtless trickster'.[50] Two decades after the Great War, Dr Mevlut suggested that the doctor needed to be on the lookout for the hysteric's '*egocentrisme*' as a giveaway sign in distinguishing hysteria from dementia praecox among his patients.[51] These comments about hysterics' neediness and desire for public attention further undermined the legitimacy of the soldiers' condition in the eyes of the profession and other military authorities.

There is good reason to suspect that the neuro-psychiatrists actively resisted blaming the war experience for the mental disorders they encountered. Given that neuro-psychiatrists were committed to the belief that war merely served to reveal pre-existing underlying conditions, wartime hysteria or other similar conditions did not register as resulting from mental and psychic trauma experienced in combat. The case of an anonymous soldier who fought in Gallipoli illustrates that this was not an infrequent occurrence. The soldier in question, upset by ever-present death and exposed corpses, had a vision during a dream of Selman-ı Pak, one of the companions of the Prophet.[52] In this dream, Selman-ı Pak told the soldier that weapons manufacturers were prolonging the war and causing the bloodletting. The only 'manufacturers' known to the illiterate peasant soldier were a few soldiers (*tüfekçi ustası* – master gun-smith) who repaired malfunctioning guns. Guided by his vision, the soldier felt compelled to remove the obstacle to peace. 'Entering the trench' at night, 'where the master gun-smith [and his helpers slept], he slit their throats with a straight razor as though he was butchering a sacrificial [sheep]'. Covered in blood, 'he exited the [gun-smith's] trench'. Once outside, he 'lifted and flapped his arms in the air as if flying, [yelled] "master, I am coming" before he was subdued by other soldiers'.[53] Because the authorities recognised the act to have been that of a mentally ill man, the perpetrator was not executed but institutionalised until his death. However, the official diagnosis for this man was religious delirium (*Sofuluk ve din hezeyanı*).⁵⁴ According to the neuro-psychiatrist who rendered the diagnosis, the case fell in the category of ignoble (*cibiliyetsiz*) degenerates (*dejenere*), whose condition could not be identified except during a seizure since they could easily pass for 'normal'. Found mostly among 'hysterics and feeble-minded types' (*isterik ve debil*), the behaviour of this man best fit the subcategory of 'pure mysticism'.⁵⁵

Reading only religious causes into the above soldier's murderous actions completely severed its connection to the context in which the delusional act was committed. Because Mazhar Osman's religious delirium diagnosis ignores the fact that this occurred within the context of the war experience, the soldier in question simply becomes a 'religious fanatic' as opposed to someone suffering from a legitimate and serious medical condition. Would it have been diagnosed as religious delirium without the mention of Selman-ı Pak? Diagnoses like these allowed the neuro-psychiatrists to make the claim that they did not encounter mental disorders caused by or related to the war.⁵⁶

Ironically, while trained professional scientists refused to recognise or record the situational conditions that produced war neurosis, some soldiers developed their own theories from on-the-scene observation. Şevket Süreyya Aydemir, an influential political and intellectual personality during the early republic, but a junior officer during the Great War, was one of them. He explained:

> The damage first starts psychologically. When the war of movement that distracts [the soldier] comes to a halt and the gloom of the trenches starts after months of inaction, a melancholy surrounds the soul at first. This melancholy starts with the person becoming introspective. When a private, a simple soldier, becomes introspective what he finds is his own material and brutal self.⁵⁷

Şevket Süreyya's service on the eastern Anatolian front against the Russians taught him that it was not trench warfare, but the intervals of action and 'lack of action' that paved the way for mental instability.

Although he admitted that he had made some diagnostic mistakes with epilepsy early on in the war, one neuro-psychiatrist, Dr Nazım Şakir, did not dismiss hysterics or those with more serious conditions as malingerers or religious fanatics. He was significantly more attentive in keeping statistics of those cases referred to him as in need of medical assistance. While serving on the eastern Anatolian front, he diagnosed at least 412 nervous (*asabi*) cases and 58 neurological (*akliye*) cases that were referred to him from the period of the beginning of the war to 1917. Of these, he diagnosed forty-nine cases with neurasthenia, two with hysteria, one with tics, one with hysterical tremors, four with progressive insanity (*cinneti manya-i inhitati*), thirty-seven with 'mental confusion' or amentia, three with convalescent mental confusion (amentia), twelve with dementia praecox (*ateh-i şubani*), two with general paralysis and thirteen with 'nostalgie' (*da-ül vatan*) or home-sickness.[58] This is certainly a small sample in comparison to Europe, but one must remember that it only represents the cases deemed worthy enough by commanding officers and battalion doctors to be referred to the specialist in the Third Army zone of operations. Reportedly, because these general practitioners and officers were conditioned to see 'malingerers everywhere', they only referred the most extreme cases for further examination by a specialist. Nazım Şakir believed malingering was not as prevalent as others assumed.[59]

It is notable that Nazım Şakir did not fall into the German and British practice of factoring in class distinctions, reserving the hysteria diagnosis for enlisted men, while officers were diagnosed with neurasthenia.[60] Of the two cases of hysteria diagnosed by Dr Nazım Şakir above, both were officers. Similarly, of the forty-nine cases of neurasthenia he diagnosed, he did not indicate that any were officers, whereas the single case of 'tics' was an officer.[61] This indicates that he was either not aware of the class distinctions made by his European colleagues in their diagnostic practices or that he believed socio-economic or educational factors were not to be trusted in diagnosing mental conditions among Ottoman soldiers and officers.

DEMENTIA PRAECOX AND SCHIZOPHRENIA

Both the European and Ottoman (and later Turkish) neuro-psychiatrists admitted that many of these psychoneuroses, a term they came to use more frequently, resembled each other and thus increased the possibility of misdiagnosis. Many in the international medical community believed that neurasthenia was an early stage of schizophrenia and could easily resemble other psychoneuroses.[62] Mevlut Doğantuğ, for example, looked for 'egocentrism' versus 'a turn inwards', in order to distinguish between hysterics and *erken bunama* (literally, 'early senility', which equated to dementia praecox or schizophrenia). Schizophrenia, a significantly more serious disorder characterised by breakdown of thought processes and by poor emotional responsiveness, had baffled even the brightest minds of European medicine.[63] European neuro-psychiatrists battled over whether schizophrenia was a psychosis or a neurosis. In the immediate post-war period, some specialists questioned the neurosis-psychosis divide and even suggested that the difference was mostly social rather than scientific. Hence, the reconfiguring of the middle ground of psychoneurosis.[64] This reconfiguring was also reflected in the writings of the Ottoman and Turkish neuro-psychiatrists.

Many repatriated Ottoman prisoners were retroactively diagnosed with schizophrenia (*erken bunama*). Non-prisoner soldiers were also diagnosed with this condition. The case of twenty-three year old engineer (sapper) officer Zihni Efendi, presented at the Şişli meetings by Şükrü Hazım, provides a good sense of how the neuro-psychiatrist viewed the disorder and gives an insight into the condition with which the prisoners were retroactively diagnosed. Zihni Efendi had been referred to Şişli hospital from Haydarpaşa military hospital, also in Istanbul. His unit commander had noted Zihni's disregard for his duties and his depressed state; other symptoms included fatigue (*ta'ab-i azli*), headaches, lack of appetite, depression (*sa'ye karşı ademi arzu*) and 'sour breath' (*tahlili nefes*). At his initial examination at Haydarpaşa, he was diagnosed with neurasthenia and given twenty days of rest. When he returned to his unit he still showed the same symptoms and was again sent back to Haydarpaşa. Şükrü Hazım observed that Zihni Efendi's face looked blank (*bima'na*), worn-out and strained; his eyes were expressionless. His physical examination did not show anything of import, but his mental examination revealed a more worrisome picture. 'His [Zihni's] only relation to his environment', Şükrü Hazım observed, 'consisted of breathing, eating and nothing more' Zihni Efendi generally sat in the same corner 'never leaving his location'. He did not talk unless he was asked a question. Occasionally, his facial expression changed and his eyes bulged as he repeated the following: 'let us leave commander [*efendim*], it has been too long', or 'let us leave commander [*efendim*], I have stayed too long'. In any case, Şükrü Hazım observed that 'when he says "let us leave", it is visible that it is only his lips that utters those words' because he showed no desire, but seemed almost paralyzed (*arzusu mefluç*). Other than these brief panic-like interludes, Zihni Efendi spent his days in a sleep-like, catatonic state.[65]

Şükrü Hazım believed that Zihni Efendi did not have neurasthenia, as diagnosed by the specialists at Haydarpaşa, but full blown dementia praecox (*ateh-i nabehengâm*). He showed no interest in his family and his surroundings. His normal attention, personality and discernment were not there. 'If the phrase had not been used for another purpose', the doctor suggested that 'he would call people like Zihni Efendi "the living dead"'.[66] Although the phrase would be applied in the post-war period to describe former prisoners of war, Şükrü Hazım was hinting at the pages of *Harb Mecmuası* (*War Magazine*), a propaganda magazine published by the Ministry of War during the war. *Harb Mecmuası* featured pictures of the war's dead as martyrs – hence the '*yaşayan ölüler*'.[67]

Şükrü Hazım tells us nothing about Zihni Efendi's war experience. Was his dementia an underlying pre-war condition as well? How did this engineering officer get through schooling and training without his condition surfacing before the war? Even when the doctor was sympathetic to the patient, as in this case, the assumed notion that these conditions had little to do with war itself prevented

Şükrü Hazım from bringing in Zihni's recent past. We do not even know where he was fighting when his commanding officer referred him to Istanbul, but being back to the front three times indicates that he was relatively close by, possibly in Gallipoli. At the risk of speculating without enough evidence, one might suggest that Zihni Efendi possibly suffered from what was called 'buried alive neurosis'.[68] If he were in Gallipoli, being an engineering officer there would have meant digging mines to undermine and explode enemy trenches, which was common on both sides. Considering Zihni's utterances and possible duties, likelihood of buried alive neurosis is not without significant plausibility.[69] Although none of the Ottoman neuro-psychiatrists were psychoanalysts, the words of Ernst Simmel, a German Freudian neurologist, provide us with some clues as to the possible condition of Zihni Efendi: 'being buried alive as a result of an explosion with its total obliteration of conscious ego . . . [was] . . . the most frequent originator of war neurosis'. Another doctor described 'burial alive neurosis' in this way: 'He loses consciousness, and on recovery . . . finds he can neither see, hear, nor speak. He is completely isolated from the external world for he is unable to either convey or receive impressions. My colleague, M. Foucault . . . tells me that these men probably think they have died'.[70] Psychoanalysts understood certain symptoms as 'a mimetic fragment, the imitation of an action that had great emotional significance to the actor'.[71] Generally, the mimetic fragment referred to a tic the soldiers might develop, but in Zihni's case his mimetic fragment might be his last words before a significant event: that is, 'let us leave commander, I stayed too long', with his eyes bulging in fear. Could Zihni be remembering his pleas to his superior officer, before a mine explosion or collapse, as a mimetic fragment? Of course, without more evidence we do not know for sure, but such an episode remains a likely possibility.

HYSTERICAL CONDITIONS

Ottoman and later Turkish neuro-psychiatrists acknowledged that fear caused or revealed a number of disorders, including schizophrenia, but it was not the only 'uncovering' factor. Dr Fahrettin Kerim suggested that hysteria was the most 'fantastical' of all nervous ailments. It was particularly marked by 'low willpower and full suggestibility [*kabiliyet-i telkin*]'.[72] Şükrü Hazım pointed to a constant in hysterics: 'if there is something fixed in hysterics, it is [characterised by] instability'. Meaning, hysterics were unstable and fickle people who lacked perseverance.[73] Dr Mustafa Hayrullah, who had studied with Babinski, was even harsher in his observation that 'for a man to be a hysteric he had above all to have hereditary and acquired mentally degenerative foundation'.[74] Because of these factors, he and others suggested that any doctor trying 'to differentiate between malingering and hysteria' needed to be on his guard against being duped by the patient.[75]

The almost invisible dividing line between malingering and hysteria is best illustrated in a case published in 1919 by Şükrü Hazım. An Ottoman enlisted man in the Ottoman expeditionary force in Romania, who suffered from paraplegia (roughly, paralysis of both of his legs), was sent to Istanbul by the Austro-Hungarian doctors who had spent a good deal of unproductive time with the soldier. Şükrü Hazım could not find any physical problems with the man. 'Since the doctors before us had fed his inclination to sickness (*meyil-i merzasını*), we believed that his condition would not be cured with simple suggestions'. In other words, since a hysteric's personality was thought to be particularly susceptible to suggestion, doctors who were not careful and asked leading questions about symptoms could actually drive the patient to imitate that sickness. Accordingly, Şükrü Hazım decided to 'apply Kaufmann style electricity' to treat the soldier. 'That is, high intensity electrical current was applied in bursts [*fazla şiddetde cereyan-ı mutakattı*]'. As a result, after one application of the Kauffman machine, all 'signs of his two-year long paraplegia disappeared'. The patient, who had come in 'with assistance from others now walked out on his own'.[76]

Because of several fatalities during 'electro-suggestion' sessions, German doctors curtailed the use of 'Kaufmannization' towards the end of the war. While the Ottoman neuro-psychiatrists acknowledged that 'there have been some heart attacks and [other] deaths while using high voltage electricity' they continued to use the Kaufmann.[77] Kaufmannization was different from earlier forms of electrotherapy. Though conceived as a suggestive treatment, it employed a 'high-voltage form of current that could be extremely painful'. Described as a 'surprise attack' to overwhelm the patient, Fritz Kaufmann's method ignored the distinction between real nervous illness and its simulation; both were treated in the same fashion.[78] Kaufmann argued that the pain of the electricity 'displaces all negative wishful ideas' of soldiers who simply wanted to be and remain ill.[79] Accordingly, Şükrü Hazım rejected the 'simple techniques' when he discovered that the symptoms had lasted for two years in this patient from Romania. Widespread Ottoman use of these machines is unlikely because a number of neuro-psychiatrists complained they did not have access to electrotherapy machines in the provinces.[80]

The electrodes of the Kaufmann machine were placed where the soldier displayed his hysterical symptoms. In the case of the paraplegic soldier above, the electrodes were attached to the legs, but on the tongue or on the eyelids for mutism and blindness.[81] Many cases required multiple sessions of Kaufmannization. As a belated critique of such methods, Nazım Şakir wrote that besides electrotherapy, other methods tantamount to torture were employed including strict isolation, restricted diet, injection of pain-causing drugs and long cold baths. All were meant to serve as 'counter-suggestion', that is to convince the patient that it was in his interest to be cured.[82] Two decades after the Great War, Nazım Şakir denounced these methods as charlatanry.

As Şükrü Hazım and other doctors decided, sometimes the electrodes of the Kauffman machine alone were not enough. The doctor also had to bring in his personality, his authority to bear. The hysteric had to be convinced 'that his ailment would be cured' and 'of the absolute power and authority of the doctor'. Only then, he said, will 'the visible manifestations of illness invented by his [patient's] imagination ... disappear'.[83] Some doctors reportedly 'cured' soldiers of their hysterical symptoms merely through verbal suggestion by appealing to their sense of honour and duty. 'Because of a minor abrasion or falling on a limb', Mazhar Osman said, 'paralysis of that limb was encountered among some soldiers'. These were, he believed, nothing more than hysterical symptoms that were completely cured with simple counter suggestions or with the question of 'are you not ashamed?'[84] This moralist approach to curing war neurosis by appealing to the individual soldiers' sense of honour and duty was also practiced by European doctors among their men.[85]

SIMULATING ILLNESS: MALINGERING

Malingering is the purposeful simulation of illness to avoid military duty or a dangerous situation. Distinguishing between hysterical symptoms and malingering continued to be a problem for all neuro-psychiatrists, Ottoman and European alike. Because no visible cause could be identified, many legitimate nervous cases were judged to be malingering and were punished rather than treated. There are no statistics concerning the number of malingering cases. Neuropsychiatrists refer only to 'many' or 'very many cases' (*çok* and *pek çok*). Ten years after the end of the war, Mazhar Osman made a reference to the 'army of malingerers', adding, 'of the tens of thousands of malingerers we witnessed during the general war [World War I], not a single one was able to trick anyone [of us]'.[86] Dr Alfred Grotjahn, in Germany, had similarly interpreted the impact of the war on soldiers: these men all became an 'army of psychopaths'.[87]

Mazhar Osman's assessment of the extent of malingering was confirmed by other doctors. Drs Nazım Şakir, Şükrü Hazım and Mevlut Doğantuğ admitted well after the end of the war that 'many injustices were committed against the enlisted men in the first half of the war especially by general practitioners serving as battalion doctors'.[88] Later on, Mevlut Doğantuğ admitted to a bleaker picture: 'it [was] difficult to recognize the pathological character of those who were demented ... Many mistakes were made in identifying those' who were or were not malingering. 'Some of these', he continued, 'met with harsh and merciless face of the law'. Some others, he added, 'were given the death penalty in the heat of the battle, while a smaller number were' rescued by experts who understood their condition.[89] The experiences of Nazım Şakir and Doğantuğ give credence to Şükrü Hazım's admission that many cases of hysteria were taken to be malingering and punished as cowardice. In short, neither Dr His nor Mazhar Osman were correct in their early wartime view that war neurosis existed only in negligible numbers in the Ottoman Empire.

As with hysterics, malingerers were believed to mimic various diseases. The medical community believed that the process of imitation seen in hysterics was on an unconscious, neuro-mimetic level, whereas malingerers consciously imitated, or simulated, diseases. Since the thing that separated the two was intent, and since intent was often impossible to diagnose, from a medical point of view telling the difference between a malingerer and a war neurotic was more of an art than a science. Even as late as World War II, Nazım Şakir, still a practicing military doctor at that time, continued to insist that 'the most difficult thing about malingering is to be able to distinguish it from hysteria'.[90]

Nazım Şakir estimated that 90 per cent of the malingering cases he encountered during the Great War involved simulated epilepsy (sara). One cannot be sure of the basis for his estimates. Nazım Şakir suggested that there were at least two reasons for epilepsy being the malingerers' disease of choice. First, 'common people believed that it was easier to simulate' than other diseases and this 'erroneous belief was passed on from father to son'. He believed that such knowledge, or how to fool the authorities, was a long standing tradition in Anatolia. Secondly, it was well known that a medical diagnosis of epilepsy completely exempted the soldier from military service. Nazım Şakir declared epilepsy to be 'the first and sometimes the only reaction to conscription and military service for those who are "weak willed"'.[91]

The rough estimate of epilepsy constituting 90 per cent of malingering cases does not mean, of course, that Ottoman men in uniform did not resort to other forms of feigning illness to get out of military service. They actually attempted both more sophisticated and also completely crude and 'ignorant' ways of feigning illness, making themselves otherwise incapable for military service.[92] While all malingering came to factor into the concerns of the neuro-psychiatrists, this chapter is more concerned with neurosis, both real and simulated. Ironically, as it turned out, it actually did not matter whether one simulated a psychoneurosis or a physical illness to get out of military service; in the end, for the neuro-psychiatrists it all pointed to the same conclusion: the nation was in real danger of degeneration.[93]

For at least twenty years after the end of the Great War, some Ottoman and later Turkish neuro-psychiatrists maintained that the act of malingering was an illness in itself. Mazhar Osman put it tersely: 'malingering of insanity is also insanity (*deliliğin temarüzüde deliliktir*). In reality', he insisted, 'if someone is not already insane or born degenerate (*soysuz*), he would neither attempt to malinger nor be capable of it (malingering)'.[94] In his experience, intelligent and well-adjusted people did not malinger. He and others convinced themselves that the brains of those who malingered in the army were not fully developed (*yaradılış itibari ile dimağı iyi tekemmül etmemiş*). Thus, a close examination of their craniums would likely reveal degenerations (*tereddi*) in shape, and this also applied to the external ear, the roof of the mouth (palate) and finger nails.[95] They could be counted on to be 'cowardly and weak-willed' (*korkak ve iradesiz*) and therefore fully open to suggestion (*telkin*). Nonetheless, they could not grasp the simplest of military instructions leading to their being reprimanded by their officers. Constantly in fear of military punishment, these weakly types unconsciously found safety in feigning sickness, or even desertion.[96] A soldier who fell into this category was a special kind of malingerer. He was not simply a malingering coward who simulated disease to deceive others, but a degenerate who deceived himself by a mechanism that he was not aware of or one that he simply could not control.[97] These, the doctors labelled the 'low degenerates'.

The neuro-psychiatrists believed that 'intelligent' malingerers were fewer in number. While physically fit and lacking the physical degenerate stigmata, they 'lacked proper character, morals, and ethics'. These were labelled 'superior degenerates' (*dejenere superiyor*) and diagnosed with 'moral insanity' (*folie morale*), or moral degeneracy. These 'superior degenerates', it was argued, 'should be taught ethics and morality by means of suggesting proper behavior, almost like some sort of a mental therapy (*ruhi bir ortopedi*)'.[98] Besides belonging to the same diagnostic category, there was a direct connection between the 'low degenerates' and 'superior degenerates'. As George Mosse argued about Germany, 'moral sickness and physical sickness were thought to be identical, for moral sickness left its imprint on the body and face'.[99] Thus, relatively soon after the war, malingering itself came to be psychologised and therefore medicalised as a pathological condition.

Most military neuro-psychiatrists, even those who went into state civil service after the war, conceived their mission to be that of reorienting soldiers from pursuing selfish or narcissitic interests to patriotic national interests.[100] According to Mazhar Osman, while 'many young men were running to the nation's borders to fight, there were those who shamelessly tried to get out of service and deny themselves the honour of carrying weapons'.[101] Thus, he moralised the behaviour of men who were perceived to be malingering as dishonourable.

PRISONERS OF WAR

Resulting from the conclusions of the Munich congress, as early as 1916, a premise of Ottoman neuro-psychiatrists was that 'hysteria is not visible among those who became prisoners of war'. The captor, Şükrü Hazım insisted, simply would not 'put up with their [prisoners] whims or listen to their complaints. Hysteria shows itself among prisoners of war only when the subject of prisoner exchange [or repatriation] comes up because, like other diseases, hysteria is [one of the ways] how limbs [and organs] protect themselves'.[102] Prisoners would succumb to it only when it was likely to produce something positive for them. Unfortunately, Şükrü Hazım had no experience with actual prisoners of war; he based his statements on the findings of German colleagues who had diagnosed negligible numbers of war neurosis among French prisoners early in the war. Busy with the men referred from the front or those who were believed to be malingering, Ottoman psychiatrists left no indications of having taken an interest in prisoners of war during the war itself. This, of course, did not mean Ottomans in Russia, Egypt or elsewhere did not suffer from various mental conditions.

In reality, prisoners were subject to traumas of both war and captivity. One enlisted man, a prisoner in Russia, left an account of something he witnessed in a Russian boxcar in transit to a prison camp from the front. The prisoners here are the survivors of the disastrous Sarıkamış campaign. The war neurotic in the story was likely a junior officer.

> In the corner of the train wagon was a man who did not talk at all and kept quiet; he did not get involved in anything; he barely moved from where he sat; in fact, you could say he sat motionless like a statute. This behaviour bothered us and we decided he was just arrogant, but he could also be some superior officer (compared to us). He never smiled, he never talked, his eyes half-closed, he always seemed to be contemplating something ... One night, just when everyone was about to asleep, this individual ... stood up and started to yell: 'attack teams, move to forward positions; fix bayonets! Attack!' ... We all got very angry at him. He was kicked numerous times while those who kicked him continued to curse him, saying 'this is not the time for joking'. [When the kicking stopped], he was back to his old ways, there was not a sound from him. In the morning, some tried to wake him up. He was dead; his body was stiff ... After thinking about it a little, we came to an agreement that this soldier, whose name we did not even know, was still under the shock of the battle of Sarıkamış. He probably continually fought the battle in his mind as he kept to himself in silence. In that condition, he did not even eat anything [while in the train]. He must have thought he

was still in the Allahüekber Mountains. And under those conditions and feelings, he attacked the enemy one last time and became a martyr.[103]

What would the neuro-psychiatrists have made of this case? The individual described fits neither their category of prisoners showing no symptoms of war neurosis, nor of those who sought to 'get attention' and to get out of war. He died, or more correctly was killed, because his comrades failed to respond sympathetically to war neurosis symptoms until it was too late. Is it really so unlikely that some men who broke down while fighting on the front could then be taken as a prisoner by the enemy before their condition was identified by doctors on his own side? Had the anonymous soldier in the above story not been inadvertently killed by his comrades in the train, he would have carried his traumatic condition into the confines of captivity in Russia. His long-term captivity without treatment most likely would have worsened his condition.

Some men broke down in captivity from mental trauma experienced prior to capture, while others were overwhelmed by the trauma of captivity itself. The evidence for this is sparsely scattered through captivity narratives and in the passing comments made by neuro-psychiatrists after the war's end. Prisoners at times noticed sometimes small, sometimes significant mental changes in themselves and in their comrades. Those who noticed the change in themselves tell us that for lengthy periods they became depressed or quick to anger.[104] Often these manifested themselves in what Chapter 1 described as 'hatred of the near'.

Given that systematic medical records of repatriated prisoners for the Ottoman Empire and the early the Turkish republic are non-existent, the work of Swiss doctor Adolf L. Vischer becomes vital. Vischer, who visited POW camps in Russia and elsewhere, and thus reasoned from first-hand observation, discovered many cases of a psychological disorder, which he called 'Barbed Wire Disease' in reference to prisons. While not speaking specifically of the Ottoman experience, he argued that psychological conditions showed themselves in various ways and in varying degrees, from easy excitability, to an introspection and apathy. 'Barbed Wire Disease' was characterised by irritability, restlessness, memory failure, difficulty in concentrating, moodiness, general depression and nightmares.

This condition was exacerbated by the impossibility of being alone, uncertainty about the duration of captivity and absent or irregular communication from home.[105] The first condition applied to prisoners everywhere, but the second and third categories applied especially to Ottoman prisoners of war. They remained in prison camps long after the war ended. In 1920, two years after the end of the war, there were still thousands of Ottomans awaiting repatriation in Egypt, while many in Russia had to wait even longer. Seeing Europeans from the same camps repatriated years before themselves had to be disheartening. Secondly, widespread illiteracy, an inefficient mail delivery system at home and the foreign occupation of Ottoman territory resulted in Ottoman POWs receiving minimal correspondence from their families.[106] Prisoners of other nations received packages from their families, while Ottomans could not even get family news. Among the Ottoman prisoners, there was a sense of having been forgotten or ignored by the state.[107] This sense of abandonment contributed to their anxiety and mental anguish.

Depression was by far the most common form of mental disorder among Ottoman prisoners, as reflected in the captivity narratives. It is clear, however, that prisoners in Russia were more prone to depression than were their counterparts in Egypt. After inspecting the Russian camps in 1918, the Danish vice-consul in Irkutsk reported to the American Legation in Russia that, among the prisoners, there was 'an abnormally high percentage of mental disturbances ... During the four and a half years of imprisonment, the greater part of the prisoners has aged from fifteen to twenty years ... The Turkish and Hungarian peasants have suffered especially in this regard'.[108]

The more astute prisoners observed signs of depression and other more serious conditions among their fellow prisoners. Halil Ataman, in Russia, methodically kept a daily diary only to later discover that for some unknown reason he had stopped making entries and could not account for the missing time until he connected it with having also lost his senses of touch, sight and hearing. At some point he became aware that his hands, feet, eyes and ears did not perform as well as they once did. After some time in captivity, he was convinced that life had no meaning and truly wished that he were dead, for 'death was true happiness'.[109] Another prisoner in Russia, Lieutenant Ahmet, observed that in his camp 'anger and nervousness among the prisoners were like a contagious disease. Everyone was a powder keg to the point that a simple word a fellow prisoner of war might say was enough to greatly infuriate another prisoner to the point of physical response'. The author of these words, Ahmet, was justifying why he had clubbed his major with a large 'cattle bar' for jokingly refusing to return a borrowed book.[110] Suicides were rare, it seems, but there are still occasional references. Lieutenant Cemil Zeki, in an Egyptian captivity narrative, noted that 'this life of captivity affected us deeply ... A few friends went insane and committed suicide ... Poor young Turks continued to be washed out in this fashion in the desert'.[111]

There exists a detailed account of one prisoner in Russia who had a seemingly serious condition which caused him to attempt suicide. In Varnavino, after the death of a fellow prisoner from illness, an officer, known as an 'outspoken freethinker', had a change of personality and joined a group of other Ottoman prisoners who performed religious prayers and *zikr* (a religious remembrance ceremony) for long hours. Soon afterwards, his behaviour changed even more markedly. After he threw his underwear and money into the toilet, other prisoners determined to keep a close watch over him so he would not hurt himself or others. 'Sometimes he was silent as death and at other times he was exuberant and aggressive ... Sometimes he would hide in the corner of a large room, close his eyes, and shout, "I closed my eyes! You can't see me"'. When he started to attack his friends and his shouting kept everyone awake, fellow prisoners asked the camp commandant to lock him in a small room, where his friends would take turns keeping an eye on him. Each day one prisoner stood at the door keeping him company and giving him cigarettes through the hole in the door.

One day, smoke appeared through the hole. 'He had lit his thin straw bed with a cigarette and wanted to start a fire ... He tried to prevent us from extinguishing the burning bed'. He was rescued from being burned alive.

> Finally ... it was decided to send him to the Moscow asylum ... [When he was being taken away] he ... began to shout very loudly, '*Enver Paşa doloy* (To Hell with Enver Paşa)! ... Enver Paşa will fuck your mothers!' ... Then he shouted, '*Kerensky ochen khorosho chelavek* (Kerensky is a very good man)'. Then he switched to Turkish, 'I shall fuck his mother too' ... [He] shouted, 'I am a Muslim. I descended from the skies. Henceforth, you shall make the sign of the cross to me and not to Jesus'.[112]

This is an interesting case. Freethinking man turns to obsessional prayers, claims to have descended from the skies, and compares himself to Jesus. Would Mazhar Osman have diagnosed him as suffering from 'religious delirium'?

Only after the end of the Great War were Ottoman neuro-psychiatrists willing to accept that prison life could be mentally devastating. However, the reporting of such cases was delivered in almost exclusively passive language as if the neuro-psychiatrists were outside observers reporting on the events they witnessed indirectly. Yet, despite the political and social chaos in the capital city from 1918 to 1922, they should have been directly involved with at least the worst cases during the prisoners' repatriation to Istanbul.[113]

By 1928, Mazhar Osman had experienced a partial conversion. 'It has come to our attention that remaining in captivity and in prisons for a long time ... results in schizophrenia (*erken bunama*) ... A majority of our soldiers, especially our officers, who came back alive from Egypt, India, and Siberia had schizophrenia and went (returned) to their families'.[114] His former student Fahrettin Kerim wrote that 'most of our officers and men returning from captivity had schizophrenia'.[115] Mazhar Osman asserted, still in 1928, that 'victims of captivity constitute the important old-timers (*demirbaş*) at the Bakırköy mental institution'. He continued: 'hundreds of beds in the Bakırköy institution are occupied by those who became schizophrenics because of captivity'.[116] Bakırköy was the newly established mental institution in Istanbul. Previously, mental patients were sent to Toptaşı Bimarhanesi, a smaller and a much older building. Strangely, in 1923–4, five years after the Great War, the Toptaşı yearbook, or roster – likely the only one ever published – listed only thirty-nine officers (5 per cent of all patients) and only ten enlisted men among the hospitalized.[117] By 1941, Mazhar Osman was espousing the line that 'the most important nervous victims of wars are prisoners of war. Nearly half of our soldiers and officers who spent years in captivity in Egypt, India, and Siberia became schizophrenics (*erken bunama*) and spent the rest of their lives in the motherland in insane asylums'.[118]

Another possible explanation for the low numbers of war veterans in Toptaşı in 1923 and a much higher unstated number five years later, is that it is highly likely that prisoners of war with various mental conditions were initially sent home undiagnosed and untreated, except in extreme cases, hence Mazhar Osman's statement that they 'dispersed among their families'. Some years later, however, these sick individuals likely were referred back to state institutions and thus constituted the large 'old timer' group in Bakırköy.[119]

Although decades after the war Mazhar Osman and others were willing to change their views on the numbers afflicted, he remained steadfast on the question as to what caused these mental disorders. In layman's terms, he still blamed these men's biology and genetics, not their experiences. He insisted that 'some of those who were imprisoned were already schizophrenic and their deliriums were noticed [only] when imprisoned'. For Mazhar Osman, prisoners' mental ailments were no different from disorders with slightly different names encountered during peacetime: 'what is called the "barbed wire disease" or "captivity psychosis" is not any different than the pathological insanities we already know'.[120] As such, schizophrenia also became a disorder that was not caused by war or captivity, but was 'revealed' by war and captivity. In this way, it was inherited and laid dormant until something 'revealed' it, or it developed on 'weak foundations' of individuals who were 'predisposed' to mental disorders.

For at least thirty years after the war, the consensus medical interpretation on causation did not change. Referencing Ernest Kretschmer's 1921 work on schizophrenia, Mevlut Doğantuğ wrote in 1946 that schizophrenia, by then called *şizofreni* in Turkish, generally developed in people who had certain 'disposition (*anıklık*) from birth' and special psychological 'temperament' (*yaradılış*) and 'constitution' (*yapılış*). Dr Mevlut reported that Kretschmer had called this 'constitution schizoid'. He defined schizoid as the type of mental state which inclined one towards schizophrenia, although this 'was not completely inevitable'. As to prisoners of war, he concluded that 'things like captivity can ease the appearance of schizophrenia in schizoid-disposed-and-constituted types'. In short, it was not 'difficult to figure out that schizophrenics are good for nothings and dangerous during wartime'.[121]

Case studies of former POWs are much too rare in the publications of the neuro-psychiatrists. The following account was published in 1931, but it describes events that took place in 1922. Serkis Kapancıyan, an Ottoman-Armenian and a former prisoner of war in Egypt, was brought to Toptaşı by the Istanbul police to be examined by Mazhar Osman. Serkis had just killed a certain doctor Hanımyan on a city tram. Since the Ministry of Justice sent no files along with Serkis, Mazhar Osman asked the patient to tell his story in his own words. Serkis was a dealer of used shoes and a cobbler before his war service for the Ottoman army. 'At first I did not have a weapon, but at the Jerusalem [Palestine] front I was given a weapon. I served for 3 years before I was captured [by the British] and sent to Port Said'.[122] After about two years in captivity, he escaped and returned to Istanbul. After a few months' stay in Istanbul during the Allied occupation, he went to Batum in the Caucasus, and briefly fought for the Armenian side in the war there. He then returned to Istanbul and went to see the doctor at the Armenian Patriarchate. Because of his complaints of intestinal problems and 'rectal prolepses', he was referred to the Yedi Kule Armenian Hospital. There, he claimed, Dr Hanımyan operated on him to relieve his condition. But this, according to Serkis, was an operation to which he did not give his consent and one which left him crippled. 'I walked in like a lion and walked out with two crutches' after forty days. Seeing so many other doctors afterwards, from 'Americans to Turks to Armenians', every one of them told him the operation had been botched. Hopeless and in pain, he spent his last few liras on a gun to take his own life. 'Sitting in a grassy area near Yedi Kule on a nice day, I ate my yogurt and drank my milk', and when it was time, 'I put the revolver to my chest but could not go through with it'. By chance, in the tram he took when heading home, he noticed doctor Hanımyan. 'I don't know how it happened; I blacked out and took out the gun and bang, bang, I shot him. I was going to shoot myself too, but [people] grabbed my arms', Serkis explained. First in Toptaşı, and later in Bakırköy, Serkis sometimes behaved peacefully, and sometimes violently. He wounded an orderly and admitted to planning to kill one of the doctors. This 'ignorant, unbalanced, cracked-brain' (*cahil, muvazenesiz, çatlak dimağ*) man was not solely to blame for his crime and current condition, Mazhar Osman wrote. Serkis's intestinal problems should have been a clue to other doctors about his mental condition, the neuro-psychiatrist thought. If noticed earlier, he stated, an early mental intervention might have prevented the crime. Second, and more importantly, he chastised the other doctors who openly blamed Dr Hanımyan for botching the operation in front of Serkis, 'a man with mental fixations'. Other doctors' blaming of Hanımyan, he concluded, served as a 'mental suggestion' to someone who was already unstable. In other words, 'doctors had a role to play in the murder' as Serkis was one of those who 'was suggestible'. In the end, Mazhar Osman diagnosed Serkis as a 'poor degenerate, psychopath, idiot of a man'.[123] He made absolutely no connection to his captivity or war experience. Staying away from retroactive diagnosis as much as possible, one might suggest that his intestinal condition and mental issues could have also been signs of pellagra, which also existed in large numbers of Armenian refugees in Egypt.[124]

A PSYCHOPATHOLOGICAL CONDITION: THE ROAD TO DEGENERACY

Because they did not believe a direct causative connection existed between war and these men's conditions, the neuro-psychiatrists only mentioned the war as a setting to construct a chronology. For the likes of Mazhar Osman, 'military service [did] not have a negative impact on nerves of men', who were originally healthy, even as prisoners.[125] 'If we remove a young man who is already mentally defective from his hometown, then put him under a [military] discipline he won't be able to get used to, then make him go through tense, nervous, and deadly experiences in snowy and stormy weather', Mazhar Osman asked, 'and then he goes mad, should we still ask if this has to with military service?'[126] The answer was obvious; the men were already defective.

While complaining about those who 'denied themselves the honour of serving' by malingering, Mazhar Osman, strangely, told his colleagues that they had to equally suspect those who volunteered to serve. In some ways, a volunteer's motives were 'especially' dubious, according to him and some European mental specialists. In other countries, he pointed out, 'those who volunteer for military service are examined just as closely' as those who were conscripted. 'This is because the specialists around the world are in agreement that eighty percent of those volunteers are degenerates who corrupt military order and orderliness'.[127] He was, in fact, saying that both the malingerers who wanted to escape military service as well as those who volunteered were degenerates. The man who had asked 'are Turks degenerate?' in 1915 and had answered with a qualified no, was already in the process of changing his answer in the early 1920s.

In his third edition of *Tababeti Ruhiye* (1941), Mazhar Osman still argued that the majority of those who suffered from 'insanity' (*tecennün*) in World War I already had 'one or two bouts of insanity in the past'. In 'these likely types, the war became the pretext of a second [or third] attack. Accordingly, this is nothing more than the reoccurrence of an established case of insanity'. Alternatively, he said, 'if the condition is more or less awakened [*mütenebbih*] or even dormant [*mağmum*], participating in the war will increase the symptoms and turn the condition into a perfect mania or melancholia'.[128] Was the comparatively more serious diagnosis of schizophrenia without stigma in the eyes of the men of medicine? Neuro-psychiatrists, Ottoman, German and British alike, believed that this disease also had no causal relation with military service. Since it was considered an endogenous illness, it was independent of external influences.[129] The neuro-psychiatrists' words above clearly imply such a medical opinion. While 'social and political crises', especially wars, invasion and captivity, might play 'an important role' in the development of schizophrenia, it could only develop on '*musaid zemin*', or favourable ground.[130]

Both Charcot's work on male hysterics in France and the German doctors' diagnosis of thousands of their soldiers with hysteria had gone a long way to de-stigmatise hysteria's effeminate connotations, but they did not disappear completely. Hence when Mazhar Osman presented the case of a male hysteric before an audience in Şişli meetings during the war, that effeteness, which was usually avoided, resurfaced. What stood out about this patient were his effete mannerisms and his 'breasts as developed as that of a girl's in puberty'.[131]

According to other neuro-psychiatrists, namely Mevlut Doğantuğ, sexual problems of a slightly different nature could also be observed among schizophrenics. In certain schizophrenics, he claimed to have encountered loss of ethics, sense of honour and shame. 'They are misfits who show their sexual organs to (exhibitionism) others'. Of course, this led to 'onanism (masturbation) in front of people unknown to them'. They might even 'attack their sisters, [or] commit rape'.[132] Yet a few pages later, contradictions in the writing of the same military neuro-psychiatrist appear: 'from a genital point of view, in schizophrenia it is characteristic of the genital organs to become frail (*ihtiyarlamak*) and old ... Because of this one observes lack of sexual appetite among schizophrenics'.[133]

At the end of the Great War, Kraepelin questioned whether degeneration had not become a cover-all diagnosis and over applied to a wide range of conditions. Yet, even as he questioned whether some conditions could be considered as signs of degeneracy, he confirmed hysterical disorders, accident or compensation neurosis and war neurosis to be sure signs of this umbrella diagnosis. In these cases, he firmly believed that hereditary weaknesses and psychopathology played an important role, even as he cautioned neuro-psychiatrists to be selective in their diagnoses. He was firm that in the case of these conditions, external influences, such as the traumatic experiences of war or captivity, were generally overestimated.[134] But the floodgates had been opened on degeneracy as an umbrella condition, and it was not easy to turn back. Even as he cautioned others about overuse of degeneracy, Kraepelin himself declared in the post-war November revolution that Germany was now in the grip of a 'dictatorship of psychopaths', led by 'weak and degenerate personalities'.[135] During the interwar period in Turkey, former Ottoman neuro-psychiatrists, now citizens of the Turkish republic, continued to use degeneracy frequently, perhaps without remembering or heeding Kraepelin's caution. In fact, they used psychopathy and degeneracy interchangeably: 'as long as schizophrenia continues one generally calls it degeneracy (*degenerescence*) or as is the tradition with us one uses the term psychopathy (*psychopathie*)'.[136] In some ways, a re-diagnosis of a sort was taking place during these years starting as early as 1919–20. Ultimately, by including a range of mental conditions they encountered among prisoners and non-prisoners alike under the large diagnostic umbrella of degeneracy and psychopathy, the Ottoman-Turkish neuro-psychiatrists re-classified these men as degenerates and psychopaths.

QUESTIONS OF ETHNICITY

In dealing with the multi-ethnic Ottoman Empire, one has to consider the question of whether the neuro-psychiatrists distinguished between ethnic and religious groups when diagnosing diseases and pseudo-diseases. Studies on European war neuroses show that doctors frequently used ethnic differences and stereotyping as gauges of soldiers' prowess and mental and physical health. The British doctors and officers alike thought, for example, that the Irish and lowland Scots were much more likely to malinger and, therefore, were not suited for manly combat. German doctors believed that Jews and Rhinelanders were especially prone to hysterical symptoms. Populations of big cities, such as the 'degenerate Viennese mob', were sometimes presented as psychically inferior.[137] This was because mental health specialists believed that there were more degenerates in urban places than in rural areas. While ethnic prejudice helped define and diagnose illness and malingering in these two countries and perhaps in others, how did the Ottoman neuro-psychiatrists feel about ethnic groups? One does not encounter any direct evidence that the Ottoman, or later Turkish, neuro-psychiatrists developed ethnic or religious stereotypes in regards to their diagnoses; they did not make any statements regarding the likeliness of one ethnic or religious group over another in terms of war neurosis, hysteria, schizophrenia or malingering. This does not mean that Ottoman-Turkish doctors may not have been subconsciously more suspicious or dismissive of various non-Turkish ethnic groups or non-Muslims in their examination of war neurotics and presumed malingerers, but simply that no evidence supporting bias or suspicion exists in the sources left behind by the neuro-psychiatrists. However, a statement Nazım Şakir makes may be interpreted to imply otherwise in the case of non-specialist doctors or commanding officers. Briefly, he says that in countries where 'reoccurring desertions were not known to generally indicate pathological conditions', many of these 'invalids' ('dements, idiots, imbeciles, stupids') were 'unjustly' given harsh punishments. 'In opposition to this, the simulations committed by the real malingerers, meaning the cunning (*biraz açık göz*) or clever sons of Anatolia and Arabia, could not be diagnosed in every instance in spite of repeated examination committees and clinical observations'.[138] There is more than one way to interpret this statement. Those who were 'unjustly punished' may have belonged to groups other than 'sons of Anatolia and Arabia'. While this is more likely, it is also possible that those 'invalids' also included 'sons of Anatolia and Arabia' who were not as 'cunning' or 'clever' as the real malingerers from the same places. The point made by Nazım Şakir is that many legitimately ill people were misdiagnosed as malingerers early in the war, while many malingerers got away with simulating disability because they had figured out how to fool medical committees.[139]

CONCLUSION

Historians of the German war neurosis experience have argued that the war neurosis and hysteria debate in Germany during and after the war was dominated more by political agenda than by medical considerations. Wartime psychiatrists, caught up in patriotism and nationalism, were less concerned with the mental health of their soldier patients than the economic and financial welfare of the state. Since they interpreted war neurosis and its aetiology in light of their nationalistic concerns, one of the questions this chapter asked is whether their attitudes and diagnostic practices influenced or were replicated by the neuro-psychiatrists in the Ottoman Empire. The answer is yes.

Yet German psychiatric diagnostics did not develop in a nationalist vacuum and were not directly copied by the Ottoman neuro-psychiatrists. European historian Ben Shepherd has argued that in terms of psychiatric medicine, the Anglo-Saxons deferred to the expertise of the Continentals.[140] Even without their own 'pension neuroses', French and British psychiatric practices did not greatly differ from those of the Germans. The theory of degeneracy also thrived in England, where one among many men of medicine claimed that they were witnessing 'the quiet collapse of the jerry-built brains under the strain of their own weight'.[141] Some British physicians went so far as to assemble family pedigrees that purported to show that soldiers who broke down in war did so because of their tainted heredity.[142] Similarly, Ottoman and Turkish neuro-psychiatrists had just as enormous a deference to German, and to a lesser degree, French neuropsychiatry.

Much of the socio-medical thinking in the Ottoman Empire had a social Darwinist and degenerationist slant. The neuro-psychiatrists themselves were clearly concerned about the nation and motivated by serving the nation and the military. These attitudes, combined with what some neuro-psychiatrists thought was lack of motivation and selfish interest among soldiers, coloured the way neurotic soldiers, malingerers, deserters and even prisoners of war were seen. The neuro-psychiatrists viewed them as constitutionally and hereditarily weak degenerates and psychopaths, rather than as victims of war.

As elsewhere, soldiers were viewed as segments, or individual cells, of a much larger organic national body. The pathological conditions they exhibited in war or captivity were thought to damage that collective national body. This is why the neuro-psychiatrists, as members of the military, were concerned with discipline, power, health and hygiene (mental and personal) of the nation in general. Their concerns, combined with their fears about how many degenerates and psychopaths must exist in the nation's much reduced post-war population, created powerful fears of a degenerating nation and a dystopian future.

NOTES

1. While psychiatry deals with mental disorders, or diseases of the mind, and neurology with the diseases of the brain and the nervous system, they are closely related fields; this was even more the case during the earlier part of the twentieth century.
2. Mustafa Hayrullah, a neurologist, for example, was sent to Paris to study under Joseph Jules Dejerine. Further information is in M. Eraksoy, 'Mustafa Hayrullah Diker', pp. 1,505–6.
3. Günsel Koptagel-İlal, 'Son 100 Yılda Türkiye'de', p. 364; Yaman Örs, 'Regional Report: Psychiatry and Philosophy in Turkey', pp. 266–7; N. Yasemin Oğuz, 'Cumhuriyet dönemi Türk Psikiyatrisine'; Özcan Köknel, *Kötü Ruhtan Ruh Sağlığına*, pp. 266–86; F. K. Gökay, 'Raşit Tahsin Hocamız', pp. 3,069–76; Ihsan Schükry [Şükrü] and Fahreddin Kerim [Gökay], 'Die Geschichte der Psychiatrie in der Türkei', pp. 405–7. For the Fahrettin Kerim and Rober Gaupp connection, see Fahrettin Kerim Gökay, '21 Ocakta München Üniversitesinde', pp. 2,083–90.
4. Yücel Yanıkdağ, '"Ill-fated Sons" of the Nation', chapter 4
5. Jose Brunner, 'Will, Desire and Experience', pp. 297–300.
6. In German, *Granatshock*, *Granatkontusion*, or *Granatkommotion*.
7. Ben Shephard, *A War of Nerves*, p. 3.
8. Eric Leed, *No Man's Land*, pp. 170–1. By 1917 both shell shock and *nervenshock* were outlawed as diagnoses. Paul Lerner, *Hysterical Men*, p. 61; Andreas Killen, *Berlin Electropolis*, p. 137.
9. Killen, *Berlin Electropolis*, p. 130.

10. Shephard, *A War of Nerves*, pp. 9–10; Killen, *Berlin Electropolis*, p. 60.
11. Peter Barnham, *Forgotten Lunatics*, pp. 3–5, 76ff.
12. Shephard, *A War of Nerves*, p. 9; Ian Hacking, *Mad Travelers*, pp. 32–3.
13. *Diathèse*'s Ottoman equivalent was '*fesâd-ı bünye*', and the condition was defined as '*bir kısım hastalıklara musâbiyet içün bünyevi isti'dat ve kabiliyet*' or 'constitutional inclination and ability to be afflicted by certain kinds of illnesses'. Türk Dil Kurumu, *Türkçe Hekimlik Terimleri Üzerine bir Deneme*, p. 250, s.v. Diathèse.
14. Lerner, *Hysterical Men*, pp. 25–7; Mark S. Micale, 'Jean-Martin Charcot', pp. 115–27. See also, Killen, *Berlin Electropolis*, pp. 71–2.
15. Lerner, *Hysterical Men*, pp. 27, 29; Mark Micale and Paul Lerner, 'Trauma, Psychiatry and History', p. 15; Killen, *Berlin Electropolis*, p. 91.
16. Lerner, *Hysterical Men*.
17. Killen, *Berlin Electropolis*, p. 131.
18. Mark S. Micale, 'The Decline of Hysteria', pp. 4–6; Marc Roudebush, 'A Battle of Nerves', pp. 260–1; Shephard, *A War of Nerves*, pp. 98–9. See also Mazhar Osman [Uzman], 'Babinki'ye Nazaran İsterya', pp. 25–7.
19. Mazhar Osman [Uzman], 'Harb Nevrozları', pp. 3–8; Brunner, 'Will, Desire and Experience', p. 303; Shephard, *A War of Nerves*, pp. 99–103; Lerner, *Hysterical Men*, pp. 120–2; Yanıkdağ, '"Ill-Fated Sons" of the Nation', pp.163–5; Killen, *Berlin Electropolis*, pp. 134, 138–44.
20. Shephard, *A War of Nerves*, pp. 99–103. Otto Binswanger locked up his patients in isolation. Paul Lerner, 'Rationalizing the Therapeutic Arsenal', pp. 122–7; Lerner, *Hysterical Men*, pp. 120–2; Yanıkdağ, '"Ill-Fated Sons" of the Nation', pp. 163–5; Killen, *Berlin Electropolis*, pp. 134, 138–44.
21. Mazhar Osman [Uzman], 'Harb Nevrozları', p. 3. Commandeered by the Ottoman state during the war, LaPaix, temporarily renamed as Şişli Müessesi, became the temporary site of scheduled talks by Ottoman neuropsychiatric specialists in Istanbul. Although it took place during wartime, only a small number of the cases presented actually related to the war.
22. Mazhar Osman [Uzman], 'Harb Nevrozları', pp. 3–8.
23. Mustafa Hayrullah, 'Harb-i Hazırın', pp. 8–17. For an examination of German influence on the Ottoman neuro-psychiatrists, see Yücel Yanıkdağ, '"Ill-Fated Sons" of the Nation', chapter 4.
24. Killen, *Berlin Electropolis*, pp. 6–7; Lerner, *Hysterical Men*.
25. Historians of medicine would wholeheartedly agree with this decision as there is no real point in discussing what these war neurotics really had. This is in part because there is no one present-day illness from which they might have suffered. Additionally, we cannot simply translate or substitute the kinds of classifications and diagnoses which existed back then but no longer exist – such as hysteria – into 'equivalent' diseases in the new disease classification system they exists now. On this issue, see Hacking, *Mad Travellers*, lecture 2, and pp. 87–8.
26. A contemporary synopsis of Benedict Morel's *Traité des dégénérescences physiques* may be found in Anon., 'The Degeneracy of the Human Species', pp. 108–9.
27. Eric Carlson, 'Medicine and Degeneration', p. 122.
28. Ibid. p. 122.
29. Mazhar Osman [Uzman], 'Türkler Mütereddimi' p. 87.
30. Herr His, 'Medizinisches aus der Türkei', p. 1463. While the article contains no first

name, the author is very like to be Wilhelm His (1864–1934). Hasan F. Batırel and Mustafa Yüksel, 'Rudolf Nissen's Years in Bosphorus', pp. 651–4.
31. His name is mentioned as 'Dr Yahop' in Mustafa Hayrullah, *Asabiye Hastalıkları*, p. 490. 'Dr Yahop' must be Yahoub Garabetyan as also mentioned by H. Hatemi, 'Balkan Harbi Yaralıları Adlı Eser', pp. 97–9.
32. Leed, *No Man's Land*, chapter 5.
33. Although they only mention the Russian troops, some historians point to the Russo-Turkish War of 1877–8 as the first major war where numerous cases of war neurosis were detected. Catherine Merridale, 'The Collective Mind', p. 40; Anthony Babington, *Shell Shock*, p. 21. For a very brief mention of war neurosis among the Ottomans, see James J. Reid, *Crisis of the Ottoman Empire*, pp. 427–38.
34. Killen, *Berlin Electropolis*, p. 130.
35. Four per cent seems to be a generally correct rate of war neurotics in relation to total war casualties. Lerner, 'Hysterical Men', p. 8; Leed, *No Man's Land*, p. 185; Yanıkdağ, '"Ill-Fated Sons" of the Nation', p. 167. There is, of course, some change and differences in these numbers. For example, in England the actual number of war neurotics diagnosed during the war was 80,000, but after the war some 200,000 men were given pensions for war-related nervous disorders: Allan Young, 'W. H. R. Rivers and the War Neurosis', p. 359. For Italy, see Bruna Bianchi, 'Psychiatrists, Soldiers, and Officers', p. 227.
36. Clearly, the argument for trench warfare is not as neat as I present it here, but other factors – constant death, visibility and smell of rotting corpses, gas, and regression to medievalism and heavier artillery – could also be found elsewhere besides the Western Front.
37. Mabel Webster Brown and Frankwood Williams (eds), *Neuropscyhiatry and the War* and *Neuropsychiatry and the War – Supplement I (October 1918)*.
38. Leed, *No Man's Land*, p. 181.
39. Foster Kennedy, 'The Nature of Nervousness in Soldiers', p. 19.
40. Mazhar Osman Uzman, *Tababeti Ruhiye*, p. 268.
41. Mazhar Osman [Uzman], *Akıl Hastalıkları*, p. 416. A similar statement can be found in Mazhar Osman Uzman, *Tababeti Ruhiye*, p. 267.
42. Hüseyin Kenan, 'Psikopatlar', p. 387.
43. Şükrü Hazım [Tiner], 'Babinskiye nazaran isteri', p. 70.
44. Ibid. p. 71.
45. Nazım Şakir [Şakar], 'Emraz-ı Asabiye ve Akliyede Teşhis', p. 182.
46. See above discussion of hysteria and Killen, *Berlin Electropolis*, p. 103.
47. Şükrü Hazım [Tiner], 'Babinskiye Nazaran İsteri', p. 71.
48. Nazım Şakir Şakar, 'Orduda Temaruz (Simulation)', p. 159.
49. Mazhar Osman [Uzman], 'Babinki'ye Nazaran İsterya', p. 26; *adeta* may be translated as 'almost' as well. In another publication he put it this way: 'hysteria is a kind of malingering, an unconscious malingering', *Akıl Hastalıkları*, p. 380.
50. Şükrü Hazım [Tiner], 'Babinskiye Nazaran İsteri', p. 70.
51. Mevlut Doğantuğ, *Erkenbunama (Şizofreni)*, p. 32.
52. This is most likely Salman al-Farisi, or Salman the Persian, one of the companions of the Prophet.
53. Mazhar Osman [Uzman], *Akıl Hastalıkları*, p. 273.
54. Ibid. p. 273. This story is reported slightly differently in *Tababeti Ruhiye*, p. 194. Almost

30 years after the event another military psychiatrist retroactively diagnosed the likely assailant with paranoid schizophrenia. Doğantuğ, *Erkenbunama (Şizofreni)*, pp. 34–5.
55. Mazhar Osman Uzman, *Tababeti Ruhiye*, p. 194.
56. Technically they were correct in that symptoms of war neurosis were the same as those of common hysterical disorders of peacetime, see Leed, *No Man's Land*, p. 163.
57. Şevket S. Aydemir, *Suyu Arayan Adam*, p. 109.
58. Nazım Şakir [Şakar], '(330–332) Üçüncü Ordu mıntıkasında beray müşahede ve muâyene', pp. 33–4; Nazım Şakir [Şakar], '(330–332) Üçüncü Ordu mıntıkasında müşahede-i seririyası tarafından icra kılınan 58 emraz-ı akliye vakayi', p. 36.
59. Yücel Yanıkdağ, 'When Cowardice became Sickness'; Nazım Şakir Şakar, 'Orduda Temaruz (Simulation)', p. 145. Rüştü Bilge, '(Temaruz) ve (Sar'a)', p. 36.
60. The classist diagnostic distinction was more evident in England; see Killen, *Berlin Electropolis*, p. 141. See also, Barnham, *Forgotten Lunatics*, pp. 76–7.
61. Nazım Şakir [Şakar], '(330–332) Üçüncü Ordu mıntıkasında beray', pp. 33–4.
62. Mazhar Osman Uzman, *Tababeti Ruhiye*, p. 23; Mustafa Hayrullah, *Asabiye Hastalıkları*, pp. 504–12; Martin Stone, 'Shellshock and the Psychologists', pp. 249–51; Young, 'W. H. R. Rivers', p. 367.
63. Doğantuğ, *Erkenbunama (Şizofreni)*, p. 32; *Erken bunama* literally means 'early senility'. This vague term was used well into the 1940s or even later. Fahrettin Kerim gives us the following equivalents: *ateh-i muaccel = erken bunama = demans prekos = şizofreni*. Gökay, *Akli Hastalıkların Teşhisi ve Tedavisi*, p. 81. Osman Cevdet, however, equates *ateh-i muaccel* with neurasthenia. Osman Cevdet, 'Nevrasteni – ateh', pp. 572–8.
64. Barnham, *Forgotten Lunatics*, p. 155.
65. Şükrü Hazım [Tiner], 'Nevrasteni ve 'Ateh-i Nabehengam', pp. 29–30.
66. Ibid. p. 30.
67. For more on the *Harb Mecmuası*, see Erol Köroğlu, *Ottoman Propaganda*, p. 81.
68. In Europe, this neurosis was observed among men who were covered, or 'buried alive', by immense amount of earth churned up and thrown about as huge artillery shells exploded around them.
69. In his 'To the Martyrs of Çanakkale', Mehmet Akif Ersoy draws attention to this issue: '*Yerin altında cehennem gibi binlerge lağım / Her lağımın yaktığı yüzlerce adam*'. Or in English: 'Under the earth thousands of hell-like mines (tunnels) / [and] hundreds of men burned by every mine'.
70. Leed, *No Man's Land*, pp. 22–3.
71. Ibid. p. 178.
72. Fahrettin Kerim [Gökay], *Yorgun Sinirler*, pp. 12, 15. See also Hüseyin Kenan on the 'fantastical' nature of hysteria, 'Akıl Hijyeni', p. 168.
73. Şükrü Hazım [Tiner], 'Babinskiye Nazaran İsteri', p. 70.
74. Mustafa Hayrullah, *Asabiye Hastalıkları*, p. 480.
75. Nazım Şakir Şakar, 'Orduda Temaruz (Simulation)', p. 145; Doğantuğ made the same point in his *Erkenbunama (Şizofreni)*, p. 32.
76. Şükrü Hazım [Tiner], 'Babinskiye Nazaran İsteri', p. 71.
77. Perhaps because of this Mazhar Osman recommended that electrotherapy be used 'twice a day ... [it] should be intense ... [used] without anesthetics ... ' Mazhar Osman [Uzman], *Akıl Hastalıkları*, pp. 392, 394.
78. Killen, *Berlin Electropolis*, p. 138.
79. Brunner, 'Will, Desire and Experience', p. 305.

80. Nazım Şakir [Şakar], 'Emraz-ı Asabiye ve Akliyede Teşhis', pp. 181–3.
81. Mazhar Osman [Uzman], *Akıl Hastalıkları*, p. 392.
82. Yanıkdağ, '"Ill-Fated Sons" of the Nation', p. 173. See also Nazım Şakir Şakar, 'Orduda Temaruz (Simulation)', p. 147. Of course, all these methods were also employed by European doctors as well.
83. Şükrü Hazım [Tiner], 'Babinskiye Nazaran İsteri', p. 71.
84. Mazhar Osman [Uzman], *Akıl Hastalıkları*, p. 381. The same statement can also be found in Mazhar Osman [Uzman], *Psychiatria*, pp. 225–6. See also, Fahrettin Kerim [Gökay], *Ruh Hastalıkları*, p. 34.
85. Leed, *No Man's Land*, p. 169.
86. Mazhar Osman [Uzman], *Akıl Hastalıkları*, p. 417. This edition of this particular work must have been printed just as the Turkish republican government changed the alphabet from Arabic to Latin as the additional outside cover gives the publication date as 1929 in Latin characters and the author's name as Massar Osman.
87. Killen, *Berlin Electropolis*, p. 121.
88. Nazım Şakir [Şakar], 'Emraz-ı Asabiye ve Akliyede Teşhis', p. 182.
89. Doğantuğ, *Erkenbunama (Şizofreni)*, p. 40.
90. Nazım Şakir Şakar, 'Orduda Temaruz (Simulation)', p. 145.
91. Nazım Şakir [Şakar], *Temaruz ve Teşhisi*, p. 32. Rüştü Bilge, '(Temaruz) ve (Sar'a)', p. 40.
92. Yanıkdağ, 'When Cowardice Became Sickness'. For further on picric acid, see also Anon., 'Picric Acid Jaundice', pp. 92–3.
93. Yücel Yanıkdağ, 'From Cowardice to Illness', pp. 205–25.
94. Mazhar Osman [Uzman], *Akıl Hastalıkları*, p. 417.
95. Yanıkdağ, 'When Cowardice Became Sickness'; Daniel Pick, *Faces of Degeneration*, p. 209. Rüştü Bilge, '(Temaruz) ve (Sar'a)', p. 36.
96. On desertion in the Ottoman military, see chapter 5 of Mehmet Beşikçi, *The Ottoman Mobilization of Manpower in the First World War*.
97. Yanıkdağ, 'From Cowardice to Illness', pp. 205–25.
98. Ibid. pp. 205–25.
99. George Mosse, *The Image of Man*, p. 80.
100. These same sentiments can be seen in the publications of German neuro-psychiatrists as well. See, for example, Jose Brunner, 'Psychiatry, Psychoanalysis', pp. 355, 361.
101. Mazhar Osman [Uzman], *Akıl Hastalıkları*, p. 416.
102. Şükrü Hazım [Tiner], 'Babinskiye Nazaran İsteri', p. 71 *'Esir olanlarda isteri kendini göstermiyor çünki esaretde o kadar naz cekecek ve feryad dinleyecek kimse yokdur [.] Üserada isteri ancak mübadele meselesi mevzu bahis olunca meydana çıkmışdır çünki isteride diğer hastalıklar gibi uzviyetin kendisini bir mudafasıdır'*.
103. Ahmet Rıza İrfanoğlu, *Allahüekber Dagları'ndan*, pp. 63–4. Of course, uniform would have indicated rank, but frequently Ottoman men and officers put on clothing they stripped off the dead without paying attention to rank or whether the uniform was Russian or Ottoman.
104. Halil Ataman, *Esaret Yılları*, pp. 152, 165. Ahmet Göze, *Rusya'da Üç Esaret Yılı*, pp. 73–4; Mehmet Feyyaz Efendi, *Hatırat*, p. 30.
105. Adolf L. Vischer, *Barbed Wire Disease*, pp. 3, 53. See also a summary of his book A. L. Vischer, 'Some Remarks on the Psychology', pp. 696–7.
106. See Yanıkdağ, '"Ill-Fated Sons" of the Nation', chapter 4. There are numerous comments in captivity narratives and POW letters about the frustration felt by the POWs

over the absence of mail from home. It is likely that illiterate soldiers from illiterate families seldom sent letters home. They likely asked comrades to write and read letters for them. Many thousands of letters never reached the addressee. Kızılay in Ankara had hundreds of sacks of undelivered POW correspondence from World War I; despite my repeated requests I was not allowed to see the letters at the time of my research for this book. For a sample POW letter sent home, see Adnan Işık, *Malatya, 1830–1919*, pp. 774–5. For the weekly number of letters written by the Ottoman POWs between 12 March 1915 and 23 October 1915, see US Department of State 'List', enclosure in 'Turkish Prisoners of War at Meadi', 763.72114/1002, 29 October 1915.

107. Yanıkdağ, '"Ill-Fated Sons" of the Nation', chapters 2 and 4.
108. US Department of State, 'General Condition of Health among the Hungarian and Austrian Prisoners in Siberia', enclosure in 763.72114/5081, 10 October 1919, p. 1. For somewhat similar statements about the POWs in Malta and Italy (interned since the Tripolitanian War) see US Department of State, 'German, Austro-Hungarian and Ottoman Subjects Interned in Malta', enclosure in 763.72114/1803, 13 July 1916, p. 2; and US Department of State, 'Note Verbale [translation] by the Sublime Porte', in 763.72114/2687, 27 March 1917, p. 1.
109. Halil Ataman, *Esaret Yılları*, pp. 141, 152, 165.
110. Göze, *Rusya'da Üç Esaret Yılı*, p. 73.
111. Cemil Zeki [Yoldaş], *Kendi Kaleminden Teğmen Cemil Zeki*, p. 26.
112. Mehmet Arif Ölçen, *Vetluga Memoir*, pp. 103–4. For other examples of mental consequences of captivity, see Rahmi Apak, *Yetmişlik Bir Subayın Hatıraları*, p. 175; Hilmi Erbuğ, 'Kaybolan Yıllar', pp. 210, 213–14; Hayri Gökçay, *Bir Türk'ün Hâtırat ve İntikamı*, pp. 112–13; Hüsamettin Tuğaç, *Bir Neslin Dramı*, p. 121.
113. Yanıkdağ, '"Ill-Fated Sons" of the Nation', chapter 4.
114. Mazhar Osman [Uzman], *Akıl Hastalıkları*, p. 271.
115. '. . . zabitan ve askerlerimizin ekserisini bu nev cinnetle malül gördük'. Fahrettin Kerim [Gökay], *Yorgun Sinirler*, pp. 46–7.
116. Mazhar Osman [Uzman], *Akıl Hastalıkları*, p. 271. Second quote is from page 417, '*Hele bugün Bakırköy müessesinin yüzlerce yatağını esaret yüzünden erken bunayanlar dolduruyor*'.
117. Of the thirty-nine officers, twelve were identified as schizophrenic. Officers constituted the second largest group by 'trade' after farm labourers or farmers (*rençberler*). While some of these farm labourers might have been discharged enlisted men listed under peace-time occupation, we have no way of confirming it. *İstanbul Emraz-ı Akliye ve Asabiye Müessesi*, pull-out table and pp. 322–3. Türkiye Cumhuriyeti, Sıhhat ve İçtimai Muavenet Vekaleti, *Sıhhiye Mecmuası Fevkalâde Nüshası* gives 650 as the maximum number of beds in all psychiatric facilities in Turkey in 1925. Meanwhile, by comparison, at about the same time 6,000 war neurotics were still in mental hospitals in England. After the Great War nearly 100 treatment centres had been opened for such men. Joanna Bourke, 'Effeminacy, Ethnicity and the End of Trauma', p. 63; Stone, 'Shellshock and the Psychologists', p. 246
118. Mazhar Osman Uzman, *Tababeti Ruhiye*, p. 270.
119. Unfortunately, with the exception of a few references to those who committed violent crimes, we do not have much more than this on the repatriated Ottoman prisoners of war. Şevket S. Aydemir gives us the account of Hüseyin Çavuş who murdered his wife in a most gruesome fashion (*akıl almaz bir cinayet*). Aydemir was not a doctor, but the

neuro-psychiatrists would have found nothing surprising in this crime as they believed that schizophrenics could easily commit (or be talked into committing) major crimes. Şevket S. Aydemir, *Suyu Arayan Adam*, pp. 398–9. Fahrettin Kerim promises to take up the question in more detail in another publication, but he never fulfilled this promise by publishing something though he may have presented a paper at a meeting. Fahrettin Kerim [Gökay], *Yorgun Sinirler*, p. 47.

120. Mazhar Osman Uzman, *Tababeti Ruhiye*, p. 268.
121. Doğantuğ, *Erkenbunama (Şizofreni)*, pp. 6–8, 39.
122. Mazhar Osman [Uzman], 'Mecnunlar Arasında Mücrim Tipleri – 8', p. 3,776. Port Said is not really known for internment of Ottoman military prisoners of war, but the British interned, or housed, some thousands of Armenian refugees there. It is possible that Serkis was separated from the military prisoners and sent to that camp, which would explain his 'escape'. It was not easy to escape from the military prison camps.
123. Mazhar Osman [Uzman], 'Mecnunlar Arasında Mücrim Tipleri – 8', p. 3,779.
124. See note above, Serkis noted that he was imprisoned in Port Said without mentioning anything else. Port Said was where the British kept the Armenian refugees.
125. Mazhar Osman Uzman, *Tababeti Ruhiye*, p. 250.
126. Mazhar Osman [Uzman], 'Sinir Hastalıkları ve Hidmeti Askeriye', p. 845–6.
127. Ibid. p. 845.
128. Mazhar Osman Uzman, *Tababeti Ruhiye*, p. 268.
129. Killen, *Berlin Electropolis*, p. 158.
130. Fahrettin Kerim [Gökay], *Yorgun Sinirler*, pp. 46–7.
131. Mazhar Osman [Uzman], 'Babinki'ye Nazaran İsterya', pp. 25–7. Because Mazhar Osman, even as a military psychiatrist, never mentions that the patient was a soldier, there is some possibility that the man in question was a civilian.
132. Doğantuğ, *Erkenbunama (Şizofreni)*, pp. 19, 21.
133. Ibid. pp. 19, 21.
134. Killen, *Berlin Electropolis*, p. 111; Carlson, 'Medicine and Degeneration, p. 130. A contemporary synopsis of Benedict Morel's may be found in Anon., 'The Degeneracy of the Human Species', pp. 108–9.
135. Barnham, *Forgotten Lunatics*, p. 140–1.
136. İzzettin Şadan, 'Schizophrenie (Erken Bunama) – E. Bleuler', p. 192.
137. George Mosse, 'Shell-shock as a Social Disease', p. 103; Bourke, 'Effeminacy and the End of Trauma, pp. 60–1; Brunner, 'Will, Desire and Experience', p. 305.
138. Nazım Şakir [Şakar], 'Emraz-ı Asabiye ve Akliyede Teşhis', p. 182.
139. If anything else should be pointed out related to this issue it is a statement made by Mazhar Osman. Many other ethnic Turks might have agreed with what he said repeatedly. He felt that the obligation of military service unduly fell on the shoulders of ethnic Turks, because, he argued, Arabs, Kurds, Albanians and non-Muslims, along with people of Istanbul and 'the turbaned ones', meaning madrasa students, managed to stay out of military service. Mazhar Osman [Uzman], 'Türkler Mütereddimi', pp. 75–6.
140. Ben Shepherd, *A War of Nerves*, p. 97.
141. Barnham, *Forgotten Lunatics*, pp. 140, 142–3; quote from p. 140.
142. Stone, 'Shellshock and the Psychologists', p. 252.

CHAPTER

6

DEGENERATIONIST PATHWAY TO EUGENICS: NEUROPSYCHIATRY, SOCIAL PATHOLOGY AND ANXIETIES OVER NATIONAL HEALTH

We saw in the previous chapter that when in August 1915 Dr Mazhar Osman posed the question 'Are Turks degenerate?', he answered the question ambiguously but with hope for the future.[1] His answer was that Turks, like the peoples of many old nations, were 'more or less' degenerate, but that they could recover from this condition. However, this was based on the ultimately incorrect perception that war neurosis and other mental disorders did not exist among Ottoman troops and prisoners. As the previous chapter showed, by 1919 and 1920 they were ready to admit that these disorders did exist in significantly greater numbers among the troops, but the disorders were not properly diagnosed during the war. We also saw that the neuro-psychiatrists diagnosed many of the repatriated prisoners of war with schizophrenia (or dementia praecox, which evolved into schizophrenia as a diagnostic category). This belated acknowledgment and recognition of so many hysterics, neurasthenics, schizophrenics, malingerers and deserters among Ottoman troops and prisoners actually prepared the way for a much more dismaying answer to the same question of whether Turks were degenerate.

This chapter argues that given the post-Great War reinterpretation of the prevalence of war neurosis among the troops and high incidence of what was perceived to be schizophrenia among the prisoners of war, the neuro-psychiatrists were seized with the fear of a much more likely and real national degeneration starting in the early 1920s. The early twentieth century was still an age when the military's performance and health was interpreted as a reflection of the health of the nation. Reflecting this tendency, Ottoman-Turkish doctors also saw the military and the nation as a whole; thus all their concerns about the military also applied to the nation. Starting in the mid-1920s, the neuro-psychiatrists projected onto the collective body of the nation the individual signs of degeneration they identified among prisoners, war neurotics, malingerers and deserters. Suddenly, the problem seemed to be much bigger than the soldiers whose underlying degenerative conditions were 'revealed' by war or captivity. Degeneration seemed to be everywhere, threatening the whole nation. The neuro-psychiatrists feared that if unchecked, degenerates and psychopaths would procreate and multiply, thus putting the gene pool of the nation in danger. As this fear continued to grow into the later 1920s and early 1930s, the neuro-psychiatrists turned to socio-medical ideas like eugenics and social engineering that offered hope for arresting the perceived national decline and degeneration.

Some new, some reinterpreted and some age-old ideas current in the international medical community at the end of the Great War made possible the leap from individual degeneracy among the soldiers to national degeneracy. One of these was a change in diagnostic practice and terminology. While the neuro-psychiatrists diagnosed all of the men's conditions as specific mental ailments such as schizophrenia, neurasthenia or hysteria, from about 1920 on they also placed these specific conditions under two larger umbrella-like diagnostic categories: degeneracy and psychopathy. In other words, being a schizophrenic or hysteric also made one a degenerate, except the former condition was seen as proof of significantly advanced degeneracy. Although we examined it in the previous chapter, a brief reminder about what degeneracy was and what it meant to the neuro-psychiatrists will be useful here.

DEGENERATING DEGENERACY

For the contemporaries, degeneracy was tied to the ideas of Benedict-Augustin Morel, a French psychiatrist of the later nineteenth century, whose theory of degeneration provided a convincing biological explanation about how abnormal mental conditions were acquired. Like others of his day, Morel assumed that acquired characteristics could be inherited. He believed that mental disorders and generally all abnormalities of human behaviour were an expression of an abnormal constitution. Combining concepts of acquired traits becoming fixed in germ plasm (roughly, chromosomes and genes) and hereditary transmission, Morel described a progressive generational degeneration toward decay. Due to the 'law of progressivity', whatever abnormality a family showed evolved into something much more serious from one generation to the next. According to Morel's laws of degeneration, if the first generation of parents was characterised by nervous temperament, then the second generation would likely experience cerebral haemorrhages, epilepsy and the neurotic disorders of hysteria and hypochondriasis. The likely outcome for the third generation was outright insanity.

In subsequent generations, infants would be born with congenital weakness of their faculties and were likely to be sterile imbeciles, or idiots.[2] If they survived to adulthood, they were likely to develop a mysterious decline, which Morel referred to as dementia praecox, or premature dementia, the disease with which Ottoman-Turkish neuro-psychiatrists diagnosed most of the repatriated prisoners of war and some of the non-prisoners.[3] Dementia praecox, still viewed as an incurable and inexplicable madness by Emil Kraepelin, would later be equated with schizophrenia, and according to degenerationist theory, this disease represented an advanced sign of degeneracy.[4] Early versions of degenerationist theory had suggested that because degenerates would eventually become sterile, they would go extinct on their own, but this idea was abandoned at the end of the nineteenth century. Suddenly, degeneracy and degenerates became a real threat, threatening the nation as a counter evolutionary force.[5]

As the previous chapter also suggested, in the later nineteenth century the object of neuropsychiatric inquiry expanded to include populations as well as individual subjects. The more war neurotics, malingerers and schizophrenics they diagnosed among soldiers and former prisoners, the more convinced the neuro-psychiatrists became that 'mental illness', (real or perceived) could no longer be seen only in the context of the individual or the military. Two things made this shift in thinking possible. First, the neuro-psychiatrists maintained the belief through the interwar period that war had not caused mental breakdowns among soldiers and prisoners of war; rather, the experience of war merely served as a catalyst to 'reveal' dormant disorders that already existed in the bodies of these men. Therefore, the neuro-psychiatrists concluded that these disorders also existed among the members of the larger body politic, whether they had served during the war or not. Second, Ottoman-Turkish neuro-psychiatrists subscribed to the theory supported by both international medical opinion and contemporary ideologies of nationalism that an army's condition, its health and performance, reflected the nation's well-being.[6] The theory seemed to make sense; these soldiers had come from the body politic and they returned to it. Even after the war, when some of neuro-psychiatrists resigned their military positions to become civil doctors in state medical institutions, they retained their strong loyalty to and fears for the future of the nation.

How the Ottoman-Turkish neuro-psychiatrists came to this conclusion can be traced to the way the original theory of degeneration devolved into something much larger than what Morel had suggested. Later disciples of degeneration theory, such as Max Nordau, expanded the list of mental and physical illnesses and changed the timing and sequence of degenerative signs; some imbued the diagnosis with both moral and biological meanings.[7] In diagnostic usage, degeneration became an umbrella term referring to the insane, prostitutes, criminals and the poor, as well as those afflicted with a wide range of conditions, including epilepsy, sterility, sexual perversion, alcoholism and eccentricity.

Thus, as the meaning of degeneration expanded, and came to encompass not only degenerate individuals, but also families, crowds and civilisations, it attracted the attention of a range of learned men of Europe. Gustave LeBon, the French sociologist and psychologist highly popular among the Young Turks, was one such person. Another was French sociologist Émile Durkheim, who employed the medical analogy of sickness and health, and used new categories of heredity, pathology and neurasthenia to explain social problems.[8] Durkheim later came to question some assumptions about degeneration. Although he 'never emancipated himself completely from the grip of biological and medical models', he rejected certain assumptions about degeneracy. The first of these was the belief that the number of degenerates was increasing as a result of policies which inhibited their elimination and encouraged their proliferation. Second, Durkheim did not believe that degenerates threatened the future health of the nation and therefore its ability to compete with other nation-states.[9] He did believe, however, that degeneration was an objective and measurable phenomenon, one that was innate and incurable, either through individual treatment or social reform.[10]

The eminent Turkish thinker and father of Turkish nationalism Ziya Gökalp was heavily influenced by Durkheim's ideas and in turn influenced other thinkers and nationalists. Gökalp believed that 'nations have nothing to do with race, organic heredity and organic degeneration', thereby rejecting the concept of national degeneration.[11] His ideas about individual degeneration and insanity were more ambiguous. A brief passage, where he quoted the influential Victorian medical-psychiatrist Henry Maudsley (1835–1918), gives insight into his stance on the issue of individual degeneration. Maudsley had asked: 'Is there anything to help rescue a man from insanity if he has inclination to insanity?' Gökalp wrote that 'if that man possesses a high ideal, he can free himself from insanity'.[12] For Gökalp this high ideal was equivalent to his concept of *mefkure* (common ideal), which he developed in the early 1920s. He wrote:

> Generally the reason for insanity is the weakening of will power in one's psyche; it is the absence (*mahrumiyet*) of a superior force that would [otherwise] establish and maintain discipline over wishes and desires. *Mefkure* (ideal) has complete capacity and determination in maintaining control and restraint over wishes and desires. The increase in the numbers of cases of insanity during times of lack of ideals and decrease in times of ideals is proof of this reality.[13]

Paraphrasing Dr Pierre Janet (1859–1947), the pioneering French psychologist, Gökalp added that psychasthenia, by which he meant both psychasthenia and neurasthenia, was caused by a weakened psyche (or willpower) in the individual. Accordingly, Gökalp noted that

> when will power weakens, those wishes and desires that are [normally] controlled become out of control. The result is the many cases of symptoms of nervousness, hypochondria, melancholy, anxiety, fears, paranoia, etc. . . . Today, what is called neurasthenia is present both in Europe and in our country in great many numbers; it seems to have been [finally] realized that its only medicine is *mefkure* . . . In summary, if a man possesses a *mefkure*, his psyche will be steady and steadfast just as his body will be strong.[14]

Gökalp argued against neuro-psychiatrists who tended to see problems like melancholy or paranoia as organic and hereditary. Disagreements notwithstanding, he did agree with the neuro-psychiatrists on some points. Like the neuro-psychiatrists, he thought that neurasthenia existed in great numbers in Turkey. Only people who possessed *mefkure* had higher goals; only such people were unselfish, non-egotistical and non-narcissistic. The Ottoman-Turkish neuro-psychiatrists had also come to believe that selfishness and narcissism, which would have run counter to *mefkure*, were at the root of some of the distressing mental conditions they encountered.

Ottoman-Turkish neuro-psychiatrists almost fully accepted the medical or pseudo-medical theories current among European scientists; sometimes they even expanded what counted for degeneracy and predisposition to mental illness. Dr Mustafa Hayrullah argued, for example, that 'life as a struggle was the same for everyone', but those who were afflicted with hereditary and transformative (*istihalevi*) neurasthenia would find themselves 'exhausted' and 'worn out' first. These types would be the first to break down not necessarily because they were hereditary neurasthenics, but 'they may be neurasthenic because they do not have [hereditary] resistance (or endurance) and therefore neurasthenia is inevitable (*mukadder*)'.[15] For him, hereditary neurasthenics were those whose parents had 'various psychological conditions' and who themselves accordingly had disposition (*istidat*) to these diseases. Even children born of parents whose bodies had been exhausted by serious physical illnesses (*ağır bünye hastalıkları*) had this predisposition. The 'nervous makeup' of these types could not withstand even the lightest of exhaustions in this 'active life of our time'.[16]

Clearly, in the eyes of the Ottoman-Turkish men of science of the time, there were multiple sources of degeneration. Heredity, 'our one and only moral and physical capital that we bring with us to this world when we are born', seemed to be the causative factor.[17] A year after the founding of the Turkish republic in 1923, Hüseyin Kenan provided anecdotal evidence for the importance of herediterian degeneration for Turkish neuro-psychiatrists: 'We see it every day in the clinic in large numbers. For example, the son of a father with syphilis and the grandson of a syphilitic becomes afflicted with *dementia praecox*. Similarly, the son of an alcoholic and syphilitic father becomes a psychopath'.[18] In this line of thinking, the schizophrenic prisoners of war represented advanced signs of degeneration. While the neuro-psychiatrists made occasional references to exogenous – external, inorganic or even environmental – factors as playing important causative roles in schizophrenia, they nearly always assumed internal causes as the underlying reason for the disease.

DEGENERACY IN THE OTTOMAN EMPIRE

How did Mazhar Osman answer his provocative question: Were Turks degenerate? Many looked to him for the definitive answer. He said 'like all nations (*milletler*), especially old nations, Turks are more or less degenerate, [and] are likely to be'. Although he used the word *ırk* (race), he was referring to ethnicity. Mazhar Osman contended that although ethnic groups (*ırklar*) degenerate due to many factors, in some cases this corruption was not advanced and, if conditions allowed, the ethnic group could be restored to health. In other cases, this was impossible. Every *ırk*, or ethnic group, had a set of physical (material) and psychological (*ruhi*) essences. Over time, some original characteristics became perfected and more pronounced (*iyileşir*), while others faded out and disappeared. 'Sometimes this losing [of specific characteristics] allowed the ethnicity to gain in better qualities (*iyilikler*). In fact, it is as if the ethnicity is put in the position of selecting certain material and moral (*maddi ve manevi*) qualities'.[19] For Mazhar Osman, history showed that Turks, having come from Central Asia, 'lived under the influence of many factors for six hundred years and acquired many qualities while losing many others'.[20] Since one of the factors in 'preservation of ethnicity' (*muhafaza-yı ırk*) was heredity, or heritage, Ottomans could not stay 'purely' as Turks in Anatolia. Because the Seljuk Turks had mixed with 'converts and non-Muslim elements, [they] brought about a generation whose morphology was better looking and more attractive'. Turks lost some of their 'evident qualities' specific to Mongol ethnicity by selection (*istifa*), which apparently Mazhar Osman did not consider physically 'appealing' or 'attractive'.[21] Revealed in a later publication in an indirect way, Mazhar Osman implied that the Turks owed their 'physical beautification' to mixing with local Anatolian Greeks.[22] In 'morphological terms', in spite of, or as a consequence of, this 'external modification' (*harici tadilata rağmen*), the *ırk*, which came from Central Asia, 'could not maintain its original toughness (*salabet*) and vigour (*tendürüst*) for very long. Especially because of [later] ignorance and indifference those strong

Turks became weaker from year to year'.[23] Did the loss of seemingly undesirable Mongol facial features balance out the loss of toughness and vigour? Not in time of war and competition among nations.

Nonetheless, in 1915 Mazhar Osman believed that further degeneration could be halted. He argued that despite the overwhelming odds, this 'most gentlemen people of the East' were more or less able to protect their innate moral qualities (*hasail-i fıtriyesi*). Turks were able to protect, to a certain extent, their seemingly 'opposing' virtues: 'from one side contentedness and humility and from the other courage and warrior-like qualities'.[24] Because, he said, he had observed first-hand the mental condition of the people of Anatolia under tremendous stress in the bungled First Balkan War, he was hopeful for the future. After all, for him, ethnicities like the French and the Magyars, who were also well-known for their warrior-like qualities, were well ahead of Turks in terms of degeneration.[25] As such, Turks had more hope than others.

What Mazhar Osman suspected in 1915 about the 'more or less' degeneration of Turks was confirmed with real statistics in 1917. At one of the medical conferences periodically organised by Mazhar Osman at the Şişli LaPaix Hospital during the Great War, Dr Nazım Şakir delivered a paper. The lone neuro-psychiatrist responsible for a whole army of men centred in Erzurum, Nazım Şakir gave the paper while he was on leave in Istanbul. His published paper, consisting exclusively of statistics, produced evidence of the most obvious degenerates he encountered in the Third Army. His tables demonstrated that among 70,000 soldiers examined in the Erzurum Central Hospital (the American Missionary Hospital, commandeered by the Ottomans during the war), 2,000 soldiers or 2.8 per cent were diagnosed as physical and mental degenerates.[26] The tables list the physical stigmas that identified a degenerate. They ranged from misshapen skulls (855 soldiers), to ears (1,166 soldiers), to irregular hands and feet (612 soldiers) and nose and mouth (863 soldiers), and 'lack of balance in genital organs' (82 soldiers).[27] The neuro-psychiatrists believed that physical appearance and mental disease were most often found together. In this way, physical stigma, as an outward 'sign', gave the 'degenerate' away even before a psychological examination. Putting it more crudely, Mazhar Osman, using German neurologist Paul Julius Möebuis as his guide, reported that 'ugliness' was the principle external symptom of degeneration.[28] As historian Daniel Pick has described it, degeneration could be 'grasped in its visual immediacy; its truth was grounded and confined in the image: "An irregular and unsymmetrical conformation of the head, a want of regularity and harmony of the features and, as Morel holds, malformations of the external ear, are sometimes observed in [the insane]"'.[29] Soldiers with more than one physical stigma were almost always degenerates.

In allowing the physical stigma to speak as evidence of degeneration in these soldiers, Nazım Şakir observed the same signs that Morel and Maudsley had seen in their subjects. According to degenerationist thinking, there were three levels of degeneracy: low (imbecility and idiocy), where degeneration was at its worst; middle, or medium (debility); and high, who were referred to as 'superior degenerates' (*muvazenesizlik*). In the low degenerates, doctors observed high incidents of mental and physical disturbance. In the middle degenerates, mental disturbance would be minor and physical appearance close to normal. Their moral and characteriological behaviour was also considered normal or close to normal. In high degenerates, mental activity and physical appearance was normal or very close to normal. However, at this level, there was thought to be disequilibrium between mental capacity and affective and moral capability. In other words, high degenerates were generally what the neuro-psychiatrists called 'moral degenerates'.[30] Moral degenerates were sociopaths who only cared about themselves and lacked self-control; they did not or could not distinguish between right and wrong. These types, Mazhar Osman added, lived among us and could not be detected easily.[31]

Nazım Şakir's statistics also identified a subgroup (numbering 1,320) that exhibited 'deficiency in intelligence, attention, memory, [and] common ideas (*iştirak-ı efkar*)'[32] (see Table 6.1). While all degenerates had mental problems, only some had physical markers of degeneration. This tells us that the remaining 680 apparently had degenerate stigma, such as misshapen skulls or ears, but no obvious signs of mental degeneration. Although unique in his precision among other neuro-psychiatrists, the usefulness of Nazım Şakir's statistics are limited from a social and cultural perspective.[33] Issues of individual and national identity were important enough for Nazım Şakir to ask about, but we do not know what questions or criteria he used. How did he measure each soldier's awareness of his own person and nation? What marked the distinction between being religious and being a fanatic? Unfortunately, such questions cannot be answered based on the information Nazım Şakir offered. However, what Nazım Şakir's tables allow for is a glimpse into of issues of identity. For example, within this smaller sample of 1,320 degenerates, he noted that the majority were completely unaware of their national identity. Only 7 per cent could identify their 'own person, nation, and nationals', while 21 per cent were only partially aware of some markers of identity.

The idea that physical attributes were representative of mental health and personality gained momentum after the Great War. In 1921, Dr Ernst Kretschmer, an assistant of Dr Robert Gaupp, who had been influential in the wartime war neurosis debate in Germany, developed a classification system for identifying predisposition to mental illness based on body type. This came to be known as the 'constitutional approach' to degeneracy. He classified three main body

Table 6.1 Distribution of 1,320 mental degenerates

Deficiency in intelligence, attention, memory, concentration (*iştirâk-ı efkârda noksaniyet*)
(Some conditions and numbers overlap)

Condition	Number	Percentage
Literate (can read and write)	25	2
Can only read	37	3
Those who recognise his own person (*şahsını*), nation and members of his nation (*milletdaş*)	96	7
Fanatic (blindly (-*körü körüne*))	984	75
Relatively aware (*az çok*) of his own person and nation	280	21
Is aware of things around him (*hakikat-ı eşyaya vakıf*)	56	4.3

Source: Nazım Şakir, 'Erzurum Santral Sertababetine Vurud Eden', p. 35.

types: asthenic (thin, small, weak), athletic (muscular, large-boned) and pyknic (stocky, round, fat).[34] According to Kretschmer, each body type was associated with certain personality traits and psychopathologies. For example, he believed that pyknic persons were normally friendly, interpersonally dependent and gregarious, but under certain conditions they were predisposed toward manic-depressive illness. Thin or asthenic types were associated with introversion, timidity and, under extreme conditions, with schizophrenia. Kretschmer further divided personality into two constitutional groups: schizothymic (schizophrenic) and cyclothymic (bipolar mood disorder). In general, the schizoids were the hyperesthetic (sensitive) and anesthetic (cold) characters, while the cycloids were depressive (or melancholic) and hypomanic (mildly manic) characters.[35]

For Turkish neuro-psychiatrists like Fahrettin Kerim, Kretschmer's typology, wedded to degeneration theory, further confirmed the connection between the body and mental disorders. The typology would allow the doctors to identify those who would easily break down under strain of war or even under pressure of daily life, and thus become a liability to the nation. Thanks to the typology, Fahrettin Kerim said, one could tell from appearance the character of patients without ever interviewing them. He confidently predicted, based on body type, what regions of Turkey would be more likely to produce specific types of mental disorders. For example, Turkish citizens living in the Black Sea area generally belonged to the cyclothymic type, thus being prone to bipolar disorders. Those in the Aegean were schizothymic, or prone to schizophrenia. The most common body type in Turkey was asthenic or thin, which was characterised by introversion, timidity and, under extreme conditions, schizophrenia.[36]

The neuro-psychiatrists were well within the mainstream of medical thinking in believing that science explained the connection between an individual's appearance and deviancy. They could now diagnose more easily than ever before what type of people would be likely to break down in wartime, or cause social and political trouble in peacetime.[37] If Kraepelin's wartime observation that war neurosis 'above all afflicted less stable, emotionally excitable, nervous and infirm personalities', then this typology now could indicate who was an emotionally well-anchored male, and who was not.[38] This construction of deviance as rooted in the body was also a process in which some imaginary model of the 'normal' body was created. Similarly, much like the 'normal' body required an 'abnormal' or deviant body, the sane minded, strong-willed and morally well-anchored types needed their Other. Yet, despite the considerable degree of overlap between body type and mental disorders, the method of identification was not completely fool proof. The judgment and expertise of the neuro-psychiatrist was required to make the crucial determination.[39] This was the critical element in the constitution of the experts' authority because only they had the experience and authority to make the final call. That expert authority could also see into the depths of the body to distinguish one dangerous type from another in the form of degenerates and psychopaths in the interest of the nation.

For a number of Ottoman and later Turkish neuro-psychiatrists, psychopathy emanated from degeneration. Just as the term degeneration became a shifting term after Morel, so did psychopathy from time to time and place to place. Ottoman-Turkish neuro-psychiatrists frequently used the two terms interchangeably. Much like degeneracy sometimes defied definition and diagnostic borders, the diagnostic border between psychopathy and complete insanity was not clear and intersected at various points. This is why for neuro-psychiatrist İzzeddin Şadan certain conditions constituted what he, following Maudsley, called a 'middle zone', between a healthy (normal) person and a mentally insane one.[40] Yet, both could say with certainty that there was also a very close connection between hysteria and psychopathy. In an argument similar to one put forth by Mazhar Osman, İzzeddin Şadan claimed that mental illnesses caused by the war did not increase during the war as much as had been expected. However, he noted that the 'half-insane *(yarı deliler)*', or psychopaths and degenerates, showed an 'astonishing' increase in numbers during the war.[41] The war, while not causing mental conditions, exposed to the neuro-psychiatrists' gaze large numbers of degenerates and psychopaths.

For the neuro-psychiatrists both degeneracy and psychopathy had certain characteristics, symptoms and signs. For example, atavism, described as an evolutionary throwback where physiognomies of remote ancestors reappeared in modern humans, was a characteristic of degeneracy. Dr İzzeddin Şadan translated and described atavism as some kind of 'animalization' *(hayvanlaşma)*, implying that bestial characteristics appeared in persons deemed to be suffering from such a condition.⁴² For Mazhar Osman, psychopaths had no 'self-control' or 'willpower' because of their intense desire for self-preservation, which amounted to 'egocentrism' or narcissism. Because of this they cared for no one or no object beyond themselves. Whereas German neuro-psychiatrists accused their war neurotics of having 'sickness of the will', Mazhar Osman argued that they had 'infantilism of the will'.⁴³ People whose will was sick, infantile or did not exist at all were no use to the nation and community. In fact, their shortcomings constituted a threat to the well-being and survival of the nation in such difficult times as the neuro-psychiatrists viewed the immediate post-Great War years.

In 1915, Mazhar Osman was optimistic that the 'more or less degenerate' nation could be diverted away from its path toward further degeneracy. But by 1918, with the war lost and many men dead, the situation did not look as optimistic. Looking only at political factors, Mazhar Osman characterised 1918 as a year when 'our [national] politics became bankrupt and our military surrendered their guns'.⁴⁴ Other neuro-psychiatrists shared his view. Dr Hüseyin Kenan saw the immediate post-war period as a time when 'a thousand disasters' faced the homeland, where 'hearths were destroyed and families and their dwellings were burnt [to the ground]'.⁴⁵ Looking at the physical destruction of the Great War and the ensuing War of Independence from their perspective, it is easy to see how they came to the conclusion that degeneration was everywhere. The neuro-psychiatrists thus stood at a crossroads: they could stand by and watch the degenerates and psychopaths 'infect' the rest of the nation and push it to its complete degeneration, or they could fight back and confront the danger. Since, in the words of Mazhar Osman, degenerates and psychopaths 'bred like rabbits' and were nothing less than a 'source of infection' (*menba-yı intan*) for society, the choice was between nothing less than the degeneration or regeneration of the nation.⁴⁶ The neuro-psychiatrists opted for regeneration, which required massive campaigns for public hygiene and closer inspection and classification of the whole population – and the experts and authorities to carry it out.

DANGER IDENTIFIED, SOLUTIONS CONSIDERED: NEUROPSYCHIATRY IN THE SERVICE OF THE NATION

Ottoman turned Turkish neuro-psychiatrists were not alone in their anxieties about degeneration. Well before 1918, it was clear that those degenerationists, who had earlier predicted the natural extinction of the degenerate through sterility, had been wrong. Henry Maudsley had abandoned the theory of eventual extinction in favour of one which understood degeneration as a counter-force to evolution.⁴⁷ If degenerates would not die out, then degeneracy was a much bigger threat to the nation than previously thought. Morel had argued that psychiatry should not concern itself with curing the incurable, but instead should attempt to change the social conditions that produced degeneration.[48] In Germany, Alfred Grotjahn, a neuro-psychiatrist, eugenicist and founder of social hygiene, called for a third of the German population, those he termed the 'army of psychopaths', to be institutionalised or prevented from reproduction in order to prevent 'national degeneration'.[49] Grotjahn was well-read and respected by his Ottoman and Turkish colleagues.

When Dr Şükrü Hazım came to a similar estimate as Grotjahn that 'roughly about a third of the population is low value individuals', he was operating within a European medical intellectual tradition. In fact, he continued, 'when we also factor in the losses in the war, [these] low value individuals, we must accept, [suddenly] become more numerous', in terms of their impact on the population.[50] From the perspective of neuro-psychiatrists, this was a frightening depiction of the nation's future. Since degeneration was a counter-force to evolution, these degenerates could in time overwhelm the nation if certain measures were not taken.

How had it become so bad? Why was this generation of neuro-psychiatrists so confused or surprised by the state of affairs? Shortly before the war, the Military Sanitary Commission (*Sıhhıyeyi Askeriye Riyaseti*) had dropped psychiatry courses and clinic training from the curriculum of military doctors in the making. The Commission had made a crucial 'mistake', which revealed its dismissive attitude towards psychiatry, but Mazhar Osman and his younger colleagues were even more determined to prove their value and to change attitudes towards psychiatry. They wanted every graduate of the military medical school to have some background in psychiatric medicine so they would be able to recognise basic signs of mental illness. In the end, due to thousands of mental breakdowns during the war, the war proved the utility of psychiatry. After the war, these clinics and courses were reinstituted in the military medical schools, with Mazhar Osman offering a new, timely and popular course on Psychopathy.[51] Yet, this was still not nearly enough for the neuro-psychiatrists; it was too late and too little. Military doctors in other specialties taking a course or two in psychiatry were a good first step, but the neuro-psychiatrists believed that reforms were needed to make it possible for closer mental examination of recruits. This was the only way to identify degenerates and psychopaths and exclude them from the military. A strong military devoid of these dangerous types would assure the political survival of the nation. Their dream was that the reforms would start within the military, and that by teaching and requiring good physical and mental qualities, they would soon expand to society at large.

The likes of Mazhar Osman complained that signs of mental deficiency, psychopathy and degeneracy were not properly identified during military recruitment – either during the empire or in the early republic. The neuro-psychiatrists could be of great help in deciding how the military selected soldiers in recruitment. Reflecting the collective voice of the neuro-psychiatrists, Mazhar Osman believed that since 'discipline and obedience as the spirit of military service are virtues only to be found in a healthy brain, then the first sign of a deviated brain is rebellion and lawlessness'. Those who rebelled against military discipline and expectations weakened the army. Taking Europe as his guide, he added, Europeans had known for the past twenty years that 'what a one-legged man means in a military parade is the same as a mental invalid in military service'.[52] It was essential to keep the 'mentally invalid' out of the military, but this would not be easily accomplished. The officers and generalist doctors who staffed the military recruitment centres, under the spell of a 'strange mentality', believed the more recruits, the stronger the army. In other countries, he maintained, every soldier – even volunteers – were put through a psychological examination by neuro-psychiatrists. In the Ottoman military, however, recruiters almost never referred recruits for psychological examinations, even those recruits who requested such an examination. This mentality continued into the early republican years in the 1920s. Because these recruiters thought that 'whatever or whoever [was] recruited from among the people was a gain' for the military, they were 'cruelly indifferent' to mental deficiencies even when acknowledged by the soldier candidates. The doctors needed to change this attitude.[53]

The neuro-psychiatrists argued that the military was not made stronger by 'randomly recruiting soldiers', but instead by carefully selecting them. They argued that it was better to recruit fewer soldiers, so long as they were healthy, rather than 'many soldiers with [various] illnesses'. Who should be excluded from military service? Of course, those who were 'insane', which all would agree at a minimum, included those who were clearly mad, or who attacked others, or randomly uttered 'ridiculous' things. Because the generalist recruitment doctors had either graduated before courses on psychiatry were required or what they took simply was not enough to change attitudes, they thought only in terms of this unsophisticated definition of insanity. The neuro-psychiatrists had 'witnessed the recruitment of many a melancholic, hypomaniac, paranoiac, schizophrenic' into the army by these generalists. Because it took an expert to identify not only those who outwardly displayed mental illness, but also those who were 'inclined to insanity (*müstaid-i cinnet*) [who] should not be conscripted without due diligence (*sellemehü's-selam*)', the neuro-psychiatrists had to be a part of the medical commissions who examined recruits. Those who were inclined to insanity were the numerous psychopaths. Because of their numbers, Mazhar Osman believed, 'the world has turned into a mental institution'.[54] Accordingly, 'those who were borderline insane [psychopaths] should be pardoned altogether' from military service. But in addition, 'lawless types, vagabonds, intensely immoral types, those who are poisoned in various ways (including alcohol), and uncommonly disagreeable persons [also] cannot be soldiers'.[55] Therefore, in the name of all neuro-psychiatrists, he recommended that these types be rejected from military service.

In a 1937 publication, Mazhar Osman repeated again what he had been saying for nearly two decades. He said that simply because a man has 'proportionate arms and legs' did not mean that he would necessarily become a good soldier and adequately perform the duties required in the military. For him, a soldier needed 'to be as sound mentally as he is physically'. However, in 1937 he went a little further, when he added: 'How do you give a task to a soldier who is more stupid than the packhorse he feeds[?] He is not even a packhorse that can carry loads'. He still believed that physically fit but mentally unfit types could be identified and removed from the military by more selective recruitment procedures in which the neuro-psychiatrists should be closely involved to eliminate the degenerates and psychopaths.[56]

To show how selective recruitment would help the Turkish military and therefore the nation, Dr Fahretin Kerim, among other neuro-psychiatrists, cited the example of the American soldiers who had served in France. The Americans, he said, made sure that every soldier went through a psychological examination, which served to exclude from service those who had a history of mental illness, but also those who were 'more or less' degenerate. Because of the elimination of degenerates from among them, the American soldiers 'joyfully went to the front like they were going to a boxing match or a rugby game', and there 'was not a single case of desertion among them', he stated. They fought 'the world's most warrior-like army (Germany)' with the same attitude. When the war was over, he observed, the American soldiers 'returned [to] their homeland with same pleasure and delight'.[57]

Of course, reality was different than this idyllic description suggested. Despite the allegedly superior mental testing of recruits, the American commander in France, General John J. Pershing, complained about the 'prevalence of mental disorders' among his men. There were too many degenerates and psychopaths in the form of 'general paretics, tabetics, psychoneurotics [and] imbeciles'.[58] Either misinformed or intentionally exaggerating, the Turkish neuro-psychiatrists were less concerned about accuracy, and more about the better selection of military recruits and the dangerousness of degenerates and psychopaths to both the military and the larger body politic. They were more interested in using this as evidence that the military of the Turkish republic needed to follow the American model of medically screening military recruits.

Because the doctors had a tendency to see the military and the nation as an inseparable whole, or the whole nation as a 'military nation', all their concerns about the military also applied to the nation. Mazhar Osman made two additional points in his 1925 article 'Nervous Disorders and Military Service'. In his first point, he connected the military to the nation by telling a story about Pyrrhus of Epirus (319–272 BCA), the ancient Greek general. Yet, he also selected this story to make a point about the importance of selective recruitment. 'Committing the whole nation to war would turn the military into that of Macedonian Papirus [sic, Pyrrhus of Epirus]. Fighting until the last man dies might make the army victorious, but there would be no nation left behind to live. In reality, wars are fought to allow the nation to live'.[59] He ended this article with the words of Dr Pellegrini, the well-known Italian military doctor, which was meant to show that the Italians had worries along the same lines. Reportedly, Pellegrini had said that 'to hand over weapons, artillery, machine guns, [and] bombs of the current century to moral imbeciles, epileptics, [and] degenerates is beyond irresponsibility; it is a blunder'.[60] These two references served to highlight Mazhar Osman's patriotism and nationalism on the one hand, and his concern about demographic problems the post-war nation faced, on the other.

The comparatively peaceful years after the Great War and the War of Independence did not calm the fears of the neuro-psychiatrists; rather, they gave them the time to extol psychiatry's usefulness in creating a healthier military and nation. Because of what they had discovered about the population during the war, the neuro-psychiatrists believed they needed to play a more direct role in the future of the nation or that future would be bleak indeed. In the 1920s, their mission was to convince those in power of the role neuro-psychiatrists must be allowed to play. Claiming to speak on behalf of all of his colleagues and the profession of psychiatry in Turkey, Mazhar Osman sought significantly expanded responsibility in almost every stage of life. He claimed that neuropsychiatry must be involved in a citizen's life from childhood – guiding children's education, their selection of a profession and even selection of partners in marriage. Obviously, military recruitment need not have been mentioned again; that was a given. In his vision of an enlightened future, doctors would be the propagandists of civilisation. They would be a source of trust for the people; they would teach the people about life and health; they would also encourage people to be devoted to the state. In short, physicians in general, but neuro-psychiatrists in particular, could serve as the connection between the state and the people. Allowing his optimism to overcome his reason, he added, 'in modern and civilized nations, states do whatever doctors recommend' in the interest of the nation.[61] Accordingly, ignoring the advice of doctors stalled modernity and civilisation.

As the neuro-psychiatrists sought expanded roles to help cure the nation, they were not at all shy about comparing the republican regime to the Ottoman state. Certainly, Mazhar Osman took to heart his assumed duty of propagandist for the state and civilisation. Going along with the current national historiographical trend at the time, he called the Ottoman state itself degenerate, as it had turned the 'homeland into a hotbed of disease'.[62] Given the situation, only the neuro-psychiatrists knew how to deal with the problem of degeneracy before it was too late. Armed by what they believed to be indisputable 'scientific truth', which frequently was nothing more than social commentary, the neuro-psychiatrists were emboldened to mentally conceive of themselves as the vanguard of the defenders of progress, health and modernisation of the nation.

MATTERS OF DEMOGRAPHY, THE GREAT WAR AND 'MILITARY SELECTION': THE PATH TO EUGENICS

Although there might have been some war enthusiasm in other quarters in the empire when the war started, for demographic reasons the Ottoman neuro-psychiatrists did not view the war in a favourable light. They agreed with those European men of science who believed that wars had a way of killing the select, strong and healthy members of society, while preserving the weakly and defective types. In other words, the strong ran to the front to fight and die for the nation, the weak ran away to save their lives. This line of thinking ran against both the war euphoria visible in some European capitals and the scientific opinion that pointed to the supposed 'positive functions of war and its redeeming features of sacrifice and racial purification'.[63] Because they believed that in wars the strong would triumph and the weak and the sick would be obliterated, many European doctors postulated that wars were eugenically beneficial for the nation.[64] In their opinion, wars would wipe out the biological dregs of society.

In his 1915 'Are Turks degenerate?' piece, Mazhar Osman made the historical case for the degenerative qualities of wars. He claimed that 'war, revolution (*ihtilal*), and [lengthy] military service' caused the 'more or less' degeneration of Turks as a people. He later charged that the lengthy military service required for the frequent wars waged by the Ottomans had produced what he called 'a social murder' (*ictimai cinayet*). Seemingly pointing directly to the regime of Abdulhamid II (*istibdat devri*; r. 1876–1909), he argued, 'the old regime failed not only to protect the Turkish ethnicity, but it seemed that it acted upon a well-planned agenda to eradicate it altogether'.[65] Due to various exemptions from military service granted to the people of Istanbul, to 'those with turbans' and to non-Muslims, he argued, the burden fell on ethnic Turks. Only they had to leave 'families and jobs behind for years'. He also excluded other Muslims of the empire because, he believed, 'nine-tenths of Kurds, Albanians, and Arabs did not serve'.[66]

For several reasons, Ottoman (pre-1908) military service had produced a demographic nightmare for Turks and for Anatolia. First, many young soldiers had died of illnesses or wounds before producing children. If they lived, they were away from home for fifteen to twenty years. By the time the soldier returned home, 'his wife's reproductive capacity would likely [have] long passed; that family was now practically extinguished'. Even those who came back alive brought deadly or incurable diseases from various frontier areas into the midst of the homeland with dire consequences.[67] In this way, lengthy military service not only extinguished many of the men who served, but also shortened the lives of those who never left Anatolia.

It is not easy to separate the demographic costs of the Great War from the War of Independence (1919–22, sometimes called the National Struggle). However, between 1914 and 1922, Anatolia had suffered a great demographic catastrophe because of wars, Armenian deportations, massacres, migration, diseases and famine, which indiscriminately took the lives of both men and women. What was already relatively clear to the psychiatrists in 1918, at the end of the Great War, became even starker by the time the War of Independence ended. Military losses were only a small part of a larger picture. For Anatolia, the losses from 1914 to the founding of the republic in 1923 'have been calculated at twenty percent lost to death, another ten percent to emigration, and up to half the survivors displaced as refugees'. For comparison, French and German wartime population losses were less than 5 per cent each.[68]

If eastern Anatolia was hardest hit during the Great War, then western Anatolia was devastated by the Greek occupation and the War of Independence. Five years after the end of the wars, the republic conducted its first census in 1927. It revealed something that must have been visible to everyone: especially among certain age groups, there were many more women than men. By extrapolating backwards from 1927, one can reconstruct what the neuro-psychiatrists saw. Adjusted for 1914, for the age group of 15 to 23 there were 18 per cent fewer men; for the 24 to 33 age group there were 33 per cent fewer men; and for the 34 to 43 age group there were 32 per cent fewer men by the end of the two wars.[69] The surviving population did not need an official census to recognise reality; it was evident all around them. The wars might have ended, but their effect on the nation's body would continue for significantly longer.

As early as 1920, the imperial government under occupation in Istanbul had seen this similarly discouraging demographic picture, and made an attempt to reverse the declining birth rate. Sultan Mehmet VI, the last Ottoman Sultan, issued an imperial decree proclaiming 1 May 1920 as 'Marriage Day' in Istanbul and what little of Anatolia remained in Ottoman control. As an incentive, couples incurred no charges for marriages performed on that day and the first children of those who wed on that day were to receive a bracelet from the local governor.[70] Unfortunately, the success of 'Marriage Day' remains unknown, but the opportunity was widely publicised. Even the Ottoman prisoners still in Egypt heard about the offer.

What the 1927 census officially confirmed was already evident to a lot of people, but the census also revealed that the country was dangerously under populated. In an age when large populations represented national power, Turkey's population density lagged significantly behind even some 'former provinces' of the Ottoman Empire. In comparison to Turkey's twenty-one people per square kilometre, Greece had fifty-two and Bulgaria had sixty. In Western Europe, Germany had 141 and Belgium had 276.[71] All this would have been no surprise to someone like Dr Tevfik Rüşdü, a member of the Nationalist Assembly in Ankara. He had argued in 1922 that relative depopulation of the empire had begun before the Great War. Nonetheless, he conceded that the war had created 'incredible holes' in the population and 'great emptiness' in the country. Tevfik Rüşdü wrote that as he travelled around the country, he encountered 'empty and naked farm fields, empty villages . . . and no signs of life anywhere'.[72] In a 1930 article titled 'We are on the Eve of Population Increase', Mazhar Osman mused, 'if only we had not entered the war, at least half a million more young men would have populated this land; more than one million children would not have died from famine'. If the young men had not died and 'each had an average of four children, they would have added three and a half million to our country's population'.[73] Those men would not come back, but in 1930 things looked a little better than they did right after the Great War.

In the aftermath of defeat, invasion and dismemberment, especially the neuro-psychiatrists but many other doctors and political leaders feared that the nation may not survive for long, based on demographic statistics and the medical conditions that affected them. In Germany, where the demographic situation was not as horrific, similar feelings led to biological nationalism and eugenic extremes. In Turkey, the birth rate was elevated into an index of national vitality. For medical professionals, other such important indicators included: decreased population, prevalent disease, the perceived number of degenerates. In the 1920s, all these indicators of national degeneration and national decline were attributed to low birth rates, coupled with prevalent deadly and maiming diseases. Those who were well aware of the situation, the physicians and neuro-psychiatrists, had come to see that it was their patriotic duty to intervene.

General loss of life during the recent wars certainly bothered all those who had been military doctors, but some saw the losses suffered by a certain segment of the war dead as significantly more unfortunate. This particular group, which reportedly suffered more than a 50 per cent casualty rate, was the educated (*münevver*) class of Ottomans – namely young graduates of civil and military lycées and universities who would have been the junior officers and officer candidates in the army. According to medical authorities, their loss was a much bigger blow to the nation because these men had been of high value to the nation. A wartime military veterinarian turned eugenicist in the late 1920s, Dr Mahmut Şemsi saw the deaths of these 'studly young men' as a heavy blow to a defeated empire at the time, but their deaths also deprived the nation of the eugenically valuable offspring they would have produced, had they lived.[74]

Because they believed modern wars worked against natural selection by assuring the deaths of the healthy and the brave, some Turkish doctors employed the term 'military selection', to refer to the destructiveness of wars on the genetically valuable portions of populations.[75] While they did not publically take responsibility, neuro-psychiatrists were privately aware of their indirect role in the destruction of the nation's superior genetic stock. Convinced that mental and physical invalids would be a burden by creating morale problems on the front, military psychiatrists had either completely exempted them from service, or had quietly reassigned them to labour duties in the rear positions where they remained safer.[76] As a result of these practices, the neuro-psychiatrists had unwittingly facilitated the survival of degenerates, psychopaths, malingerers and deserters, while the best specimens of the nation lost their lives by the tens of thousands. Şükrü Hazım outlined the neuro-psychiatrists' collective concerns:

> During war, [fighting] fronts obliterate the select and strong members of the population while a filter is established behind the front lines. Those seen as weakly, sickly, invalids, and defectives are not conscripted . . . [sent to the battle, but are] and left behind. Among the conscripted, those who display physical or psychological damage, [and] those degenerates and psychopaths are sent back as well. And added to this are the deserters [who remain behind] the lines.[77]

For Şükrü Hazım, it was not enough that the 'degenerates' had largely survived, his overwhelming concern was that 'they [were likely to] marry and become fathers. They are the ones who would increase the population'.[78] Into this environment came the post-war repatriation of the 'living dead' and 'schizophrenic' prisoners. Although these men had done their wartime duty by fighting, the mental diseases among them were a source of anxiety for the neuro-psychiatrists. Since modern medicine had identified and thus disproportionately preserved the unfit from the front's juggernaut, it was only right that modern medicine serve to counter the harm dysgenics and their offspring would bring on the nation.[79]

THE DEGENERATE DANGER AND THE STERILISATION OPTION IN EUGENICS

Scholars have argued that eugenic thinking was a fundamental aspect of some of the most important cultural and social movements of the twentieth century.[80] In varying degrees, it was connected to ideologies of race, nation and gender; it also meshed with population control and social hygiene. While the US and Germany led the way in adopting and institutionalising extensive eugenic practices, this new (pseudo-)science assumed different forms in different nations.[81] Practiced negatively, eugenics took the form of sterilising, castrating, segregating and even euthanising populations deemed undesirable or dysgenic. The aim of positive eugenics was to increase the desirable, or eugenic, segments of society while discouraging the procreation of the undesirables, or dysgenics, through the use of intrusive methods.[82]

In Turkey as elsewhere, neuro-psychiatrists led the way in the discussion and promotion, or balancing, of eugenic ideas.[83] The discussion that follows examines their discourse about and practice of eugenics and demographic policies in the post-war empire and the Turkish republic until 1939 Examining only the neuro-psychiatrists and not other doctors or social scientists means that only a partial account of the eugenics movement in Turkey is presented here.[84] Nonetheless, the critical role of the neuro-psychiatrists in this context cannot be overestimated. The eugenic practices they championed became the official policy adopted by the state, which served to marginalise more radical and non-interventionist proposals. They attempted to evaluate the more radical practices, such as sterilisation and castration, within the context of their experiences and loss of life as a result of the Great War. On the whole, neuro-psychiatrists were both the most ardent supporters of limited eugenics, and seemingly the most sceptical of extensive negative eugenics. Only a couple took a slightly different path.

Among those who survived the war were 'degenerates and psychopaths' who had escaped, or malingered, or deserted as a result of a mental condition, or broken down at the front or in captivity. With so many healthy men now dead and widowhood reaching 30–35 per cent in some areas of the country, the neuro-psychiatrists' immediate concern became what they termed 'unsupervised' marriages. With the hereditarily valuable men in short supply, they envisioned degenerates and psychopaths having a much better chance of finding a healthy, 'unsuspecting mate'.[85] Given this danger, neuro-psychiatrists had to intervene for the good of the nation. Expressing the collective fears of his colleagues, as he always did, Mazhar Osman declared that in order to 'reduce the number of insane people', psychiatry needed to 'intervene in matters of marriage'. Because psychiatric illnesses were hereditary, 'the marriage of nervous [or neuropathic] people' had to be prevented. He advocated for greater involvement of neuro-psychiatrists in the screening and selection of potential marriage partners.[86]

Since a portion of the 'unfit' had evaded detection by specialists, women could not be expected to tell the difference between a eugenic and dysgenic man. Given that there were so few men available in the post-war period, women acting 'with their emotions' would be willing to marry almost any men who seemed 'normal'. Yet it was not only emotional women who could not be trusted with such decisions. Likely referring to arranged marriages, Dr Fahrettin Kerim cautioned about an 'incorrect tradition among our people' of marrying off young people with mental conditions as a way 'to cure' them.[87] That is to say, these families believed marriage would fix things. For these doctors, marriage was not something that could be left to emotions; nor could it be left to unfounded assumptions and folk traditions. It was much too important for the nation's survival and, as such, it constituted a state matter.

For the neuro-psychiatrists, the idea of healthy women marrying degenerates and psychopaths presented a horrifying scenario. Since human failings such as insanity, criminality, alcoholism and schizophrenia, among others, were considered hereditary defects, procreation between a healthy person and an unfit person would result in similarly congenitally inferior offspring.[88] If both parents had such tendencies, the degenerationist theory suggested, the offspring would be worse off than the parents themselves. Such possibilities further convinced the neuro-psychiatrists that the problem was bigger than what it seemed on the surface.

Neuro-psychiatrists and others who promoted eugenics in Turkey closely followed the scholarship and practices of those countries that were considered advanced and where eugenics was practiced. As they became more informed about the policies and practices in other countries, they engaged in both public and medical debates about relative merits of various eugenic measures: sterilisation, castration, internment and institutionalisation. Especially after the passing of the 1933 eugenic laws in Germany, German theories and practices often came up in Turkish publications concerning eugenics, which usually featured a list of physical and mental conditions that qualified one for sterilisation in Nazi Germany. That list included schizophrenia and a number of other mental conditions.[89] As the two who were most outspoken, both Fahrettin Kerim and Mazhar Osman made statements which appear both to give tacit support to sterilisation and at the same time oppose this policy. For example, Mazhar Osman reiterated the need for 'encouraging and mandating' procreation among the healthy, while telling the 'rotten' that 'you are enough; there is no need of a generation of you'. The doctors' 'expectation' from implementing eugenics was to bar the increase of the unhealthy. As Mazhar Osman wrote, 'our beloved homeland, which was acquired and established only by spilling litres (*okka*) of blood for its every handful, is in need of healthy arms to work for its defence, comfort, rebuilding, and progress'. Individuals with 'unhealthy arms and warped heads' would be of no help. They simply comprised 'useless crowds' (*kuru kalabalık*), or even worse, for 'they are the parasites of society' (*cemiyetin tufeylisi*).[90] An ambivalent Fahrettin Kerim explained that German eugenicists 'say: sterilization is a social vaccination, just like when a state vaccinates its citizens in the face of a contagious disease to protect the healthy. [Sterilisation] is carried out for the interest of the society'.[91] He also acknowledged that recent advances in medicine proved the possibility of 'getting a healthy generation from those half-diseased types'. Because the threat was not great, he concluded that 'it was not necessary to [completely] remove [the possibility of reproduction] from that generation' (*nesil*).[92] Nonetheless, since it was just as likely that the half-diseased types would produce yet another 'degenerate', sterilisation remained on the table as an option in Turkey.

In their cautiousness as reflected in a number of public talks and publications, the Turkish neuro-psychiatrists seemed to divert from their former German teachers and colleagues – Kraepelin, Hoche, Gaupp, and others – who fully and openly supported negative eugenics in Germany.[93] They continued to discuss eugenics and considered the applicability of each of these measures for a country like Turkey. Some of these were discussed in more public publications; others were only brought up in specialised medical publications with limited circulation.

Perhaps more than any others who were involved in the eugenics debate, neuro-psychiatrists debated what they saw as the danger inherent to sterilising women, particularly those with 'questionable morals'. They argued that since sterilisation did not remove sexual desire but only made pregnancy impossible, 'prostitution would increase rapidly'.[94] According to this misogynist idea, the most important barrier to keeping women chaste was their fear of becoming pregnant. The doctors reasoned that sterilisation would remove that fear and women would then become promiscuous. In this way, promiscuity and prostitution became closely linked; women would not only have sex in greater numbers, but they would also charge for it. The idea that many women would immediately turn to prostitution is likely based on Cesare Lombroso's late nineteenth-century study *The Female Offender*. Lombroso had argued that since women were not capable of committing serious crimes, any inborn criminality among them would be expressed in prostitution.[95] The Turkish neuro-psychiatrists thought that prostitution and promiscuity would increase the number of syphilis cases and for these Turkish specialists, syphilis was the most significant culprit in the degeneration of the nation.[96] During the Great War the number of syphilis cases had already increased significantly among soldiers from Anatolia.[97] These physicians wanted to prevent, not create, yet another condition that was sure to result in more syphilis.

The legalisation of sterilisation could have other unintended consequences. The neuro-psychiatrists worried that educated and healthy individuals would volunteer for sterilisation in order to protect family financial assets. If used as a form of birth control, the 'fittest' would only have as many children as they could afford, thereby depriving the nation of their offspring. Mazhar Osman argued that only the intelligent could make such intricate calculations, while the 'degenerates, less intelligent types' and 'imbeciles', who already procreated 'like rabbits', would go on procreating.[98] Thus, a sterilisation practice could backfire and serve to magnify the existing demographic problem. The Turkish neuro-psychiatrists decided that the answer was to allow sterilisation only of individuals with proven hereditary disorders.[99] A nation as under-populated as Turkey could not afford to allow mistakes of this sort. The doctors devised this solution because they were already concerned about the nation's under-population. The nation could not afford to leave sterilisation decisions to civilians; this included the healthy and the imbeciles.

Similarly, Mazhar Osman did not seem to oppose Western governments' policy of partial castration for repeat offenders of 'moral and sexual' crimes (*ahlâkî cürüm*, dangerous moral criminals), but he opposed the practice for any other reason.[100] He argued that a more 'humanitarian' alternative to castration needed to be found, especially 'at a time when we are attempting to get rid of the death penalty both because of a general sense of human compassion and because of the possibility of mistakes made in rendering judgment'. Therefore, he reasoned, it did not make sense to implement a policy that would 'create an army of eunuchs'.[101]

The neuro-psychiatrists' concerns about sterilisation and castration emanated from their concerns about the country's significant depopulation. Recent medical advances had cured many diseases, and others once thought to be hereditary were found to be acquired. Therefore, the neuro-psychiatrists, as medical professionals, were uneasy about the finality of sterilising women or castrating men.[102] They were not willing to remove any possibility that some of these people could be cured and returned to health, thus become candidates in helping the nation increase its healthy population.[103]

Degrees of belief in negative eugenics varied even among the neuro-psychiatrists, but the differences were clearer in comparison to doctors specialising in other branches of medicine. When at a 1935 medical conference in Istanbul, a group of various specialists came together to discuss the benefits and dangers of eugenics, dividing lines became more visible. After Emil Orfanidis, a dermapathology specialist in Istanbul, delivered his talk 'Struggle against Racial Degeneration', neuro-psychiatrist Hüseyin Kenan commented on what he had just heard. Hüseyin Kenan found the sterilisation option to be the 'correct idea' in the case of hereditary diseases. He argued that the policy of sterilisation for hereditary diseases had been 'very successful in Denmark', well before it was adopted in Germany.[104] This was not in opposition to Orfanidis, who thought that sterilisation was only a small part of 'a larger struggle' against degeneration. Moreover, Orfanidis argued in his paper that a certain Dr Lowenthal, who completely opposed sterilisation, had exaggerated the downsides of this eugenic practice and was, in fact, 'wrong about them'.[105] In short, both Emil Orfanidis and Hüseyin Kenan were similarly minded. At the same conference, Dr Bağdasar Manuelyan, likely a surgeon, commented on a paper delivered by Mazhar Osman on sterilisation. Manuelyan cautioned in that 'there was no reason to rush' into and 'attach high hopes to eugenics', like some other 'extremist eugenicists' in Europe had.[106] He seconded Mazhar Osman's point that uncertainties about the hereditary nature of certain mental diseases required caution. Dr Osman Şerafeddin Çelik, a bacteriologist, also cautioned against being stampeded onto the eugenics bandwagon. 'The reason why so much attention is paid to this problem in Germany', he insightfully asserted, 'is not because of scientific investigation, but because of the agenda and problems of the group who have captured the government [there]'.[107] In some ways, he saw what some others failed to see. It was important, and possible, to separate eugenics from Nazi ideology.

The internment and institutionalisation of the congenitally unfit was also considered as a viable solution to the problem of degeneracy. European doctors estimated that, on average 1,200 people in every 100,000 were invalids. Turkish neuro-psychiatrists used this proportion to estimate that with a 1927 population of 14 million, Turkey could have as many as 170.000 mental invalids.[108] Applying German and American expenditures per patient as a guide, Turkey's neuro-psychiatrists estimated that the internment of 170,000 dysgenics in Turkey would cost the state about 140 million lira annually; this was a number which nearly equalled the republic's 1928 total national budget. Turkey never interred people deemed to be dysgenics. For the neuro-psychiatrists, its inadvisability was not just about the cost, but also about fairness. Money spent institutionalising defectives was money that would be used for 'limiting of imbeciles, not for rebuilding the country'. Under such a policy, 'taxes of those who work will be used to feed these idiots; while the children of those who work will go hungry, these [idiots] will live and eat in palaces'.[109] Some physicians did not like the financial cost of institutionalisation and believed that the monies could be better used to encourage the procreation of fit members of the nation.

The neuro-psychiatrists were admittedly confusing and sometimes misleading in that they made contradictory statements that both supported and opposed aspects of negative eugenics.[110] We can see this as proof that they were cautiously debating the merits and dangers of positive and negative eugenics. However, we also need to be aware that eugenics was a controversial topic. Publicly expressed opinions sometimes differed from private opinions as expressed in medico-academic discourse. Publically, Mazhar Osman opposed negative eugenics far more often than he favoured it. However, he also complained that even what he considered an 'academic discussion' of eugenics was enough to bring anonymous death threats against those who advocated any form of eugenics or dared to write about it.[111] Unfortunately, Mazhar Osman did not say any more than this on the topic and there is no mention in the sources of an anti-eugenics movement. As late as 1939, Mazhar Osman publicly repeated his familiar statement: 'we find our law [which bars those with hereditary diseases from marrying] to be adequate at this point'.

'POSITIVE' EUGENICS

The neuro-psychiatrists mostly agreed that the limited state funds available should be used to promote positive eugenics. The first step in implementing a policy of positive eugenics was to increase the number of marriages. As far as the neuro-psychiatrists were concerned, 'from a eugenic point of view, marriage is not a personal decision, but a racial, stately matter ... They [couples] have to understand that they are taking on a sacred duty for their generation, race, and country'.[112] Therefore, marriage could not be left to chance. The imperial government had offered no-fee marriage and little bracelets for the children born, but members of the nationalist parliament went much farther by legislating marriage. In 1922, the Nationalist Assembly in Ankara considered making marriage compulsory for healthy men, just as military service was. In this proposition any man who did not marry by the age of twenty-five, some members reportedly suggested, should be treated like a military deserter. Unlike the real desertion from the military, however, the marriage deserter would lose his job and civil liberties. This bill did not become a law in 1922, but similar laws with lesser financial punishments were later adopted.[113]

The republic's Marriage Hygiene Law of 1930 was largely embraced by the neuro-psychiatrists because they thought it would achieve their goals while avoiding the finality expressed in other nations' eugenics policies. The Law required a pre-nuptial medical examination, and barred people with certain physical and mental diseases from obtaining a marriage licence.[114] For example, those with syphilis and tuberculosis could not marry until they had been treated and certified healthy enough for marriage and reproduction. Mental diseases was a general category, but included a number of conditions, namely schizophrenia, which the neuro-psychiatrists placed under the umbrella of degeneracy and psychopathy.[115] Mazhar Osman positively noted that the law did not recognise 'a mental invalid as a full person', and thus denied him or her the right to legal marriage. In the eyes of the neuro-psychiatrists, the Marriage Hygiene Law held the possibility of larger positive gains for the health of the nation than did negative eugenic practices employed in other countries. Without the law, a marriage between a healthy and a dysgenic person was still possible. Even if the dysgenic partner were sterilised, this only guaranteed that there were no unhealthy offspring. The neuro-psychiatrists viewed 'fruitless' marriages between healthy and dysgenic people as damaging to the nation. This was the genius of the Marriage Hygiene Law. In addition to regulating marriage partners, it also guaranteed that no healthy person would have to bear the burden of a dysgenic spouse. More importantly, barring these marriages made the healthy individual available to marry another healthy person and thus produce healthy offspring. As compared to invasive eugenics, some neuro-psychiatrists praised the Marriage Law as a 'much better policy for any under-populated country like ours'.[116]

Getting healthy couples to marry was the first step toward increasing the healthy population of the country, but the neuro-psychiatrists believed that the second was to make sure that these marriages became as 'fruitful' as possible. For Fahrettin Kerim, Mazhar Osman and a few others, marriage was not about love or companionship, it was about procreation to increase the population. Fahrettin Kerim even proposed that women who intended to work rather than to have children should not get married at all. There was no reason to waste scarce healthy men in fruitless marriages.[117] Everyone needed to be reminded that marriage was not a selfish union based on emotion; prospective couples had to be made aware that the future of the nation was in danger and they were needed in this struggle against degeneracy.[118] The accepted belief among European and Turkish doctors was that if typical families had only two children, a nation would completely collapse in less than 300 years.[119] Some German doctors also identified the two-child practice as having 'enemy characteristics'.[120] Given the higher infant mortality in Turkey, the 'collapse' would occur sooner there. In this light, two-children families were 'hurting' the nation's future. Thus, the solution was to encourage families with 'hereditarily valuable genes' to have as many children as possible. The bottom line was to strictly enforce the Marriage Law to bar any increase in the number of the unfit and to increase the number of fit children.

To accomplish their goals, the neuro-psychiatrists urged that the state inaugurate a project of social and demographic engineering. They and other Turkish eugenicists suggested that the government strongly encourage its civil servants and the intelligentsia to have four or five children.[121] There were, admittedly, obstacles. First, they feared that some educated people did not want to have large families for reasons like personal financial concerns, which the neuro-psychiatrists and other doctors judged to be selfish, egotistical and unpatriotic. Second, there was abundant evidence that the enlightened class sought to raise children of quality rather than quantity. Therefore, after their second child, such couples practiced birth control.[122]

Suggestions for social and demographic engineering projects did not only come from the neuro-psychiatrists. In a book published by the government's Military Press, which gave it at least a semi-official status, Mahmut Şemsi, a military veterinarian turned eugenicist, proposed state-arranged marriages among specific groups. His idea was that the state should immediately begin to arrange marriages between mentally healthy veterans and the 'daughters of families who were known to have a reputation for their bravery, patriotism and devotion to the nation, especially those who had a long pedigree of such qualities'. Most importantly, the state must arrange marriages for unmarried military officers. In case an officer could not be matched with an eligible girl from a family with a military pedigree, the next best option was to locate healthy young girls from families that were financially well off. The writer contended that such matchmaking would increase the likelihood that the children born to such marriages would be brave, selfless, intelligent, resourceful and valiant. To make the effort worthwhile, such couples had to be mandated to have more than three children.[123]

Less manipulative, and far more practical, were suggestions from neuro-psychiatrists that the state offer financial incentives, rather than mandates, to encourage families to have their third, fourth or fifth child. The idea, as Fahrettin Kerim put it, was to make sure these healthy individuals felt that 'to produce healthy and numerous children was an important national duty'.[124] Other suggestions included that civil servant salaries should be determined by the person's marital status. Anyone who was married would receive a significantly higher salary than a single person. A raise of 25 per cent would be awarded after the second child was born, and could increase with additional births by 200 per cent. Another option was to offer tax breaks to families with more than two children.[125] Since the state was financially challenged, the eugenicists suggested that the monetary awards for the multi-child families could be financed by special taxes imposed on those who were single or did not have children. Putting rhetoric to practice, in the late 1920s and early 1930s, the state began to offer both small cash awards and medals to mothers who had six or more children. From 1931 to 1948, 132,892 mothers were granted cash awards, the sum of which reached over 4 million Turkish lira.[126]

The neuro-psychiatrists' concern for the health of the under-populated nation was evident in other projects meant to arrest further degeneration of the national body. They viewed heredity as the most important factor in degeneration, but environmental factors such as alcoholism and drug use could also turn people or their offspring into degenerates. Therefore, the neuro-psychiatrists attempted to attack those environmental and social factors.

Much like their German colleagues, particularly Alfred Grotjahn, the Turkish neuro-psychiatrists started to expand their knowledge and area of interest into other specialties. In fact, they became what Grotjahn called social pathologists, combining the sciences of hygiene, psychiatry, criminology, eugenics and *puericulture* (the rearing and hygienic care of children).[127] Turkish neuro-psychiatrists' writings are peppered with references ranging from Caesar Lombroso's criminological theory of the born criminal, to how best to raise a child and what kind of life a woman should lead. According to the neuro-psychiatrists, so many things needed to be considered before marriage and pregnancy that the people could not be left on their own to make these important decisions without considering what it meant for the nation. For example, even the timing of pregnancy was important; the neuro-psychiatrists argued that children of mothers who became pregnant 'during wartime [grew up] to be exceedingly neuropathic types'.[128] Thus, the doctors asserted that their authority was needed in many arenas of life to arrest further degeneration of the nation either because of 'improperly timed' pregnancies or environmental poisons from pornography to alcohol.

As social pathologists, they wanted to decide what was good for the health of the nation and what was not. In this role, they supported what might be called positive eugenic measures, ranging from prohibition to censorship. Alcohol was one of those environmental poisons that led to degeneracy even among healthy populations. In 1919, doctors Mazhar Osman and Fahrettin Kerim founded the Green Crescent Society (Turkish Temperance Society) in order to discourage the use of alcohol. They fully supported the nationalist government's prohibition of alcohol in 1920 as an enlightened and necessary reform.[129] Although the prohibition did not last very long, a decade later, the same two doctors founded the Society of Mental Hygiene (*Hijyen Mental Sosyetesi*). They convinced the state to censor newspapers from publishing accounts of and statistics about suicide, especially in Istanbul. Committing suicide, besides being a symptom of a degenerate mind, was a selfish and unpatriotic act from a eugenic perspective. The neuro-psychiatrists were convinced that newspaper stories about suicide romanticised the act and thus encouraged others. Similarly, concerned about their dysgenic effects, they also managed to prohibit the publication of pornographic material for a brief period.[130] All these positive eugenic measures they suggested as policy show the level of influence the neuro-psychiatrists had with state authorities. A significant number of these suggestions were readily adopted by ministries and other agencies.

The Society of Mental Hygiene sought to influence the selection of school texts, insisting that they promoted good mental hygiene, or the science of maintaining mental health and preventing disorders. Because these men promoted themselves as the spokespersons of the nation's mental health, the Ministry of Education accepted their proposal. It is not known whether their next suggestion to the same Ministry about creating 'characterology files' on each student found similarly receptive ears.[131] The idea was to create, from an early age, a paper trail on students who showed signs of mental retardation or psychopathic tendencies. In this way, early medical intervention, whether in the form of 'mental orthopaedics' or something more drastic, would be possible. In order to show that physical examination alone was not adequate, Fahrettin Kerim and others went to one of the boarding schools in Istanbul. After examining 200 students, they found some of whom they were convinced an academic education would be wasted on, due to the students' 'lacking in intelligence'. They recommended students such as these should be sent to a trade school. They also suggested that similar assessments should be extended beyond that particular school by widely administering the Binet-Simon intelligence tests.[132] As they worked with state agencies to test school children, some of the neuro-psychiatrists also turned to other avenues to directly inform the people and other professionals of the benefits of positive eugenics and social hygiene. They did this in the form of publishing journals.

Mazhar Osman and Fahrettin Kerim published medical journals to provide a platform for themselves and like-minded people to promote hygienic reform, eugenic ideas and discussion of more professional issues. Mazhar Osman published two journals concurrently. *Sıhhi Sahifeler* was clearly intended for the educated, or literate, public where he and other doctors frequently published articles on pronatalism and personal and public hygiene. His other journal, *İstanbul Seririyati*, however, was significantly more medico-technical. The intended audience was other professionals. Fahrettin Kerim published *Tıp Dünyası*, which appealed to both audiences. All three journals featured articles on a broad range of issues from the two editors, other neuro-psychiatrists and medical professionals.

Accordingly, their names were publically recognised as their influence steadily expanded. When they needed or wanted something for the nation, they appealed to the many members of the parliament and ministers who had medical backgrounds. The neuro-psychiatrists had the ear of Dr Refik Saydam, who headed the Ministry of Health from 1921 to 1937 almost without any interruption in office.[133] With his help, they received permission to move the mental institution from Toptaşı to Bakırköy. An expert on infectious diseases, Dr Refik Saydam had served as a military doctor during the Great War and was a friend of Mustafa Kemal. He would first become the Minister of the Interior, then the Prime Minister after Mustafa Kemal's death in 1938. How the neuro-psychiatrists exercised influence on national policies is difficult to document, but their legislative role in getting the National Assembly to pass their social hygiene laws – marriage laws, the prohibition of alcohol, the censoring of suicide news – point to a political influence that far exceeded their small numbers.

The year 1939, when German armies invaded Poland and inaugurated another world war, was a tense time period for the neuro-psychiatrists concerned about eugenics. Because they feared that Turkish participation would produce another demographic catastrophe, the neuro-psychiatrists hoped that the President of the Republic, İsmet İnönü, who had been a colonel in the Ottoman army and general in the republican army, understood the potential dysgenic consequences of entering another war. He had shown his interest in matters of national health and population growth and had just confirmed Dr Refik Saydam as the new Prime Minister (1939–42). While the 1935 census showed that the population had increased 18.7 per cent since 1927, through the interwar years, they frequently referred to recent wars of the Ottoman Empire as 'social suicide'.[134] Therefore, when Turkey declared neutrality in World War II, the psychiatrists-turned-eugenicists agreed that it was an important victory for eugenics. Mazhar Osman repeated in 1940 what he had first said in 1915: war is a 'slaughter' that 'mows down' in the space of a month or two all those young men a nation raised in twenty years.[135]

EXPLORING THE DARK SIDE: NEGATIVE EUGENICS IN TURKEY

Although the date of its actual meeting is not without some dispute, in 1938–9 the Seventh Turkish National Congress of Medicine convened in Ankara.[136] The major theme of the Congress was eugenics, and this theme made it a particularly important congress. The meeting was attended by İsmet İnönü, various ministers and members of the National Assembly, many of whom were actually former civilian or military doctors. General and Dr Abdülkadir Noyan, an internist and veteran of the Great War, presided over the Congress, a good portion of which had been designed to influence his thinking on eugenics. Unfortunately, not all papers presented made it into the published proceedings.[137] Some evidence suggests that the medical professionals and scientists who were promoting negative eugenic policies invited Noyan to a separate meeting to lobby for the application of negative eugenics in Turkey. What the pro-eugenics group privately proposed to General Noyan is not known; it logically had to be more extensive or more extreme than what was already practiced in Turkey. Reportedly, after the meeting Noyan announced in the name of the Turkish government that 'eugenic ideas are not suitable for us'.[138]

It needs to be noted that a number of Turkish publications on eugenics, including articles by the neuro-psychiatrists, included drawings or pictures of how to sterilise men and women, sometimes describing in detail the steps in the operation. One publication by Mazhar Osman contains more than a dozen pictures of sterilisation operations. The accurate knowledge the authors employed indicate that eugenic sterilisations were already being practiced in one way or another.

The wording of some of the publication titles indicates something more than a medico-academic debate. One example of such a title was 'Application (or practice) of Eugenics', by Ali Esat Birol (1901–99), a doctor specialising in women's diseases at the Gülhane Military Medical Academy. His paper, given at the same Congress, was published separately. Containing twenty-seven pictures and drawings showing sterilisation procedures on both man and woman, this forty-six-page publication began with the following statement: 'However sorely we desire an increase in population in our policy, from the point of quality we have the same level of need in needing high quality citizens who are beneficial to the nation'. What followed next championed the benefits of sterilisation and insisted that 'sterilization operations have no health effect on man and women. In fact, in cases of sterilization due to eugenic reasons, equilibrium and improvement are visible in the patients' sexual sensations'.[139] He also took up the subject from a legal angle: 'There have been many discussions about whether states have the right or not to mandatorily interfere, by law, in the integrity of the individual's body and being. Many eugenicists liken this method to inoculation and quarantine-like health measures'.[140] Despite some ambiguous statements he made in the same presentation, Dr Ali Esat Birol wanted to introduce negative eugenics in a measured way.

As he recommended future gradual expansion towards negative eugenics, Dr Ali Esat maintained that positive eugenic measures already in place were not sufficient. They should be expanded and 'we should get started on negative eugenic measures limited to heavy hereditary diseases'. For now, he recommended, it was 'sufficient to make sterilization mandatory on degenerate murderers, schizophrenics, hereditary idiots, and those with psychosis as they are released from prisons, mental institutions, and hospitals'. Over time, he added, 'more serious and organized' prenuptial examinations would reveal others with hereditary diseases. These should be prevented, not merely discouraged, from marrying and those who are already married should be prevented from having children.[141]

Fahrettin Kerim wrote, in a 1940-published conference paper, 'in cases where it was absolutely clear that a disease was hereditary, sterilization should be carried out'. He offered the example of a mother and daughter. The mother had muscular dystrophy and the daughter started to show signs of the same disease. He referred the case to the hospital's medical committee, which approved sterilisation for the child-bearing-age daughter. Fahrettin Kerim requested that Professor Wilhelm Liepmann, one of the émigré doctors who escaped Nazi Germany, conduct the sterilisation operation. It is not known if the patient or the mother were asked for consent or even consulted, but the operation was performed. Fahrettin Kerim opposed sterilisations in popular publications, but in a specialist professional journal, *Türk Tıb Cemiyeti Mecmuası (The Journal of the Turkish Medical Society)*, he admitted to actively facilitating the sterilisation mentioned above. Justifying the action in patriotic terms, he added, sterilisation 'is a matter not of savagery, but of respect for the good of the country. It is, of course, necessary to cut off the family that always produces degenerates'.[142] Feeling obliged to provide cover for his support of sterilisation, he made the following convoluted statement: 'I am not absolutely against sterilization, but I am not in favour of it in every instance. Cases should be examined carefully and diagnosed with absolute certainty'. He added that because there were no sterilisation laws in Turkey, some medical institutions had an 'open door [policy] on this issue'.[143] Apparently, this could mean that institutions complied with whatever orders the medical committees or individual doctors made. Thus, Ali Esat Birol stated that he had conducted five sterilisations for 'medical reasons'.[144] Ali Esat Birol closed his lengthy paper with the following: 'In order to find our deserved place in the world as a strong and cultured [country], it is necessary to follow and apply a population policy based on new scientific foundations'.[145]

Based on the foregoing, it is clear that negative eugenics were practiced in the Turkish republic for reasons doctors identified as 'medical'. Whether what was practiced constitutes a eugenics programme is another matter that has to wait for further research. However, no matter what the numbers were, sterilisations without the knowledge and consent of the patient because they might produce degenerate offspring cannot be anything else but negative eugenics. In many ways, the 'open door policy' mentioned by Fahrettin Kerim indicates such a hidden programme. It is likely that in this 'open door policy', women were much more likely to be the victims of sterilisation than men.[146] One cannot even venture a guess at how many women were sterilised by doctors purposefully or inadvertently. As some European and American doctors did, Turkish doctors may even have used x-rays to sterilise women without surgery.

ADVANCING NEUROPSYCHIATRY THROUGH DEGENERATION

The theory that more than a third of the national population could be degenerate and had to be dealt with by medical means remained in vogue long after the war that gave rise to it had ended. The Great War, by causing the end of the Ottoman Empire, actually reinforced the arguments of the degenerationists. During the chaotic years of 1918–23, this idea was further strengthened. The rise of eugenic policies in a number of countries in the 1920s gave it further life. A 1946 military psychiatry book still talked about degeneration.[147] However, in the post-World War II United States, the word 'degeneration' disappeared from the *American Encyclopaedia of the Social Sciences*, which in the 1930s had looked to the Germans with some admiration. In 1945 and afterwards, degeneration was identified with fascism, the Final Solution and the Nazi doctors.[148] In Turkey, it would take a few more years before the final demise of the theory of degeneration.

First the war neurotics, then the 'living dead' prisoners of war, and finally the degeneration thesis allowed the neuro-psychiatrists to advance their professional cause. They laid medical claim to more than one-third of the nation's population. Mostly visible only to the neuro-psychiatrists, these problems allowed them to demand expanded powers and responsibilities in making the national health policy. They inserted themselves into issues ranging from who should be conscripted to who should be allowed to marry. In fact, at least two of the neuro-psychiatrists examined here, namely Mazhar Osman and Fahrettin Kerim Gökay, became household names and powerful figures in the inter-war and post-World War II years.[149] However, it would be a colossal mistake to view all this only in the context of a medical 'will to power' or professionalisation argument. Such a one-sided argument would overlook the social, political and cultural anxieties and fears at the time.[150]

During the Great War and the early republican period, Ottoman and Turkish neuro-psychiatrists, as agents of the state, felt fear, anxiety and powerlessness against the perceived danger of degeneracy. Of course, this is not meant to 'justify' their discriminatory and misogynist, classist discourse and actions which resulted in physical and mental violence against others deemed unhealthy and unfit. In many ways, fear of degeneration coalesced with the chaos of national history and fight for national existence. By means of their writings, speeches and radio talks they passed on the fear of degeneration and benefit of eugenics to the political elites. Both Fahrettin Kerim and Mazhar Osman were invited by the Republican People's Party, the ruling party from 1923 to until after World War II, to talk about eugenics. From the mid-1920s onward, the republican regime began to address nearly all reasons listed as causes of degeneracy that the neuro-psychiatrists had identified, beginning with Mazhar Osman's 1915 article.

The achievement of modernisation and civilisation was the aim of the Kemalist republic. Along with other nationalists and patriots, neuro-psychiatrists wanted to see the nation modernised and civilised. Paradoxically, however, they believed that modernisation and civilisation tended to increase mental disorders. The increase in the number of mental disorders served as modernity's arrival on the one hand, but the increased numbers of degenerates and psychopaths also pointed to a turn away from modernity and toward atavism on the other. Therefore, the degenerates not only threatened the gene pool of the nation, but also its progress towards modern civilisation.

CONCLUSION

It is unlikely that without the 'living dead' schizophrenic prisoners of war, war neurotics, malingerers and deserters during the Great War as witnessed, treated and diagnosed by the neuro-psychiatrists, there would not have been such deep fear of degeneration and psychopathy in the last few years of the Ottoman Empire and the early Turkish republic. Efforts to explain wartime and prison camp breakdown in terms of pre-existing, hidden conditions surfacing during wartime were all attempts to locate these differences or 'deviance' deeply in biology. If these men who supposedly passed a cursory physical and mental examination broke down, malingered or deserted, what was the physical and mental health of the rest of the population like? The neuro-psychiatrists interpreted mental problems of both the enlisted men and the officers as advanced signs of degeneracy and psychopathy. Then, in an age when the military's health was taken to be a reflection of the nation's health, they projected this worrisome picture onto the nation at large. From the neuro-psychiatrists' perspective, the Great War revealed not only the poor health of the nation, but also its degeneration.

In this environment, where degeneration seemed to be everywhere, they turned to eugenics with hopeful eyes, and believed it would offer an opportunity for national survival. In attempting to find a solution to reversing the degeneration of the nation, they ended up pathologising more than a third of the population. The knowledge and anxieties resulting from this were used to define and identify who was normal and who was abnormal, and therefore dangerous to the national body. Degenerates, psychopaths and others with certain mental and physical illnesses were not deemed worthy of full membership in the wider body politic and their rights were curtailed, or worse. Significantly, those who were deemed degenerate, psychopathic, eugenic or dysgenic were not so determined by ethnicity, but purely by biology, or as they would have said by 'constitution'.

In this way, the Other was the dysgenic degenerate and psychopath. And that Other threatened the nation and was the cause of its less than healthy condition. Without the Other, the nation could regenerate and become healthy again.

As they turned to eugenics to arrest the degeneration of the nation, the neuro-psychiatrists felt the tension between quantitative and qualitative population. In Europe, the Great War had precipitated a shift to the qualitative, but from the neuro-psychiatrists' view, post-war Turkey simply did not have a large enough population to concentrate only on quality. Therefore, while working on the quality, they could never let go of the quantity issue. Partially, this is what held them back in terms of the extent of the eugenics they favoured. Once the nation was populous enough, they could turn more and more to quality.

While science and medicine influence culture and history, science and medicine are in turn influenced by culture and historical experiences. There can, in fact, be a close relationship between social life and historical experience on the one hand, and medical research and inquiry on the other. The relationship is reciprocal and mutually dependent, but was not always direct. In Turkey from 1914 to 1939, some medical questions emerged because of social anxieties, but sometimes those social anxieties were created at least partially by the medical and scientific knowledge at that time.

NOTES

1. Mazhar Osman [Uzman], 'Türkler Mütereddimi', p. 72.
2. These are actual categories of diagnoses.
3. See Daniel Pick, *Faces of Degeneration* for a much fuller examination the process of degeneration. Also, Julia Rodriguez, *Civilizing Argentina*, p. 72; Eric Carlson, 'Medicine and Degeneration', p. 122.
4. Carlson, 'Medicine and Degeneration', pp. 122–4.
5. Pick, *Faces of Degeneration*, pp. 51, 209, 154.
6. Daniel Pick, *War Machine*, pp. 80–1.
7. Carlson, 'Medicine and Degeneration', pp. 122–4.
8. Pick, *Faces of Degeneration*, pp. 95, 97–8. However, see also Mike Hawkins, 'Durkheim's Sociology and Theories of Degeneration', pp. 138–48.
9. Hawkins, 'Durkheim's Sociology', pp. 132, 124. See also Pick, *Faces of Degeneration*, who seems to think that Durkheim was more of a believer in degeneration than Hawkins suggests.
10. Hawkins, 'Durkheim's Sociology', p. 124.
11. Ziya Gökalp, *Yeni Türkiye'nin Hedefleri*, p. 11.
12. Ziya Gökalp, 'Mefkurenin Harikaları', pp. 63–4.
13. Ibid. pp. 64–5.
14. Ibid. pp. 64–6.
15. Mustafa Hayrullah, *Asabiye Hastalıkları*, pp. 491–2.
16. Ibid. p. 492.

17. Hüseyin Kenan, 'Psikopatlar', p. 386.
18. Ibid. p. 386. Fahrettin Kerim also noted the important role of heredity in what they identified as schizophrenia and various other mental disorders. Fahrettin Kerim [Gökay], *Yorgun Sinirler*, p. 49; Fahrettin Kerim [Gökay], *Ruh Hastalıkları*, pp. 24, 97.
19. Mazhar Osman [Uzman], 'Türkler Mütereddimi', p. 72.
20. Ibid. p. 72.
21. Ibid. p. 73. The word morphology is used in the biological sense here to mean form and structure of organisms.
22. Mazhar Osman Uzman, *Tababeti Ruhiye*, p. 202. He mentions '*Rumların kadimden beri güzelliği ve çenebazlığı*', or 'Greeks' beauty and chattiness since the ancient times'.
23. Mazhar Osman [Uzman], 'Türkler Mütereddimi', p. 73.
24. Ibid. p. 73.
25. Ibid. p. 74.
26. Nazım Şakir [şakar], 'Erzurum Santral Sertababetine Vurud Eden', p. 35
27. Ibid. p. 35; İzzeddin Şadan on these physical markers, 'Bünyevi Psikopatilere dair', p. 1,290.
28. Mazhar Osman Uzman, *Tababeti Ruhiye*, p. 224.
29. Pick, *Faces of Degeneration*, p. 209, quoting H. Maudsley, *Body and Mind*, pp. 62–3.
30. Mevlut Doğantuğ, 'Ruh Hastalıklarında Anormal Reaksiyonlar', p. 103. Also in Yücel Yanıkdağ, 'When Cowardice Became Sickness'; İzzeddin Şadan, 'Bünyevi Psikopatlara Dair', p. 1,292.
31. Mazhar Osman [Uzman], *Akıl Hastalıkları*, p. 423.
32. *Redhouse Sözlüğü* gives the meaning of *Hakikat-i eşya* as 'noumenon', which originates from ancient Greek 'I think, I mean'. I translated this as cognition or understanding of oneself. Nazım Şakir [şakar], 'Erzurum Santral Sertababetine Vurud Eden', p. 35.
33. Unfortunately, the table does not even provide basic information about the Ottoman soldiers. Tainted at least by the psychiatrist's identification of them as degenerate, therefore not 'average' Ottoman soldiers, we cannot even use it to determine rate of literary or appeal of religion among Ottoman enlisted men.
34. The athletic category was later combined into the category of asthenic.
35. Mazhar Osman [Uzman], *Akıl Hastalıkları*, p. 425. Kretschmer's book was translated more than once and went through at least a couple of editions. See, for example, Kretschmer, *(Kretschmer)' in karakter ve beden yapısı ölçüleri*.
36. Fahrettin Kerim Gökay, 'Ruh Hastalıklarının Tekevvününde İrsiyet ve Bünye', pp. 285–6. See also his *Beden Yapılışı ve Karakter Münasebeti*.
37. The belief that one's moral character was rooted in the body was a well-established Western idea, but August Morel, Cesare Lombroso and Ernst Kretschmer carried it even further in order to establish a closer link between the body and 'deviancy'. For more on moral character and the body, see Jacqueline Urla and Jennifer Terry, 'Introduction: Mapping Embodied Deviance', p. 6.
38. Emil Kraepelin, 'Psychiatric Observations', p. 248.
39. Gökay, 'Ruh Hastalıklarının Tekevvününde İrsiyet ve Bünye', pp. 284–5.
40. Mazhar Osman [Uzman], *Akıl Hastalıkları*, pp. 422, 424–5; İzzeddin Şadan, 'Bünyevi Psikopatilere dair', pp. 1,288–9.
41. İzzeddin Şadan, 'Bünyevi Psikopatilere dair', p. 1,292.
42. Ibid. p. 1,290.
43. Mazhar Osman [Uzman], *Akıl Hastalıkları*, p. 426.

44. Mazhar Osman [Uzman], 'Tababet-i Akliye ve Asabiye Kongresi', p. 135.
45. Hüseyin Kenan, 'Psikopatlar', p. 385.
46. Mazhar Osman [Uzman], *Akıl Hastalıkları*, pp. 426–7.
47. Pick, *Faces of Degeneration*, pp. 209, 154.
48. Ibid. p. 54.
49. Andreas Killen, *Berlin Electropolis*, p. 38. For more on Grotjahn, see S. Milton Rabson, 'Alfred Grotjahn, Founder of Social Hygiene', pp. 43–58; Myron Kantorovitz, 'Alfred Grotjan as a Eugenist', pp. 155–9.
50. Şükrü Hazım Tiner, *Eugenik Bahsine Umumi Bir Bakış*, p. 30.
51. Mazhar Osman [Uzman], 'Sinir Hastalıkları ve Hidmeti Askeriye', p. 845. Just before the war when the course was removed, Mazhar Osman actually had to resign his position from the military, but when the Ottoman Empire mobilised he was reappointed. In 'Üçüncü Emraz-ı Asabiye ve Akliye Kongresi', p. 124, he gives slightly different information.
52. Mazhar Osman [Uzman], 'Sinir Hastalıkları ve Hidmeti Askeriye', p. 844.
53. Ibid. p. 845.
54. Ibid. pp. 845–48; Mazhar Osman [Uzman], *Akıl Hastalıkları*, p. 423.
55. Mazhar Osman [Uzman], 'Sinir Hastalıkları ve Hidmeti Askeriye', p. 848.
56. Mazhar Osman [Uzman], 'Ruh Tıbbının İçtimaiyatta Rolü', p. 205.
57. Fahrettin Kerim Gökay, 'Harb ve Sinir', p. 4, 606–7. See also Mazhar Osman [Uzman], 'Sinir Hastalıkları ve Hidmeti Askeriye', p. 849, for similar observations.
58. Ben Shephard, *A War of Nerves*, p. 126.
59. Mazhar Osman [Uzman], 'Sinir Hastalıkları ve Hidmeti Askeriye', p. 847. Although phonetically, Mazhar Osman's text reads 'Papirus', it really should be Pyrrhus of Epirus as it is close phonetically and even closer contextually. Pyrrhus, considered one of the greatest commanders of his time, is famous for the term 'Pyrrhic victory', a victory with devastating costs to the victor.
60. Mazhar Osman [Uzman], 'Sinir Hastalıkları ve Hidmeti Askeriye', p. 849.
61. Mazhar Osman Uzman, 'Ord. Prof. Mazhar Osman'ın Söylevi', pp. 1,068–9.
62. Mazhar Osman Uzman, 'Konferans', p. 57.
63. Marius Turda, *Modernism and Eugenics*, p. 41.
64. Pick, *War Machine*, pp. 80–2.
65. Mazhar Osman [Uzman], 'Türkler Mütereddimi', p. 75; Mazhar Osman Uzman, 'Konferans', p. 59.
66. Mazhar Osman Uzman, 'Konferans', p. 59. The accuracy of this statement, which is unlikely to be true, is not as important in this context as it is used to reflect his perception.
67. Ibid. p. 60; Mazhar Osman [Uzman], 'Türkler Mütereddimi', p. 76.
68. Carter V. Findley, *Turkey, Islam, Nationalism, and Modernity*, p. 233.
69. Tabulated from the 1927 census. Devlet İstatistik Enstitüsü, *Genel Nufus Sayımı, 1927*. See also Başvekalet İstatistik Genel Direktörlüğü, *1935 20 İlkteşrin Genel Nufus Sayımı*, p. 4.
70. Anon., 'Marriage Day in Turkey', p. 43.
71. Yaşar Nabi, 'Nufus Meselesi Karşısında Türkiye', p. 35. I did not confirm the accuracy of these numbers since what they thought was the situation is more important.
72. Tevfik Rüşdü, 'Teksir-i Nufus', pp. 101, 104.
73. Mazhar Osman [Uzman], 'Nufus Bereketi Arefesindeyiz', p. 3. Clearly, Mazhar Osman is referring only to the direct casualties of war.

74. Mahmut Şemsi, *Harbin İstifai Tesirleri*, p. 24.
75. Following Ernest Haeckel, Dr Manuelyan in particular used the phrase 'military selection'. See Dr Manuelyan's comment on Mazhar Osman's conference paper in Mazhar Osman Uzman 'Kısır ve Idiş Etme', p. 251; Tiner, *Eugenik Bahsine Umumi Bir Bakış*, pp. 29–31.
76. Mazhar Osman Uzman, 'Öjenik', pp. 3, 5.
77. Tiner, *Eugenik Bahsine Umumi Bir Bakış*, p. 30.
78. Ibid. p. 30.
79. Mahmut Şemsi, *Harbin İstifai Tesirleri*, p. 25.
80. The word eugenics comes from the Greek for good and generation (or origin); it was used in the late nineteenth century to refer to the 'science' of heredity and good breeding. Eugenics is generally separated into two categories: positive and negative eugenics.
81. Frank Dikötter, 'Race Culture: Recent Perspectives on the History of Eugenics', pp. 467–78. For a comparative and brief look at the eugenic practices in England, the US, Germany, France and Belgium, see Server Kamil Tokgöz, *Öjenism, 'Irk Islahı'*, pp. 8–9.
82. Another term used for dysgenics was cacogenics.
83. Perihan Çambel, *Ögenik (Eugenics) Hakkında Düşünceler*, p. 24.
84. See Nazan Maksudyan, *Türklüğü Ölçmek: Bilimkurgusal Antropoloji ve Türk Milliyetçiliğinin Irkçı Çehresi, 1925–1939* on social scientists as eugenicists.
85. Mazhar Osman Uzman, 'Kısır ve İdiş', p. 249; Mahmut Şemsi, *Harbin İstifai Tesirleri*, p. 23–5.
86. Mazhar Osman [Uzman], 'Üçüncü Emraz-ı Asabiye ve Akliye Kongresi', p. 114.
87. Fahrettin Kerim Gökay, 'Irk Hıfzısıhhasında İrsiyetin Rolü' p. 14; idem, Milli Nüfus Siyasetinde (Eugenique) Meselesinin Mahiyeti', p. 211–12.
88. Mazhar Osman Uzman, 'Kısır ve İdiş', p. 249; Mahmut Şemsi, *Harbin İstifai Tesirleri*, pp. 23–5.
89. Mazhar Osman Uzman, 'Ruh tbbının içtimayiatta rolü', p. 204. Fahrettin Kerim Gökay, *Akıl Hastalıklarının Tekevvününde İrsiyet ve Alkolün Tesiri*, p. 3.
90. Mazhar Osman Uzman, 'Öjenik', pp. 2–5.
91. Gökay, *Kısırlaştırılmanın Rolü*, p. 4
92. Gökay, 'Ruh Hastalıklarının tekevvününde irsiyet ve bünye', p. 304.
93. Mazhar Osman's mentor, Emil Kraepelin, favoured direct state intervention. Paul Lerner, *Hysterical Men*, p. 22. Mazhar Osman Uzman, 'İdiş ve Kısır etme', in *Eugenic İdiş, Kısır ve Eyi Çocuk Yetişdirme Hakkında İki Konferans*, pp. 15, 18.
94. Mazhar Osman Uzman, *İdiş ve Kısır Etme*, p. 19–20; Uzman, 'Kısır ve İdiş Etme', p. 249. In the former work, a longer version of the latter article, Mazhar Osman's statements are less gender specific to women. Here 'women' is replaced with 'young people', but he makes a stronger statement about sterilisation leading to 'excessive' or 'limitless' sex.
95. Rodriguez, *Civilizing Argentina*, p. 35. See also, Caesar Lombroso, *The Female Offender*.
96. Mazhar Osman Uzman, 'Kısır ve İdiş', p. 249; Mazhar Osman Uzman, 'Öjenik', p. 10; Mazhar Osman Uzman, *Tababeti Ruhiye*, p. 219; Mahmut Şemsi, *Terbiyenin Biyolojik Temelleri*, p. 35.
97. Mazhar Osman Uzman, *Tababeti Ruhiye*, p. 336; see also, Zafer Toprak, 'Istanbul'da Fuhuş ve Zührevi Hastalıklar, 1914–1933', pp. 31–40.
98. Mazhar Osman [Uzman], *Akıl Hastalıkları*, pp. 426–7; Mazhar Osman Uzman, *İdiş ve Kısır Etme*, p. 17. Paul Weindling reports similar charges (egoism and personal

indulgence) against those who did not want to have children. Paul Weindling, 'Social Hygiene and the Birth Rate in Wartime Germany', pp. 428–31.
99. Tiner, *Eugenik Bahsine Umumi*, p. 69.
100. Mazhar Osman Uzman, 'Kısır ve İdiş Etme', p. 250; idem 'İdiş ve Kısır Etme', pp. 20, 33.
101. Ibid. p. 33.
102. Ibid. p. 20.
103. Mazhar Osman Uzman, 'Öjenik', p. 9; Mazhar Osman Uzman, 'Ruh tıbbının içtimayiatta rolü', p. 205.
104. Emil Orfanidis, 'Irkın Tereddisine Karşı Mücadele', p. 466, when Hüseyin Kenan comments on Orfanidis's presentation.
105. Ibid. p. 467.
106. Mazhar Osman Uzman, 'Kısır ve İdiş Etme', pp. 252–3. Manuelyan commenting on Mazhar Osman.
107. Ibid. p. 253. Osman Şerafeddin commenting on Mazhar Osman.
108. Clearly, this was a lot less than what Dr Şükrü Hazım estimated when he referred to more than one-third of the country being degenerate and psychopathic. He had had in mind various degrees of degeneracy and psychopathy, whereas the smaller number represented those who were completely without any hope and a burden on society.
109. Mazhar Osman Uzman, 'Kısır ve İdiş Etme', p. 248–9. See also, Mahmut Şemsi, *Harbin İstifai Tesirleri*, p. 12; for other arguments against the financial possibility of such a policy, see Fahrettin Kerim [Gökay], 'Milli Nüfus Siyasetinde (Eugenique) Meselesinin Mahiyeti', p. 207; Mazhar Osman Uzman, *Tababeti Ruhiye*, p. 20.
110. For further reading and different angles on eugenics see Sanem Güvenç-Salgırlı, 'Eugenics as Science of the Social: a Case from 1930s Istanbul'. Güvenç-Salgırlı rightly calls Mazhar Osman the 'most outspoken eugenicist' in Turkey' (p. 179). He hardly gave other neuro-psychiatrist-turned-eugenicists a chance to speak their mind. One exception, of course, was Fahrettin Kerim. See also, Ahmet Yıldız, *Ne Mutlu Türküm Diyebilene*, p. 171. There are a few other works which focus on eugenics in Turkey and they all come to the same conclusion – that no negative eugenics were practiced: Ayça Alemdaroğlu, 'Politics of the Body and Eugenics Discourse in Early Republican Turkey', pp. 61–76; Murat Ergin, 'Biometrics and Anthropometrics: Twins of Turkish Modernity', pp. 281–304; B. Arda and C. H. Güvercin, 'Eugenics Concept: From Plato to Present', pp. 20–6.
111. I could find no other evidence or mention of these death threats. Mazhar Osman Uzman, *İdiş ve Kısır Etme*, p. 16.
112. Mazhar Osman Uzman, 'Öjenik', p. 7. Only a few years earlier, for him marriage was less of a stately matter. For comparison, see his *Eugenic, İdiş, Kısır, Eyi Çocuk Yetiştirme Hakkında İki Konferans*, p. 35.
113. The proposed law also recommended that if the man refusing to marry had private means, a quarter of his fortune would be confiscated by the state. The only exceptions were students, who could postpone marriage until they completed their degrees. *The Lancet* found the proposed legislation 'sound' as it also insisted on medical examination, which 'should, therefore, prevent the . . . marriage of the unfit'. Anon., 'Compulsory Matrimony in Turkey', pp. 22–3.
114. The 1930 law actually says 'syphilis, gonorrhoea, soft chancre, leprosy, or mental disease', 7th chapter, items 123 and 124.
115. Mazhar Osman Uzman, 'Öjenik', p. 9; Naci Somersan, 'Prenuptial Medical Examination

in Turkey', pp. 261–3. On the specific schizophrenia comment, see Fahrettin Kerim Gökay, *Kısırlaştırmanın Rolü*, p. 7.
116. Mazhar Osman Uzman, 'Ruh tıbbının içtimayiatta rolü', p. 205; also Fahrettin Kerim Gökay, 'Irk Hıfzısıhhasında İrsiyetin Rolü ve Nesli Tereddiden Korumak Çareleri', p. 14.
117. Fahrettin Kerim Gökay, 'Milli Nüfus Siyasetinde (Eugenique) Meselesinin Mahiyeti', p. 211.
118. Mazhar Osman Uzman, 'Öjenik', p. 4.
119. Ibid. p. 9; Ali Esat Birol, *Öjenik Tatbikatı*, p. 9.
120. Weindling, 'Social Hygiene', p. 429.
121. Mazhar Osman Uzman, 'Öjenik', p. 4. Mazhar Osman thought that there was no reason to encourage procreation in the countryside as he 'knew of many women who gave birth to 8–10 children but only 2–3 lived' in the end, but the 'educated classes' needed encouragement in this regard. 'Öjenik', p. 6.
122. Birol, *Öjenik Tatbikatı*, p. 9.
123. Mahmut Şemsi, *Harbin İstifai Tesirleri*, pp. 25–30. There were similar encouragements in Germany for the civil servants to have larger families. Weindling, 'Social Hygiene', p. 429.
124. Fahreddin Kerim Gökay, 'Irk Hıfzısıhhasında İrsiyetin Rolü', p. 14.
125. Mahmut Şemsi, *Harbin İstifai Tesirleri*, p. 17; Mazhar Osman Uzman, 'Öjenik', pp. 7–8.
126. Mazhar Osman Uzman, 'Öjenik', pp. 7–8; Mazhar Osman [Uzman], 'Cumhuriyetin Sıhhat Siyaseti', p. 41; Orhan Aybers citing 'Çok Çocuklu Annelere Yardım', *Sağlık Dergisi*, number 10–11 (1948), p. 52, in Aybers, 'What did the Governmental Apparatus Comprehend', p. 183.
127. Killen, *Berlin Electropolis*, p 120; Rodriguez, *Civilizing Argentina*, p. 30. Mazhar Osman gave a 'Radio Conference' in 1935 'By the Order of the Ministry of Health', the text of which was published as 'Siniri Sağlam Çocuk Yetiştirme', in *Eugenic, Idiş, Kısır ve Eyi Çocuk Yetiştirme Hakkında İki Konferans*.
128. Mazhar Osman Uzman, *Tababeti Ruhiye*, p. 198. Among the neuro-psychiatrists, Hüseyin Kenan and İzzeddin Şadan deal more with Lombroso. Hüseyin Kenan, 'Psikopatlar', pp. 385–90.
129. See also Mazhar Osman Uzman, *Tababeti Ruhiye*, pp. 220–3. On the prohibition law, see Onur Karahanoğulları, *Birinci Meclisin İçki Yasağı ve Men-i Müskirat Kanunu*.
130. Çambel, *Ögenik (Eugenics) Hakkında Düşünceler*, pp. 29–30; Fahrettin Kerim Gökay, İrade ve Sinir Sağlamlığı', p. 14; Fahrettin Kerim Gökay, 'Milli Nüfus', pp. 208–9; Fahrettin Kerim Gökay, 'Türkiyenin Hijyen Mental ve Psişiyatri Sahasındaki Hizmetleri', p. 3; the 'Press Law' was passed in 1931.
131. Fahrettin Kerim Gökay, *Türkiyenin Hijyen Mental ve Psişiyatri Sahasındaki Hizmetleri* (reprint of an article from *Tıb Dünyası*, number 135, 1939), p. 3.
132. Fahrettin Kerim [Gökay], *Akıl Hıfzıssıhhası 'Hygiene Mentale' Noktai Nazarından Ruhi Tetkikler*, pp. 5–6. For Stephen Jay Gould's criticism of the Binet-Simon tests, see his *The Mismeasure of Man*, pp. 176–87.
133. Mazhar Osman [Uzman], 'Nufus Bereketi Arefesindeyiz II', p. 33.
134. Başvekalet İstatistik Genel Direktörlüğü, *1935 20 İlkteşrin Genel Nufus Sayımı*, p. 4. Mazhar Osman Uzman, 'Konferans', p. 60.
135. Çambel, *Ögenik (Eugenics) Hakkında Düşünceler*, p. 33. Mazhar Osman Uzman,

'Konferans', p. 59. Frederic Shorter argued that demographically World War II was devastating anyway because child death rates rose and fertility dropped: Frederic Shorter, 'Turkish Population in the Great Depression', p. 104. However, we should remember that entry into the war would have only increased the demographic cost.
136. According to one researcher, the Congress was to take place in October 1938 but it was postponed to 1939. Aybers, 'What did the Governmental Apparatus Comprehend from a Healthy Society during the 1930s in Turkey?', pp. 154–5, indicates, after interviewing a doctor who attended, that the Congress was postponed to 1939 due to Mustafa Kemal's illness, who died on 10 November 1938. Even though publication carries the year 1939, it was likely published early enough to be ready for the perusal of the Congress attendees, as some conference proceedings still tend to be in Turkey.
137. This also supports the publication appearing before the actual Congress. Apparently, some papers could not make the deadline.
138. Aybers, 'What did the Governmental Apparatus Comprehend', pp. 154–5. However, this statement is not in the 1939 publication of the proceedings.
139. Birol, *Öjenik Tatbikatı*, p. 3, 44–5.
140. Ibid. p. 45.
141. Ibid. p. 45.
142. Fahrettin Kerim Gökay, 'Ruh Hastalıklarının Tekevvününde irsiyet ve bünye', p. 303. On Wilhelm Liepmann (1878–1939), see Arın Nemal, 'Jin. Ord. Prof. Dr Wilhelm Gustav Liepmann', pp. 153–62.
143. Fahrettin Kerim Gökay, 'Ruh Hastalıklarının Tekevvününde irsiyet ve bünye', p. 304. There is some controversy on this point. In his work on Turkish demographics in this period, Frederick Shorter argued that the state technically prohibited sterilisation in 1936, but this law was 'interpreted' to mean 'no information could be disseminated concerning birth control methods'. Shorter, 'Turkish Population in the Great Depression', p. 114.
144. Birol, *Öjenik Tatbikatı*, pp. 18, 44.
145. Ibid. p. 46.
146. There is no hard evidence for this, but it seems more likely based on the frequency of descriptions of female sterilisations in books and articles about eugenics. One can consult G. Gürkan Öztan, 'Türkiye'de Öjeni Düşüncesi', pp. 265–82 about women and eugenics in Turkey, but the article does not offer hard evidence. One is more likely also to encounter articles like the following: Kenan Tevfik, 'Kadınları Kısırlaştırma Usulleri', pp. 92–7.
147. Münif Sanan, 'Asabi ve Ruhi Muayene', p. 103.
148. Pick, *Faces of Degeneration*, p. 237.
149. Fahrettin Kerim Gökay became both the Governor and Mayor of Istanbul for about a stretch of a decade. He also served as MP and Ambassador to Switzerland.
150. Pick makes a similar argument. He says that the professionalisation argument and power and knowledge equation overlooks felt fears and anxieties of the degenerationists. For Pick, the fear of degeneration also meant 'a felt historical and historiographical *powerlessness*', in reference to Foucault's power/knowledge equation. *Faces of Degeneration*, pp. 236–7.

EPILOGUE

THE SEARCH FOR A USEABLE PAST: PRISONERS OF WAR, THE OTTOMAN GREAT WAR AND TURKISH NATIONALISM

In 1951, some thirty-three years after the end of the Great War and twenty-three years after first referring to the 'living dead' prisoners of war, Dr Mazhar Osman passed away at the age of sixty-seven. Despite the fact that in this book we have encountered his harsh views on prisoners of war, war neurotics, malingerers, women and other groups, he had done a great deal during his lifetime to advance the science of psychiatry and public hygiene in Turkey. Among other accomplishments, he created the first modern psychiatric hospital, founded the Green Crescent (Temperance Society) to curtail alcohol use, and played an important role in the establishing of serology, neuro-pathology and experimental psychology labs. On 27 May 1960, nine years after Mazhar Osman's death, the Turkish republic witnessed its first military coup, which toppled the *Demokrat* Party in power since 1950. This coup started a chain reaction of events that brought to positions of great power and influence three generals of the Turkish military. Had he lived to see the coup, it is possible that Dr Mazhar Osman may have noticed something familiar about those three generals.

Because the coup was planned and led by colonels, some generals were not happy at all about a group of subordinates attempting to take charge. It was rumoured that upon receiving the news of the coup, General Ragıp Gümüşpala (1897–1964), the commander of the Third Army in Erzurum – the same army which had fought against the Russians during the Great War and gave up many of its own as prisoners of war – threatened to march his soldiers to Ankara and to crush the coup. They would only remain in Erzurum if Gümüşpala's one demand was met: he asked that the leader of the coup be someone above his own rank. Presumably, this was because, as a general, he did not want to take orders from colonels, who had just overthrown the first democratically elected government of the Turkish republic. Whether the rumours had truth to them or not is less important than what happened next. The colonels decided to ask Cemal Gürsel (1895–1966), a three-star general who had just gone into voluntary retirement, to be their leader. Just before his retirement, in a famous letter, Gürsel had urged the military to stay out of politics. Gürsel accepted and as the new leader of the junta, he promoted Ragıp Gümüşpala to be the Chief of Staff of the Turkish military forces. However, General Gümüşpala did not stay in that position for very long; within months of his appointment, he went into voluntary retirement. If rumours are true, Gürsel had secretly given Gümüşpala another task: to establish a new political party in place of the abolished *Demokrat* Party. Gümüşpala and a few others founded the *Adalet* Party (Justice Party), which would become the main opposition party to the Republican People's Party (RPP), originally established by Mustafa Kemal himself. The RPP had dominated politics until the 1950 elections. To the position of Chief of Staff vacated by Gümüşpala, Gürsel appointed General Cevdet Sunay (1899–1982).

Generals Cemal Gürsel, Ragıp Gümüşpala and Cevdet Sunay were veterans of the Ottoman Great War; they had either served as newly appointed junior officers or cadets of the imperial military academy. These men had something else in common: they had spent time as prisoners of war. Captured just as the Ottoman fronts were slowly collapsing towards the end of the war, Gürsel and Sunay were prisoners in Egypt. Gümüşpala was captured by Russians. We do not know if Gürsel and Sunay knew each other in Egypt, but the latter had the distinction of being in the same British prison camp as his father.[1] When civilian rule returned in 1961, Gürsel was elected as the fourth president of the republic.[2] Three years later Gümüşpala died. Having served as president of the republic for five years, Gürsel died in office in 1966. Now retired from the military, Cevdet Sunay succeeded Gürsel as the fifth president of the republic from 1966 until 1973.[3]

As it were, 1960 might have been the year of the former prisoners of war. That year, just a couple months before the May coup, Said Nursi, an ethnic Kurd and citizen of the Turkish republic, died while in internal exile as imposed by the RPP administration. As an Ottoman soldier, Said Nursi had spent long years as a prisoner of war in Russia's Kostroma province, not too far away from Vetluga. Unlike the three generals, from the republican state's perspective, this particular former prisoner had been nothing but a thorn in its side. After his repatriation, Said Nursi, known as *Bediüzzaman* or 'the wonder of the age' among his followers, became the 'most influential religious figure in Ottoman and Turkish culture' since the late eighteenth and early nineteenth century.[4]

These men – and many others – had other things in common as well. None of them fitted the description of schizophrenic 'living dead' prisoners of war.

Admittedly, Mazhar Osman and Fahrettin Kerim had identified 'only' half of the repatriated prisoners as such. Some of these men had stayed in military service and rose through the ranks to become top-ranking generals, chiefs of staff, and finally presidents of the republic; others became influential and long-time members of the National Assembly, governors, ministers, judges and governors. And, of course, one became a religious reformer, who had followers who had also been prisoners of war, either with him or in other locations.

The common denominator among nearly all of these politically influential men is that they did not leave behind comprehensive accounts of their captivity experiences.[5] Former prisoner of war Said Nursi left behind a memoir, but he only briefly mentioned his captivity experience, mainly to make the point that while even the Russians allowed him to preach in captivity, the Turkish republic denied him the same right.[6] Similarly, a handful of high-ranking officers who published memoirs of their experiences in World War I chose not to mention their captivity. Asım Gündüz, former POW and Chief of Staff of the Turkish armed forces during the republican period, published his war memoirs, but they did not include a word about being taken captive by the British.[7] Another interesting case is that of Colonel Arif [Baytin], the highest-ranking Ottoman in Krasnoyarsk, discussed in Chapter 2 and 3. Baytin published his war memoirs, but the narrative ends just before he is captured.[8] But what makes Baytin's case interesting is that he is believed to be the same person as A. Süleyman, who published his captivity narrative in a serialised form in the Turkish daily *Vakit*.[9] While he was commonly known as Arif Bey among the troops, he chose to initialise his first name when he published the *Vakit* narratives. It is fortunate for historians that a significant number of former prisoners who did not rise to power and influence did leave behind diaries and memoirs of their captivity. In a number of cases, those diaries or memoirs were published posthumously by family members rather than the prisoners themselves. Since so many kept a diary or wrote a memoir without publishing them, it is clear that the prisoners wanted to keep the memory of their captivity alive in some way, even if they did not share it publicly. But what prevented these men from writing and speaking about their experiences?

In his examination of British war narratives, scholar Samuel Hynes argues that, in most of the belligerent countries, captivity experience did not become a significant part of how the Great War was remembered. In *The Soldiers' Tale*, he points out that former British POWs either did not write about their experiences at all, or they placed them parenthetically in long narratives.[10] Hynes suggests some possible reasons for this silence among Europeans. First, for European POWs, captivity was short or not significant enough of an experience to write about. Second, he argues that the 'disgrace of captivity' may have helped to maintain a silence around the experience.[11]

A hint of 'disgrace of captivity' may have encouraged some Ottoman prisoners of war to maintain silence as well. We are not really talking about a societal, cultural shame, but a personal one. While other nations and peoples might have felt differently, there are no similar concrete public or military examples of shame being attached to being a prisoner in Turkish or Islamic culture.[12] However, a few publications appeared before or during the war that should be mentioned in this connection, for they certainly present certain opinions. The short book, *Mehmetcigin Esareti-Yahut Esir Olma!!!* (*Little Mehmet's Captivity, or Don't become a Prisoner of War!!!*) by H. Cemal, as the title indicates, is one such work.[13] While the title of the book might imply a much stronger message, the text simply recounts the story of a group of Ottoman soldiers who became prisoners in the hands of the Bulgarians during the Balkan Wars.[14] It portrays life in captivity as miserable and very difficult. *Şanlı Asker Ali Çavuş* (*Sergeant Ali, Illustrious Soldier*) is somewhat similar, but much more simplistic. The story is full of not-so-subtle messages about how an ideal Ottoman soldier should behave. Just in case the 'simple' Anatolian soldier does not get the message, each paragraph ends with a phrase that gives the moral of the paragraph. For example, in one instance, during the Russo-Turkish War of 1877–8, overwhelming numbers of Russians surround the outmatched Ottomans and call on them to surrender. But the Ottoman officers and soldiers respond together with 'we would rather die than surrender'.[15] Ottoman headquarters urged the officers to read this work to their men while in training.[16] However, at least one former prisoner of war objected to such words. This was A. Süleyman: 'The ordinary [empty] words expended on how it is preferable to choose death instead of captivity cannot be acceptable in our opinion'. Furthermore, the former POW argued, to pass such a severe sentence on a warrior who becomes a prisoner, simply because of preordained luck, cannot be within the bounds of humanity.[17] Despite the sternly cautionary words in simple stories read to the enlisted men, the idea was not that one should choose death over captivity, but that a soldier should fight until captivity becomes the last option.[18] After all, even one such overly patriotic and cautionary tale put it this way: one must 'fight until the last bullet is spent, the bayonet broken, the sword bent'.[19] The message conveyed in the above books are not so much that there is shame in captivity, but that it is a terrible experience and one should do his best not to be captured, 'for captivity is an unbearable misfortune and trouble. Captivity does not take away one's life quickly like *Azrael* [the Angel of Death]; it eats away at one's conscience and dignity like a parasite'.[20]

While there may not have been specific cultural norms concerning captivity in Ottoman and Turkish cultures, personal shame should not be discounted completely. In one case, for example, an Ottoman, İbrahim Sorguç, who was captured by the British and spent some time in Egypt, kept mementoes from his captivity, especially photographs. Curiously, however, he scratched his own image out of these group photos of his captivity friends, who included his older brother. Thirty-five years after his captivity, İbrahim Sorguç decided to write down his memoirs of captivity and his role in the War of Independence in which he participated after his repatriation. His son, who prepared the work for printing approximately forty-four years later, added that his father 'could not digest his captivity'. The former prisoner of war, who presumably returned from Egypt with his head bent down, returned from the War of Independence with his head 'high and full of pride'.[21]

What did it mean to be a prisoner of war to the prisoners themselves, while they were still in the prison camps, before they had a 'chance' to fight in the nationalist army and 'recover' their pride? Although more than one POW claimed that no one who had not been a prisoner of war could understand what the experience meant, we might attempt to understand what they said it was.[22] Writing to a government office in Istanbul to complain about not being able receive news from his family, one prisoner claimed that 'life in captivity is more dangerous than being in the Gallipoli campaign, but you cannot understand it because you have not experienced this kind of oppression (*müzahim*) and suffering (*meşakki*)'.[23] Under the deplorable (*elim*) and melancholic (*hazin*) grief (*ekdar*) of captivity,[24] said an Ottoman doctor in captivity, 'our oppressed (*ezilmiş*) and worn-out (*yıpranmış*) minds enter a vegetative state (*hububat*)'.[25] Captivity for one was a 'crisis of uncertainty' (*buhran-ı müphemiyet*) of one's surroundings that exhausted one's heart and soul with deep sorrow.[26] While the prisoners were clearly overwhelmed with feelings of sorrow and wasted years of precious life, they interpreted their captivity as bad luck, faith, as *kısmet*, a test from God. 'Oh my God!' said one, 'What a humiliating experience it was. Our hands clasped behind our necks, rank and file and officers together, we were herded by the bayonet-wielding Russian soldiers. As if we had all committed some grave sin, the men could not bring themselves to look at the faces of officers, as neither could the officers look at their men'.[27] 'What could we do?' another asked in a letter to his family, 'It is divine whim (*cilve-i ilahi*)'.[28] He was seconded by yet another who characterised his captivity creatively as having been 'grasped by the iron claws of cruel fate and thrown into a deep and dangerous whirlpool of despair and calamity'.[29] As is clear from the expressions used by the prisoners to explain their experiences, captivity itself was seen as an unfortunate fate. Seeing their captivity in this light must have served to ease the weight of being imprisoned; after all, if it was fate, no one could escape it.

Healing the Nation has made use a significant number of captivity diaries and memoirs. Considering that the literacy rate in the empire was about 5 per cent, the number of personal stories we have is remarkable. A significant majority of the captivity memoirs and diaries used in this book were published by family members or sometimes unrelated individuals after the former prisoner passed away. Personal shame may have kept many former prisoners from seeking publication themselves, but most likely it only played a minor part. The rest of this Epilogue will suggest that there were other political, social and ideological reasons for their reluctance.

To understand this, one needs to examine the nationalist historical narrative of the 1920s and 1930s and even beyond. So far, *Healing the Nation* examined how people imagined their community and how they discursively and legally included or excluded groups or individuals from the collective community called the nation; but there was yet another form of inclusion and exclusion. Looking at nationalist discourse, history, school books and literature in the early republican period, the rest of the Epilogue first examines how the Ottoman Great War was largely excluded, marginalised, and finally only selectively included in the early republican national narrative. The aim is to investigate what effect this had on the former prisoners of war who possibly wanted to tell their story of captivity in what turned into a marginalised war. Finally, and in connection, it briefly examines how the images of 'living dead' former prisoners, 'hysterical men' and the 'army of malingerers' fit into the nationalist discourse that viewed Turks as constituting a 'military nation'. In other words, how could Turks be a 'military nation' if there were so many of these degenerates?

Following Fatma Müge Göçek's point about the nature of nationalist historiography in another context, this Epilogue concurs that 'the main components' of the nationalist narrative and historiography – namely, its time frame, selective privileging of certain events and historical sequencing or chronology – allowed certain events to be 'intentionally highlighted', others to be 'suppressed', forgotten, reinterpreted, and 'still others fabricated' or embellished. This reimagining and reinterpreting of the past made possible what might be called selective nostalgia, or a politically and ideologically determined reordering, representation and forgetting of the Ottoman past to serve the needs of the republican present.[30]

Unlike other nations and empires that took part in the Great War, the Ottoman Empire and Turkey experienced wars both before and after World War I. Russia, which experienced a revolution and civil war during and after the Great War, might be the lone exception. While in Europe the Great War was a major point of crisis and a peak of tensions, in the Ottoman Empire it represented a middle ground in what has sometimes been called the 'Ten-Year War'. In this vision, the 'Ten-Year War' started with the Balkan Wars in 1912–13, continued with World War I (1914–18), and ended with the War of Independence, also known as 'the National Struggle' (1919–22).³¹ In this context, the National Struggle, as the last stage of this long period of warfare, came to be viewed as the major crisis point. The Great War brought defeat and the end of the empire, whereas the other ended in victory and made the 'rebirth' of a new nation and state possible. In the emergent teleological nationalist narrative, the Great War and the destruction it caused became a dark, destructive, unfortunate, but nevertheless necessary event that paved the way for the rebirth of the nation.³²

Well before the republican nationalist narrative came into existence, the Great War was made 'unnecessary' both by the post-war Ottoman government (1918–22) and in literature of the period. Just as the empire was surrendering in 1918, most of the members of the wartime Ottoman cabinet – namely, the triumvirate of Enver, Talat and Cemal Pashas; Minister of War, Grand Vizier and Minister of the Interior, and Minister of Navy respectively – fled what remained of the Ottoman Empire. They feared prosecution by the Entente after the armistice and were justified in their assumptions. In addition, post-war Ottoman administrations established tribunals to investigate the reason for entry into the Great War and the deportation and murdering of Armenians during the war.³³ These investigations concluded that the war had been the work of a few reckless individuals and therefore a mistake.

This new narrative – that Ottoman entry into the war had been the work of a small group of men and, therefore, a mistake – continued into the republican period. The republican period was also characterised by the new leaders' attempts to distance themselves from the policies and leaders of the Committee of Union and Progress, which had led the wartime cabinet. One common theme in these accounts was the 'guilt' of the inner circle of the Young Turk leadership (Talat, Enver and Cemal Pasha, especially). The war was ascribed to the harebrained ideas of the same group of people who had hijacked Ottoman policy.³⁴ Some argued that Enver Pasha, the Minister of War, 'in thrall to Germany, more or less single-handedly pushed the empire into a war it did not want'.³⁵

Soon enough, the narrative about the decision to enter the war morphed into something more sinister. Meant to discredit the wartime leaders, this interpretation portrayed them as men who 'sold' the country to the Germans. Such a view, already present in the nation-state's discourse, even appeared in the epic poetry of Nazım Hikmet, who was periodically jailed as a communist by the republican government in the 1930s and 1940s.³⁶ The passage below describes the immediate post-war period:

> We saw the fire and betrayal.
> And in the market of the bloody bankers
> those who sold the country to the Germans

and rested on the bodies of those who had died [in war]
now worried about their own lives.
And to save their heads from the people's wrath
They fled in the dark.
Wounded, tired, and poor was the nation, but
it was [still] fighting the most ferocious countries.
It was fighting still so that it was not enslaved twice,
so that it was not robbed twice.[37]

Nazım Hikmet was anti-war and anti-imperialist, rather than anti-Young Turk leadership. A line in a folk song, or a lament, went: 'Foolish people believed in German promises'.[38] Once portrayed as the work of those unscrupulous leaders who dragged the country into war – either for their own benefit or for the benefit of Germany – and fled the country after the defeat to save themselves while leaving the country in the hands of the invading Entente, the war itself became constructed as illegitimate and, therefore, unworthy of the sacrifices it claimed.

From history books to works of literature, World War I was portrayed in the republican period as an unnecessary war. However, it was also required to set the scene for the rebirth of the nation-state. Besides making the War of Independence possible, the Great War was needed to provide a comparison. The defeat in the Great War gave way to the Entente invasion of the motherland by French, Italian, English and Greek armies, the War of Independence resulted in the expulsion of those imperialist armies. Seen as resolving the wrongs and injustices of the Great War, the War of Independence became:

> [a] war that was fought, on the one hand, against conservative, reactionary, traditionalist, utopian internal opposition forces, and on the other, against imperialist, capitalist, colonialist and opportunist outside forces in order to separate the Turkish people from their political, social, economic, legal, cultural, philosophical past in all kinds of areas and direct them towards life in a modern world. [It is also] a war that was the vanguard and an example to the rebellions of oppressed peoples and thus a universally-qualified war of freedom that opened new phases both in Turkish history and in world history.[39]

The Ottoman Great War simply could not compete with this image of the War of Independence. Yet it had still been needed, though only in its specific episodes.

As historian George Mosse argued, the number of fallen soldiers during the war was of crucial importance to Germany because, without the dead, there would have been no myth at all.[40] That is, the greater the sacrifice, the easier the event played into the myth of the war experience. Without getting too far into the macabre task of comparing numbers, we might ask how the War of Independence compares to the Great War in terms of the sacrifices it claimed. In the nationalist discourse, the battle scenes of the War of Independence are described as having claimed the greatest of the sacrifices from all members of the nation; thus, in this war, fought as the last stand of a nation facing extinction, the 'plains and hills were full of dead soldiers'.[41] Yet, in reality, the actual battle casualties of the War of Independence are no more than a fraction of the dead in the Great War.[42] Obviously, the story was not about the numbers per se, but about the worthiness of the sacrifice for the cause at hand.

Viewed as the war that resulted in the rebirth of the nation, the War of Independence also represented a clear break with the Ottoman past, and thus historians generally adopted the year 1923 as the starting date for the history of modern Turkey.[43] Although this was most common in the early republican period, according to one critic the practice was continuing in the late 1990s.[44] Thus, when middle and high school education was reorganised in 1923-4, a class called *Malumat-ı Vataniyye* (National Information) was introduced for the seventh and eighth grades in which students learned about the 'new' Turkish nation, starting with the War of Independence, to the exclusion of the Ottomans.[45] Starting in the mid-to-late 1920s, the history of the Turkish republic in junior-high and high school history textbooks began with the conclusion of the Treaty of Mudros in 1918. The Great War was completely ignored, with the exception of a brief and limited review when the life of Mustafa Kemal was discussed. In these textbooks, the War of Independence and the Turkish revolution were established as topics of the greatest importance.[46]

Scholars generally agree that in its nation-building project, the young republic attempted at first to reject and exclude its Ottoman past.[47] The virtual exclusion of the Great War and the Ottoman Empire was characteristic of the early years of the Turkish republic. As time passed, however, the Great War became separated from Ottoman history and was selectively integrated into the history of the republic. However, this inclusion was limited. For example, the official *Türk Ansiklopedisi* published by the Ministry of Education, devoted 5.5 pages to the Great War, with a majority of that space going to the battle of Gallipoli, where Mustafa Kemal fought. The War of Independence received 31.5 pages.[48]

The complete or partial exclusion of the Great War from the nationalist historiography, nationalist discourse and even social memory became even more obvious as the anniversaries of the founding of the republic tended to be marked and celebrated with publications of all sorts on the War of Independence. Some of these works were general histories of the war, but numerous others covered local aspects. An early example of this was *İstiklal Harbinde Kastamonu* (*The Role of the Province of Kastamonu in the War of Independence*) published in

1933, but many other similar works were produced which covered nearly every province in the newly established republic.[49] Soon this tendency showed itself in extraordinary forms. Besides histories that highlighted the role of a certain city, town or even village in the War of Independence, there appeared professional and amateur histories of the roles of teachers,[50] women,[51] people of religion,[52] or ethnic and religious minority groups[53] who played some part in the War of Independence. These histories, detailing the roles of various places and groups, constituted nothing less than a process of legitimation, of belonging through having taken some part, however small or large, in a war that came to define the Turkish nation. While likely thousands of these mainly amateur histories have appeared since the 1930s, serious studies and memoirs of the Great War did not begin to appear until the late 1980s and 1990s.[54]

This lack of interest in the Great War is also visible in works of literature; that is to say, the Great War is nearly invisible in literature. There are numerous novels and scholarly studies of these novels on the War of Independence, but there is no category of World War I novels in Turkish literature. However, this did not mean that the Great War was never mentioned. It was. Subjects relating to the Great War sometimes entered into the novels, collectively known as the 'War of Independence genre' during the late 1930s, the period known as 'National Literature'. One could also find the Great War mentioned in leftist leaning novels of the 1960s. Erol Köroğlu notes that in these works the Great War had a specific role to play – to function as a prop in the construction of national identity.[55]

Although others also exist, a good example of the Great War as a rhetorical tool is one of Yakup Kadri's essays originally published in 1922. Here, the reference to the Great War, which had ended only four years earlier, is meant to highlight how everything was different during the War of Independence. This passage also illustrates the separation from the empire:

> I now fully believe that a sense of power resulting from the courageousness of one's spirit and soul is enough to do anything. But, only in this way; one should not blindly expect courage from moral power. That kind of a wrong belief, which was prevalent during the General War [World War I], pushed us from one adventure to another; it brought the failure of the Egyptian expedition and the tragedy of the Battle of Sarıkamış. This time, every soldier knows why and for whom he is fighting, and every commanding officer possesses the understanding of limits of his capabilities. Today's National Anatolian Army is nothing like – neither in spirit, nor in shape – the imperial army of yesterday.[56]

Yakup Kadri saw an almost instantaneous change in almost everything from the imperial to the national period. Here, as in his other writings, Ottoman officers lacked souls, scruples, initiative and other important qualities, but the officers of the National Army are the idealist types; they are assertive people who have cut off their ties to the recent past and are ready to welcome the new – at all costs.[57]

As hinted at above, there is one exception to the exclusion of the Great War from republican history. In this re-visioning, the Battle of Gallipoli, which took place in 1915 and where Mustafa Kemal made his name as a victorious commander, was actually separated from the Great War to serve as a prototype for the War of Independence.[58] This is why many works of literature on the Battle of Gallipoli were included in various anthologies with generic titles such as 'Turkish literature and the War of Independence'.[59] The Battle of Gallipoli was removed with surgical precision and appropriated into the republican history as part of the National Struggle.

As one of the things that makes a nation is its past, that past can be used selectively if it is for the good of the national community. National histories sanctify what is felt to unify the community. In this project, selective events from the past are presented as '"facts" outside of relations of time and space'.[60] Therefore, similar to the anthologies mentioned, this selective inclusion even influenced works of juvenile literature. *Bu Yurdu Bize Verenler (Those Who Gave us This Land)* serves as an instructive example. In this short work from 1975, the author traces the lives of four heroes, each of whom is introduced with a bold caption that reads 'From Among the Heroes of Our War of Independence'. Two of these heroes served in the Gallipoli campaign during the Great War, and later joined the War of Independence, which forms the major part of the story, while the other two are associated only with the War of Independence.[61] Clearly, the implication here is that participation in the War of Independence was a constitutive experience for those who 'gave us this land'.[62]

Writing about the memory of World War I in Europe, the late George L. Mosse argued that, especially in the defeated nations, there was a general feeling of pride at having taken part in, and sacrificed for, a noble cause mixed with the mourning that dominated the memory of that war. Thus, the reality of the war experience was transformed into what he calls the myth of the war experience, which looked back upon the Great War as a meaningful and even sacred event.[63] In this way, in the interwar years, Europeans attempted, on the one hand, to forget the war experience and, on the other, to remember and to give some semblance of having suffered for a worthy cause. As the foregoing showed, if remembrance and myth-building involves the conferring of a certain status on the event and the bereaved, and the formation of dignified narratives to explain the necessity and value of the losses, then the subject of the myth of the war experience in Turkey has been not World War I, but the subsequent War of Independence.[64]

There were yet more factors in the specific post-war environment of Istanbul and the Anatolian peninsula that kept the former prisoners from telling their stories. As horrible as the captivity experience might have been for the prisoners, especially for those in Russia, a majority of people on the home front probably lived through even worse experiences than the prisoners. As Chapter 6 discussed, the demographic losses of Anatolia were staggering. Istanbul also suffered, but not as much as most regions of Anatolia. Most civilian deaths took place in Anatolia, as it had served as the operating ground for Turkish and Russian armies, site deportations, massacres, Greek invasion, further war, famine and disease. The wars disrupted the infrastructure and caused a major labour shortage, which in turn led to famine and epidemics of cholera and typhus, and even the plague.[65] Even then, people remembered that during the war and afterwards, when walking through the streets of Istanbul, one could hear nothing but the grieving voices of mothers, wives and sisters who had lost their sons, husbands and brothers.[66] Thus, in comparison, the former prisoners of war felt as if they were the 'fortunate' ones.

Even as some people became the war rich, making immense amounts of money from the economy and finance, the majority of the people of the homeland were devastated. During the Great War, prices had risen by about 400 per cent, and they would quadruple once again after the Allied occupation of Istanbul. There were severe shortages of coal and wheat.[67] Even when Istanbul was not as bad comparably, the suicide rates there went up 400 per cent from 1916 to 1921, with a major increase from 1918 to 1919 – that is, at the end of the Great War.[68] There is no official explanation for this, but undoubtedly, with the large upsurge coming at the end of the war, one explanation is that it was related to the war and its devastation. The poet Nazım Hikmet recounts the deplorable situation of Istanbul at the end of the war in his epic *Kuvayı Milliye* in this way:

> Sugar was distant and unreachable like jewels
> Kerosene was equal to the value of molten gold
> And honest, hard-working, poor Istanbulites
> Burned their urine in their number five kerosene lamps
> What they ate was corn cob and barley
> and seeds of broom-straw
> And the children's necks were thin as straw.[69]

In short, there was and had been much suffering, death, disease, war, destruction and poverty in the homeland while the prisoners were in captivity. The returning prisoners came back to a country full of civilians who had suffered more than they had. Even if the prisoners did not think that way, contemporary observers on the home front did. In fact, at least some prisoners in Egypt believed that the people on the home front thought of them as having a comparatively easy life in captivity.⁷⁰

This imagery appeared in popular literature produced in the post-war years. In a short story about post-war Istanbul by Yakub Kadri, a repatriated POW, Namık, goes to see his friends from pre-war days. Every time he sees one of them, he is disappointed by their reaction. They do not appear interested in hearing Namık talk about his captivity experience. In fact, they tell him that he should have stayed there, for life in captivity could not have been worse than it was in Istanbul.⁷¹ So how could the former prisoners of war tell their stories in this environment, when the entire country had suffered from wars and everything they brought upon the people of Anatolia? Public compassion was monopolised by the tide of refugees and the anguish of bereaved families who had lost their loved ones to war, disease and famine. In this environment, even if the former prisoners still believed that they had suffered more than the people on the home front, who would have sympathy for their stories of suffering in captivity? After all, did not the prisoners add to the people's suffering and misery by being disease carriers and bringing home trachoma and other ailments?

Clearly, then, the prisoners, upon repatriation, found themselves in an environment where the home front seemed to have suffered more from the indignities of war. And some of the repatriated prisoners, much like the three generals we met at the beginning of this Epilogue, found themselves fighting for the War of Independence. A few years later, the political and ideological environment in the republican years made it even more difficult for the prisoners to tell their story. If most of the Great War had been excluded from the history and historiography of the new republic, any prisoner attempting to tell their story would have been going against the tide. Scholars working on war and remembrance have argued that 'the nature of warfare is a critical determinant of the activity of remembrance. A succession of wars or other kinds of violent disruptions present a different challenge to remembrance in the case of one single war, however large'. In other words, if an upheaval is followed by other dramatic events, the latter posed 'retroactive interferences' to the remembrance of the former upheaval.⁷² While a similar and natural 'retroactive interference' was certainly at work here, in the case of the Turkish republic, the foregoing showed that there were other interferences that resulted from both deliberate and unintentional ways of writing, representing and remembering recent history.

If the myth of the War of Independence and other factors marginalised the Ottoman Great War and captivity experience, another discourse relating to the supreme soldierly characteristics of Turks seemingly undermined the neuropsychiatrists' conclusions about the many hundreds of thousands soldiers as schizophrenics, hysterics, malingerers and deserters, or overall degenerates and psychopaths. Although the origin of the concept went back to the late nineteenth century, in the 1930s, a reinvigorated version of it argued forcefully that Turks were a 'military nation', where every Turk was 'born a soldier'. The idea was based on the concept originally suggested by German General Wilhelm Leopold Colmar von der Goltz in his influential 1883 work, *Das Volk in Waffen* (*The Nation in Arms*). This work was translated into Ottoman as *Millet-i Müsellaha* within a year.[73] Goltz Pasha had spent over a decade in the Ottoman Empire reforming the military. His ideas, therefore, became very influential among the students of the Ottoman military academy, which included Mustafa Kemal. Most of them graduates of the military medical academy, the neuro-psychiatrists were also fully aware of the concept. From the 1930s on, state-building and military service came to be defined as 'cultural/national/racial characteristics' of Turkish people. What made this possible especially at that time was the publication of *Askerlik Vazifesi* (*Military Service/Duty*), authored by Afet İnan and Mustafa Kemal Atatürk himself, and the creation of what has been called Turkish History Thesis, an official, nationalist account of Turkish history. This discursive move created a myth that established military service as a 'cultural practice', rather than a citizenship obligation, or a duty for the nation-state.[74] The discourse also 'slowly divorced military service from the recent wars and the Ottoman past'. State ideology produced and maintained the myth that compulsory military service for men was the essential condition of Turkishness. Accordingly, the concept of Turks as soldiers became inseparable from the idea of nationalism. Further, the military became an institution for the education and nationalising of Turkish men in the early republican period.[75]

What made this a worthwhile project was the immense increase in the size of the Turkish military in the later 1930s. Immediately after the 1927 census, the first modern census of the republic, the state passed a new conscription law, which eventually made the increase in the size of the military possible. While the size of the military in 1932 was estimated to be only 'little greater than that existing in 1922' at 78,000, by 1939–40 it had jumped to 800,000. This represented a 900 per cent increase.[76] The coming of World War II surely was an important factor in this increase. However, the numbers did not go down after the war. Could the only reason for this have been 'education and nationalization' of the enlisted men in the largest numbers possible?

When the Turkish Historical Thesis openly stated that 'The Turk is the best soldier ... Turks are the nation whose military spirit is the most evolved', how could the neuro-psychiatrists go on during the interwar years about schizophrenics, hysterics, malingerers, deserters and psychopaths without clearly contradicting the Thesis?[77] If more than one-third of the nation was estimated to be what amounted to dysgenics, how could Turks be a military nation? Since the fear of national degeneration extended well into the late 1930s, it was not the case that there was change in this neuro-psychiatric discourse before 'military-nation' ideology could take root. Since they also did not scapegoat any ethnic or religious groups with these shortcomings they observed among the members of the military and the nation, there was little chance that the degenerates and psychopaths who committed these not so soldierly acts could be easily explained away as belonging to other ethnic and religious groups.

Use of a dual or layered discourse allowed the neuro-psychiatrists to talk both about Turks as a military and warrior-like nation, on the one hand, and a partially degenerate nation whose degenerative conditions were uncovered during military service, on the other. Of the two, one was a public discourse meant for the ears of lay people and the populace in general. This discourse allowed Fahrettin Kerim to say such things as: 'weakness of the nerves is not something to be seen among Turkish soldiers'.[78] For the Turkish soldiers 'the rumbling sounds of advancing tanks and the piercing sounds of war planes have as much influence as the sounds of village drum and *zurna* (a musical instrument) and the buzzing of a mosquito'.[79] In this way, horrifying noises of industrialised war were made both familiar and inconsequential.

Fahrettin Kerim had forgotten neither his own statements nor those of Mazhar Osman about the shameless 'army of malingerers' or those others who developed hysterical symptoms as a result of simple falls or injuries; they talked about these in what might be called a more medico-technical discourse meant for the ears of medical colleagues, and possibly for the educated political elite who would have been capable of understanding such a discourse. In this way, it was not a contradiction for the neuro-psychiatrists to laud the steel nerves of the Turkish soldiers in public and still argue that 'schizophrenia is encountered frequently during military service' in a medical book without undermining the nationalist discourse.[80]

Other works where degenerates and psychopaths came up had even more limited circulation. For example, Nazım Şakir's work on malingering was published by the military Medical Academy Press in Istanbul and was meant for internal military circulation only. Similarly, *Ordu Doktorunun Nöropsişiyatri Kılavuzu (Military Doctor's Neuro-Psychiatry Guide)*, a later work published by the Turkish General Staff, also had a limited circulation, meant for military doctors, namely the neuro-psychiatrists.[81] In public discourse, they had to be discrete, but in private discourse within the confines of the medical community, they could talk about dangerous degenerates and the army of malingerers. In short, the use of a dual discourse allowed a strategically induced amnesia, where the living dead, malingerers, deserters and the rest of the individuals contributing to one-third of the nation being degenerate, were excluded from the public version of the nation's meaning because they disrupted the nationalist narrative. These degenerates did not disappear or fade from memory, but they were rendered invisible to the public, while remaining visible – and dangerous – to the trained gaze.

While identification of military service with national culture and a 'distancing of military service from wars' was an important part of the nationalist discourse in the 1930s, in the writings of Mazhar Osman one can see the blooming of a very similar line of thinking as early as the middle of the Great War. By 1915, Mazhar Osman was already condemning lengthy military service and wars as two of the 'most important' causes of 'more or less degeneration' of Turks. Because ethnic Turks were the backbone of the military, military service (especially during the pre-Young Turk period) amounted to an ethnic suicide mandated by the Ottoman state. In this view, Turks' innate 'warrior-like' (*cengâver*) qualities undermined them from a demographic point of view because they ended up dying in large numbers and bringing home diseases from distant frontiers.[82] This may explain why Mazhar Osman advocated short military service without frequent wars as beneficial for the individual, the family and the nation:

> If made universal (*umuma şamil*) and limited to a few years, military service is the most healthful and beneficial method to get young people to adopt habits of orderliness, physical exercise, and to toughen them up. [Military service], just as it is the most sacred occupation from a moral (*ahlak*) point of view, it is also the most beneficial fraternity (*ocak*) for the soundness of the body and the psyche . . . Psychological and physical exercises learned there are not limited to [duration of] military service; we are in favour of not limiting the psychological and physical exercises learned during military service to the duration of service, but to extending them to nation's children to the elderly. The military nation (*asker bir millet*) that will result from all this, will show seriousness and orderliness in every matter.[83]

Certainly, military service was meant not only to provide physical and mental exercise, but also to teach 'every member of the nation to be capable of protection of life and honour, and if necessary to die honourably and willingly'.[84] Learning to die for the 'protection of life and honour' if necessary did not necessarily amount to justifying war in advance. Consequently, military service of this kind would get rid of the peasant or the urbanite, and create soldiers 'out of formless clay', by nationalising and masculinising them.[85]

The kind of weakening of Turks from their earliest *cengâver* (warrior-like) days to the early twentieth century was noticed by people who were much more powerful than the likes of Mazhar Osman, Fahrettin Kerim and other neuro-psychiatrists. In 1926, Mustafa Kemal told a group of sports administrators that he saw 'inauspicious, negative, and meaningless marks on Turkish race of its past'. He added that in comparison to the 'world-conquering great Turkish nation of the past', he found today's generation 'a little feeble, a little sick, and a little weak'.[86] Mustafa Kemal's statement here, and in other places, quickly led to the republican state's attempted militarisation of sports. Accordingly, the state promoted sports as if it were a military duty for children who had not yet come of age for military service. Aside from military service, Mazhar Osman had also recommended sports as a must: 'sports life must be resuscitated. From the cities to the villages disciplining of the body (*riyazat-ı bedeniyye*) must be considered extremely important'.[87] The similarities between Mustafa Kemal's directive in 1926 and what Mazhar Osman suggested in 1915 are clear.[88]

While the militarisation of sports and the nationalising function of military service have been examined, one can also suggest that military service was a mostly positive eugenic measure meant to strengthen the individual and the national body politic. This idea was certainly current in the early twentieth century.[89] As Mazhar Osman did, European eugenicists saw the value of military training lasting beyond the duration of the service. Military service as a eugenic measure would serve two purposes. First, it would masculinise and strengthen the feeble men of the nation. Secondly, it would allow for the identification of those who were feeble, both physically and mentally. Chapter 6 outlined the kind of role neuro-psychiatrists demanded for their profession especially in the recruitment of soldier-candidates for military service. Because a 'soldier had to be as mentally fit as he was physically', the military had to be 'cleaned up' during peace time. 'A nation must have each soldier individually examined by doctors of mental medicine. [This should] not be only in the form of hospital observations, but a psychiatrist should examine the written opinions of the unit officers and doctors to judge the situation most correctly'.[90] No doubt, what Mazhar Osman was suggesting here was beyond what the medical infrastructure could manage, especially when the size of the military grew to 800,000 strong. However, military service could still serve the purposes of positive eugenics without much involvement of the neuro-psychiatrists. How much direct mental intervention these or a younger generation of military neuro-psychiatrists in the 1930s and 1940s managed, we simply do not know.[91]

Other forms of direct medical intervention, however, took place in the military. In his paper on eugenics at the Seventh Turkish National Congress of Medicine convened in Ankara, Dr Ali Esat Birol uttered the following curious brief passage: 'We see individual and more general greater advantages in mandatory operations on soldier candidates who carry illnesses that can only be cured by operations, which have been successfully practiced for many years in our country'. He provided no examples of what exactly these operations were, but highlighted their general benefits as he saw them:

> Citizens who become healthier in this way [through operations] continue to do their military service and increase the country's defensive capability. Sterilizations for eugenic indications have started in various countries after they have been studied by private and official organizations.[92]

Buried between two brief paragraphs about eugenics in a forty-five-page booklet on eugenics is a statement about operations conducted on soldiers in the army. In the absence of any additional information, what can be inferred from the context is that Dr Ali Esat was referring to operations that allowed the patient to recover from whatever was ailing him. What were the conditions that made this mandatory operation a possibility? Did he include this statement in a paper on eugenics to demonstrate that the military was successfully carrying out operations on soldiers already and expanding them to various eugenic measures would not constitute a problem? We do not know. The context does not indicate anything sinister. Yet, it does not mean that some soldiers and soldier candidates were not suspicious of the operations all the same, and remembered their intent differently.[93]

Other events in the late 1930s and early 1940s point to military service as a time when practices identified with curtailed eugenics-like measures could be employed. In his paper given at the Seventh National Medical Congress, neuro-psychiatrist Şükrü Hazım Tiner raised the issue of Alpha testing soldiers in the American army as developed by Robert Yerkes, a Harvard psychologist. Yerkes had done psychological testing of 1.7 million American soldiers during World War I, which identified 37 per cent of whites and 89 per cent of blacks as 'morons'. Overlooking the racist implications of his test, after the war Yerkes claimed that this testing 'helped to win the war'.[94] Chapter 6 has already showed that the Turkish neuro-psychiatrists were fascinated with the role American psychiatrists played in the selection of the men sent to Europe, assuming wrongly that they had managed to eliminate degenerates and psychopaths from overseas service. If Alpha testing worked for Americans, it would also work for Turks. By the early 1940s, the tests were being translated into Turkish.[95]

Universal conscription of all males which enlarged the military, also made biopolitics of the state more extensive. The state may not have had the infrastructure to examine, discipline, masculinise and make healthy and fit the whole nation, but it could manage to do it through military service for 800,000 men at a time. The nation's health had finally become the concern of the republican state, in contrast to the empire, which was portrayed as not caring about the health of its soldiers and the people in general. All this was in addition to the military service's role in nationalising the men.

When the Great War itself was only selectively included in the history of the republic, the war's psychological impact on the prisoners and other veterans could be used strategically as well. Schizophrenic prisoners, hysterics, malingerers and deserters as psychopaths disrupted the discourse of every Turk 'born a soldier'; therefore they were excluded from the official public narrative. Privately, they could serve to paint a picture of enormously dangerous times and a likely 'national degeneration', and be used to justify eugenics. In that, they would not only be excluded from the history of the nation, but also from its body politic.

CONCLUDING REMARKS

Healing the Nation showed that two closely related but distinct groups believed that the nation was on the edge of a deep precipice facing further decline and destruction. If the prisoners witnessed what they thought was the cultural, social, intellectual and civilisational decay of the national community, then the neuro-psychiatrists perceived a biological (both physical and mental) decay and degeneration of the nation. The officer prisoners noticed the decay most among the ignorant peasants who lacked national identification and civilisation, but also among other groups, including fellow officers, who did not seem concerned about nation, tradition and culture. Even as they pointed to 'biological' reasons, the medical men concluded early during the war that wartime mental breakdown was not causally connected to the circumstances of war, but was the result of weak-willed individuals unwilling or unable to put the collective, national interest above their narcissistic desires. While the neuro-psychiatrists first noticed the decay among the soldiers – prisoners, non-prisoners, enlisted men and officers – after the Great War, they projected it to the whole national body, estimating more than one-third to be 'low-value' individuals, or psychopaths and degenerates. In this way, a relationship was established between lack of 'collective consciousness', on the one hand, and degeneracy and psychopathy, on the other. For both groups, the nation was in need of their intervention to stop further decay and regenerate. One defined the nation as a community of individuals and groups around shared cultural characteristics that united around a *gaye*, an aim. The other paid more attention to biological characteristics and heredity even as their concerns transcended those of medicine and biology and operated within a nationalist discourse.

Officer prisoners searched for ways to regenerate the nation socially, culturally, politically and intellectually. In some ways, this amounted to nothing less than a social and cultural regeneration, because they wanted to change the mentality of the men, to get rid of their other worldly dogmatic beliefs, to give them a common identity and *gaye*. On the other hand, the neuro-psychiatrists also aimed at the regeneration of the nation, but a regeneration that was biological – physical and psychiatric. When the officer prisoners wanted to use education as their instrument, the neuro-psychiatrists turned to eugenics for national regeneration, or a national rebirth. Biological characteristics and heredity became important for the latter. However, their deep interest in biology and heredity should not be taken as a sign of institutional racism, or at least racism in the traditional sense. The neuro-psychiatrists discriminated against and wanted to exclude from the nation those they deemed to be degenerate or psychopathic. This study found no evidence that ethnicity or religion was a determinant for such diagnoses or exclusion. In order to stop the nation's further decline, as about a quarter of the nation faced blindness through trachoma and more than a third was degenerate, the neuro-psychiatrists and other doctors suggested bio-political ideologies and models of biological and social engineering. They attempted to transform the nation into an object of scientific regulation and expertise. The result was the biologisation of national belonging without necessarily its racialisation. The nation views of the prisoners and the neuro-psychiatrists both differed and overlapped in significant ways, but they had similar aims.

NOTES

1. His father was a battalion *mufti* or Islamic legal scholar. For more information on Sunay, see http://www.tccb.gov.tr/sayfa/cumhurbaskanlarimiz/cevdet_sunay/ accessed on 18 August 2011.
2. A 59-minute video documentary on Cemal Gürsel does not mention that he was a prisoner of war. There is simply a gap. 'After Gallipoli, he was sent to Syria front to Gaza. In 1919, he returned to the homeland': http://www.tccb.gov.tr/sayfa/cumhurbaskanlarimiz/cemal_gursel/ accessed on 18 August 2011.
3. Abdurrahman Nafiz Gürman, the fifth Chief of Staff of the republican military (1949–50), was also a former prisoner of war. He became a prisoner when he was a general staff officer of the Ottoman Africa Corps.
4. Carter V. Findley, *Turkey, Islam, Nationalism, and Modernity*, p. 287.
5. Gürsel's short biography by Mustafa Atalay does not even mention that his subject was a prisoner of war. Mustafa Atalay, *Cemal Gürsel ve Hayatı*; *Türk Ansiklopedisi*, s.v. 'Gürsel, Cemal' and 'Sunay, Cevdet'.
6. Bediüzzaman Said Nursi, *Hayatı-Mesleki-Tercüme-i Hâli*.
7. Asım Gündüz, *Hatıralarım*; Genelkurmay Harp Tarihi Başkanlığı, *Türk İstiklâl Harbine Katılan Tümen*, p. 125.
8. Arif Baytin, *İlk Dünya Harbinde Kafkas Cephesi: 29. Tümen ve 3. Alay Sancağı Hatıraları*. Kaymakam Şerif Bey's memoirs of Sarıkamış are the same: the volume ends when the author is captured. Ironically, the last chapter of the memoir is titled 'Our Last

Epilogue 269

Day'. Şerif Bey, *Sarıkamış İhata Manevrası ve Meydan Muharebesi*. Samuel Hynes noticed a similar pattern among European and American war memoirs – that war memoirs end as soon as captivity begins. Samuel Hynes, *The Soldiers' Tale*, p. 234.

9. Cemil Kutlu, 'I. Dünya Savaşında Rusya'daki Türk Savaş Esirleri ve Bunların Yurda Döndürülmeleri Faaliyetleri', p. xviii. Kutlu noticed that some passages from Baytin's *İlk Dünya Harbinde* were verbatim to the *Vakit* narrative.
10. Hynes, *The Soldiers' Tale*, pp. 234–5.
11. Ibid. pp. 234–6.
12. Antoine Prost, 'The Algerian War in French Collective Memory', pp. 172–3. Ikuhiko Hata, 'Japanese Military and Popular Perceptions of POWs', pp. 253–76.
13. H. Cemal, *Mehmetçiğin Esareti-Yahut Esir Olma!!!*
14. For POWs in the Balkan Wars, see Carnegie Endowment for International Peace, *Report of the International Commission to Inquire into the Causes and Conduct of the Balkan Wars*, passim.
15. İsmail Hakkı, *Şanlı Asker Ali Çavuş*, p. 75. A very similar message is also given in İsmail Hakkı, *Yiğitlere Öğütler-Gazilere Armağan*.
16. İsmail Hakkı, *Şanlı Asker Ali Çavuş*, p. 4.
17. A. Süleyman, 'Esaret Hatıraları', *Vakit*, 21 September 1920, p. 2.
18. Ottoman military authorities were concerned about the issue of 'legitimate' captivity versus desertion to the enemy. When the POWs escaped and returned, they were asked to answer a number of questions, which were concerned with determining whether the former POW deserted (*firar ve iltica*) to the enemy side or whether his capture was genuine (*duçar-ı esaret*). ATASE, World War I, K348, D1391, F1-1.
19. İsmail Hakkı, *Yiğitlere Öğütler–Gazilere Armağan*, p. 42.
20. H. Cemal, *Tekrar Başımıza Gelenler*, pp. 9–10.
21. İbrahim Sorguç, *Kaybolan Filistin*, pp. 16, 59.
22. Mustafa Arıkan, 'Asker Mektupları', p. 165.
23. Ibid. p. 165.
24. *Vaveyla*, 1–3 Mart 1333/1–3 March 1917, number 63, special issue, p. 7.
25. Ibid. p. 7.
26. Ibid. pp. 8–9.
27. Başkatipzade Ragıp Bey, *Tarih-i Hayatım*, p. 80.
28. Arıkan, 'Asker Mektupları', p. 32.
29. '*Gaddar feleğin pençe-i ahenini arasında*', *Vaveyla*, 1–3 Mart 1333/1–3 March 1917, number 63, special issue, p. 9. Another one was caught because of 'luck and destiny (*mukadderat*)'. Rahmi Apak, *Yetmişlik bir Subayın*, p. 159.
30. Fatma Müge Göçek, 'Defining Parameters of a post-nationalist Turkish Historiography', p. 87. In his examination of the German Great War literature, scholar Wolfgang Natter, using Freud's notion of 'belatedness', has argued that 'relating the concept of belatedness to the problems encountered in thinking about the works that fictionalize or historicize the war, one might think of the undeniably real event as being less an origin from which interpretation proceeds, as it is already its result ... [F]ragments that could not be integrated or that were censored from integration into a context of significance at the time of the event were, after a period of forgetting, reordered according to later experiences': Wolfgang Natter, *Literature at War, 1914–1940*, p. 5. I gratefully acknowledge the urging of my friend and colleague Erol Köroğlu to read Natter's work. See also, Umut Özkırımlı, *Contemporary Debates on Nationalism*.

31. The older generation of Turks, especially those who received no schooling, simply referred to this period as *'Seferberlik'*, without distinguishing one war from the other. *Safarbarlik* in Arabic means 'travel by land'.
32. Erol Köroğlu, 'Retorik bir Araç Olarah Tarih', pp. 5–6.
33. Fatma Müge Göçek, 'Reading Genocide', pp. 101–27.
34. Mustafa Aksakal, *The Ottoman Road to War in 1914*; Mahmut Şemsi, *Harbin Istıfaî Tesirleri*, p. 26; Âfet [İnan], 'Türk İstiklâli ve Lozan Muahedesi', pp. 277–8; Şükrü Günbulut, *Neydi Bu İşlerin Aslı?* pp. 140–5; Ahmet Kıymaz, *1918–1928 Arası Romanda Milli Mücadele*, p. 251; Erik Zürcher, *The Unionist Factor*, p. 27; Ahmet Eskicumalı, 'Ideology and Education', p. 192; Aykut Kansu, *Revolution of 1908*, pp. 1–27, passim.
35. Aksakal, *The Ottoman Road to War*, p. 1.
36. His last trial was in 1938. He was sentenced to twenty-eight years' imprisonment on trumped-up charges of organising a revolt in the armed forces. He was finally released in 1950 as part of a general amnesty.
37. Nazım Hikmet [Ran], *Kuvâyı Milliye*, lines 62–73.
38. Şükrü Günbulut, *Neydi Bu İşlerin Aslı?* p. 140. This lament song was 'collected' by M. Sarıözen. Although the original is *'Ahmak millet uydu Alman sözüne'*, M. Sarıözen wrote on his notes of this song that 'millet' here is not the nation but those 'people' or the leadership, who made 'us' a tool for German aims.
39. Nejat Kaymaz, 'Türk Kurtuluş Savaşının Tarihsel Konumu', p. 616. Similar images of the War of Independence exist in various types of publications. See, among others, Tanıl Bora, 'İnşa Döneminde Türk Kimliği', p. 176. Bora cites others: Suat İlhan, 'Türk Kurtuluş Hareketinin Safhaları ve Çağdaşlaşmaya Etkileri', pp. 319–26.
40. George Mosse, *Fallen Soldiers*, p. 72.
41. The above quotation is in Enver B. Şapolyo, *Türkiye Cumhuriyeti Tarihi*, p. 84.
42. The War of Independence claimed 9,167 combat dead and 31,173 wounded as cited in Anon., *Anıtlarımız, Şehitlerimiz*, p. 71. Other sources put the combat dead at roughly 13,000 and the wounded at about 35,000.
43. Attempting to give a historical and political background to the founding of the Turkish republic, some works start with the year 1918. In this way a contrast also becomes possible between a chaotic Ottoman Empire and an orderly republic that replaces it. Obviously, this has been changing in recent years.
44. Kansu, *Revolution of 1908*, pp. 1–27, especially 7–8.
45. Mustafa Ergün, *Atatürk Devri Türk Eğitimi*, pp. 79ff.
46. See Enver Ziya Karal, *Türkiye Cumhuriyeti Tarihi (1918–1960)*. This book was accepted as a history textbook for high schools by the Ministry of Education. It went through several editions, but no major change was made with the exception of bringing it up to date; a very similar case is found in Enver B. Şapolyo, *Türkiye Cumhuriyeti Tarihi*; Erdal Aslan, 'Devrim Tarihi Ders Kitapları', pp. 296–8; Eskicumalı, 'Ideology and Education', pp. 27–8, 38, 152–3, 211.
47. Christoph K. Neumann, 'Tarihin Yararı ve Zararı Olarak Türk Kimliği: Bir Akademik Deneme', pp. 103–4; Aslan, 'Devrim Tarihi Ders Kitapları', pp. 296–8; S. Eyüboğlu, *Sanat Üzerine Denemeler, Eleştiriler*, p. 133; Eskicumalı, 'Ideology and Education', p. 27; Ahmet Oktay, *Cumhuriyet Dönemi Edebiyatı*, pp. 6, 48; Levent Köker, *Modernleşme, Kemalizm ve Demokrasi*, pp. 88–9; Ergün, *Atatürk Devri*, p. 79; Artun Ünsal, 'Kayıp Kimliğin Peşinde Türkiye', p. 187; Ayşe Kadıoğlu, 'Milletini Arayan Devlet: Türk Milliyetçiliğinin Açmazları', p. 202–3.

48. *Türk Ansiklopedisi*, s.v. 'Dünya Harbi, I' and 'İstiklal Harbi'. The larger article on World War I itself is 24.5 pages, which includes the 5.5 pages on the Ottoman participation. In other words, the article provided nearly five times more coverage to the European side of the war.
49. Hüsnü Açıksözcü, *İstiklal Harbinde Kastamonu*. Another example of the same genre is Faruk Yılmaz, *Kurtuluş Savaşı ve Sonrasında Niğde*.
50. See İsmail Göldaş, *Milli Kurtuluş Savaşında Öğretmenler*.
51. See İnci Enginün, 'Milli Mücadelede Türk Kadını', pp. 618–24, 688–94; Fevziye Tansel, 'İstiklal Harbi'nin Anadolu'lu Mücahit Kadınları', pp. 81–90; Nilüfer Efendieva, 'Milli Kurtuluş Mücadelesine Kadınların', pp. 1,979–84.
52. See Kadir Mısıroğlu, *Kurtuluş Savaşında Sarıklı Mücahitler*; Cemal Kutay, *Kurtuluşun 'Kuvvâcı' Din Adamları*.
53. See Muhittin Ünal, *Kurtuluş Savaşında Çerkeslerin Rolü*; Baki Öz, *Kurtuluş Savaşında Alevi-Bektaşiler*.
54. Since 2000, but especially more recently, there has been an 'explosion' of memoir literature relating to World War I as suddenly people 'rediscovered' the memoirs and diaries of their soldier relatives and are eager to get them published.
55. Erol Köroğlu, 'Retorik bir Araç Olarak Tarih', p. 5.
56. Yakup Kadri Karaosmanoğlu, *Ergenekon*, p. 114–15. I would like to thank Erol Köroğlu for this point. Köroğlu, 'Retorik bir Araç Olarak Tarih', p. 5.
57. Köroğlu, 'Retorik bir Araç Olarak Tarih', p. 9; Erol Köroğlu, 'Mahzendeki Geçmiş', pp. 39–73.
58. Erol Köroğlu, 'Tarih, İdeoloji ve Popüler Roman'.
59. Among others, see İnci Enginün, Zeynep Kerman and Selim İleri, *Kurtuluş Savaşı ve Edebiyatımız*.
60. Umut Özkırımlı, *Contemporary Debates on Nationalism*, p. 133.
61. Each hero – Koca Seyit, Borazan Çavuş, Köprülü Hamdi Bey and Hasan Tahsin Bey – is introduced as *'Ulusal Kurtuluş Savaşımızın Kahramanlarından'* (one of the heroes of our national War of Independence): Aziz Nesin, *Bu Yurdu Bize Verenler*. The first edition of this worked appeared in 1975, while I used the fifth edition.
62. Similar attitudes towards the Great War also appeared in the Turkish film industry as it started to develop in the interwar years. During this time, various stages of the National Struggle and the War of Independence were the most popular film subjects. Footage from the War of Independence, sometimes featuring Mustafa Kemal, was shown to the public as 'documentary' films. Using war footage made these films that were not documentaries more realistic, and thus more authoritative. The earliest of them, *Ateşten Gömlek* (*Trial by Fire*), appeared in 1923, which was an adaptation of Halide Edip's memoir of the War of Independence of the same name. Others films followed: *Ankara Postası* (*Courier of Ankara*) in 1928; *Bir Millet Uyanıyor* (*A Nation Awakens*) in 1932; *Vatan İçin* (*For the Motherland*) and *Yüzbaşı Tahsin* (*Captain Tahsin*) in 1951. Ağah Özgüç, *Başlangıcından Bu Güne*, pp. 33, 104–5; Ağah Özgüç (ed.), *80. Yılında Türk Sineması*, pp. 33–41; Erman Şener, *Kurtuluş Savaşı ve Sinemamız* (n.p.: Dizi Yayınları, 1970), pp. 23–50. Although one cannot tell how many people in total watched these films, in the early decades of the republic they had the potential to reach a large number of people in a society where the rate of literacy was still very low. The American Consul in Istanbul reported that about 50,000 people in that city alone visited cinemas each day during the week, and that approximately 100,000 went to the cinemas on the weekends. US Department of State,

867.4061/3, 'A Report by Consul in Istanbul on Turkish Motion Picture Theaters', 24 October 1924.
63. Mosse, *Fallen Soldiers*, pp. 3–7; see also, Catherine Merridale, 'War, Death, and Remembrance', p. 73, paraphrasing George Mosse.
64. Ayşe Gül Altınay and Tanıl Bora point more specifically within the War of National Liberation to the Battle of Sakarya: 'Ordu, Militarizm ve Milliyetçilik', in *Milliyetçilik*, p. 140.
65. Justin McCarthy, *Muslims and Minorities*, pp. 135–9; Erik Jan Zürcher, *Turkey: a Modern History*, p. 171. See also, Mehmet Temel, *İşgal Yıllarında İstanbul'un Sosyal Durumu*, pp. 239–53.
66. Vamık Volkan, *Blood Lines*, p. 133.
67. Zürcher, *Turkey: a Modern History*, p. 146; Ahmed Emin [Yalman], *Turkey in the World War*, pp. 144–56; Nur Bilge Criss, *Istanbul Under Allied Occupation*, pp. 81–93. See also, Ahmet Özgiray, '1918–1920 Senelerinde İstanbul'un', pp. 319–22.
68. Fahreddin Kerim [Gökay], *Türkiye'de İntiharlar Meselesi*, p. 23.
69. Nazım Hikmet [Ran], *Kuvâyi Milliye: Destan*, p. 23.
70. *Hatıra-yı Esaret*, 1336/1920, no page numbers.
71. Yakub Kadri [Karaosmanoğlu], 'Hasretten Hasrete', pp. 76–81.
72. Jay Winter and Emmanuel Sivan, 'Setting the Framework', p. 34; Emmanuel Sivan, 'Private Pain and Public Remembrance in Israel', pp. 177–204, especially pp. 196–7; Merridale, 'War, Death, and Remembrance in Soviet Russia', pp. 61–83, especially 62–3.
73. Ayşe Gül Altınay, *The Myth of the Military-Nation*, p. 14; see also Altınay and Bora, 'Ordu, Militarizm ve Milliyetçilik'.
74. Altınay, *The Myth of the Military-Nation*, pp. 6–7.
75. Ibid. pp. 28–30; Altınay and Bora, 'Ordu, Militarizm ve Milliyetçilik'.
76. Altınay, *The Myth of the Military-Nation*, pp. 27–8; original wording in David Lerner and Richard Robinson, 'Swords and Ploughshares', p. 27.
77. Altınay and Bora, 'Ordu, Militarizm ve Milliyetçilik', p. 142.
78. Fahrettin Kerim Gökay, 'Harb ve Sinir', p. 4,607.
79. Ibid. p. 4,607; *zurna* is made of reed and resembles an oboe. It is played in improvisational style.
80. Mazhar Osman Uzman, *Tababeti Ruhiye*, p. 251.
81. Nazım Şakir [Şakar], *Temaruz ve Teşhisi*; Nazım Şakir Şakar, *Ordu Doktorunun Nöropsişiyatri Kılavuzu* was most likely meant for internal military-medical use since it also talks about how to catch malingerers.
82. Mazhar Osman [Uzman], 'Türkler Mütereddimi', p. 85. Of course, he argued that wars took the healthiest and strongest away and left behind the rotten (*çürükler*).
83. Ibid. p. 77.
84. Ibid. p. 77.
85. Michel Foucault, *Discipline and Punish*, p. 135; Altınay, *The Myth of the Military-Nation*, p. 63. In fact, my 'Educating the Peasants: the Ottoman Army and Enlisted Men in Uniform' argued along those lines, though admittedly without much interrogation of the intentions of the state in this process. It suggested that right at the end of the empire, military service was meant to inculcate everything from personal hygiene to national identity and obedience as the state attempted to create 'docile bodies'.
86. Yiğit Akın, *Gürbüz ve Yavuz Evlatlar*, p. 98.
87. Mazhar Osman [Uzman], 'Türkler Mütereddimi', p. 96.

88. I am not pointing to a direct connection but only suggesting that the ideas were similar, which could be the result of both men, and others of their generation, reading similar works.
89. Eugenic literature certainly suggested short military service as a eugenic measure as 'military training certainly makes men more strong and healthy for the time being, and probably permanently ...': Leonard Darwin, 'Eugenics During and After the War', p. 97. This was the presidential address delivered at the Annual Meeting of the Eugenic Education Society in 1915.
90. Mazhar Osman Uzman, 'Ruh Tıbbının İçtimaiyatta Rolü', pp. 205–6.
91. I am not suggesting that the size of the army was kept as large as it was simply because military service was seen as a positive eugenic measure. It was only an additional factor. For example, the Soviet threat after World War II may have been another factor.
92. Ali Esat Birol, *Öjenik Tatbikatı*, p. 45.
93. Obviously, this is only anecdotal evidence. When re-reading Ali Esat's piece, my father happened to be nearby. When I read the passage to him, he finished my sentence: 'yes, of course, sterilization operations'. Intrigued by his statement, I asked him to explain what he meant. He explained that when he was getting ready to do his military service in the late 1950s, he and others of his generation had heard from individuals who did their military service earlier that 'some soldiers were sterilized when serving in the military'. While the actual phrase he used was '*hadım etmek*' (castrate, or literally 'turn into a eunuch'), he meant sterilisation. Whether it was true or not, it is important to note that such a fear was etched in the memories of a younger generation of soldier candidates getting ready to do their service in the 1950s and 1960s. Personal conversation with Kadir Yanıkdağ on 29 March 2010 in Armutlu, Yalova.
94. Şükrü Hazım Tiner, *Eugenik Bahsine Umumi bir Bakış*, p. 33. See also Robert M. Yerkes, 'Psychological Examining in the United States Army', pp. 1–890. For the test's criticism, see Stephen Jay Gould, *The Mismeasure of Man*, pp. 222ff.
95. Refia Uğurel-Şemin, *Ordu Alfa Testleri 'Army Alpha Tests'*; Refia Uğurel-Şemin, *Stanford-Binet Ölçeğinin İstanbul Çocuklarına Uygulanması*.

BIBLIOGRAPHY

ARCHIVAL SOURCES
England

Public Record Office, London:
 Foreign Office, 371 and 383
 War Office, 95
 Cabinet, 21/60
British Library, India Office, London:
 Secret and Political Files, L/P&S/11
Imperial War Museum, London:
 Lt Col H. A. Strachan Papers
 Lt J. F. B. O'Sullivan Papers
 Sir Gerard Clauson Papers

Turkey

Askeri Tarih ve Stratejik Etüd Başkanlığı (ATASE), Ankara:
 Birinci Dünya Harbi Kolleksiyonu (World War I Collection)
Başbakanlık Osmanlı Arşivi (Prime Ministry Ottoman Archives), Istanbul:
 HR-HMŞ- Dahiliye Hukuk Müşavirliği
 DH-İUM- Dahiliye İdare-i Umumiye Evrakı
 DH-SYS- Dahiliye Siyasi Evrakı
 DH-KMS- Dahiliye Kalem-i Mahsus
Başbakanlık Cumhuriyet Arşivi (Prime Ministry Republican Archives), Ankara:
 General Collection
İnkilap Tarihi Arşivi (Archives of the Turkish Revolution), Ankara:
 General Collection

United States

United States Department of State, Documents Relating to Internal Affairs of Turkey, 1910–1928.
United States Department of State, Records of the Department of State Relating to World War I and its Termination, Record Group 59, Microfilm Publication M367, Washington, DC, National Archives, 1972.
University Archives, University of Illinois:
Donald A. Lowrie Papers

PRISONER OF WAR CAMP NEWSPAPERS (IN MANUSCRIPT)

Badiye
Esaret
Esaret Albümü
Esaret Hatırası
Garnizon
Hatıra-yı Esaret
Işık
İzmir
Kızıl Elma
Ne Munasebet
Nilüfer
Türk Varlığı
Vaveyla
Yarın
Zincir

OTHER PRIMARY SOURCES

A. Rıza, 'Pellagra ve Vitaminler', *İstanbul Seririyatı* 13 (1932), pp. 128–32.
A. Süleyman, 'Esaret Hatıraları', *Vakit* (various dates in 1920).
Adasal, Rasim, 'Sinir İhtilâçları ve Bayılmaları', in Nazım Şakir Şakar (ed.), *Ordu Doktorunun Nöropsişiatri Kılavuzu* (Istanbul: Askeri Basımevi, 1946), pp. 58–79.
Akçura, Yusuf, *Osmanlı Hilal-i Ahmer Cemiyeti Rusya Üsera Murahhası Yusuf Akçura Bey'in Raporu* (Dersaadet/Istanbul: Matbaa-yı Orhaniye, 1335/1919).
al-Aref, Aref, *Aref al-Aref: a Biographical Sketch, 1892–1964* (Jerusalem: al-Ma'aref Press, n.d.).
Altınay, Ahmet, *Katran Kazanında Sterilize: Bir Türk Subayı'nın İngiliz Esir Kampında Üç Yılı* (Istanbul: Tarih Düşünce Kitapları, 2004).
Anon., 'Esaret günlerinin hatırası', *Sabah* (various dates in 1918).
Anon., 'Pellagra in Egypt in 1918'. *The Lancet* (8 May 1920), p. 1,027.
Anon., 'Recent Researches on Pellagra in Egypt', *The Lancet* (1921), pp. 189–90.
Apak, Rahmi, *Yetmişlik Bir Subayın Hatıraları* (Ankara: Türk Tarih Kurumu, 1988).
Ataman, Halil, *Esaret Yılları: Bir Yedek Subayın I. Dünya Savaşı Şark Cephesi Hatıraları* (Istanbul: Kardeşler Matbaası, 1990).
Atay, Falih Rıfkı, *Zeytindağı* (Istanbul: Pozitif, 2004).

Ayberk, Nuri Fehmi, 'Türkiye Trahom Mücadelesi Tarihçesine ait Hatıralarım', *İstanbul Göz Kliniği Bülteni* 19 (October 1961), pp. 127–8.

[Ayberk], Nuri Fehmi, *Trahom* (Istanbul: Milli Matbaa, 1927).

Aydemir, Şevket Süreyya, *Suyu Arayan Adam* (Istanbul: Remzi Kitabevi, 1997).

Aydın, Hüseyin, *Acı Hatıralar* (Istanbul: Sinan Matbaası, 1965).

Aziz Samih, *Büyük Harpte Kafkas Cephesi Hatıraları: Zividen Peteriçe* (Ankara: Erkanıharbiye Matbaası, 1934).

Baki, Miralay, *Yurt Müdafaası, Seferde ve Hazarda Zabit ve Zabitlik* (Ankara: Köyhocası Matbaası, 1932).

Başkatipzade Ragıp Bey, *Tarih-i Hayatım: Tahsil-Harp-Esaret-Kurtuluş Anıları* (Ankara: Kebikeç, 1996).

Baytin, Arif, *İlk Dünya Harbinde Kafkas Cephesi: 29. Tümen ve 3. Alay Sancağı Hatıraları* (Istanbul: Vakit, 1946).

Bediüzzaman Said Nursi, *Hayatı-Mesleki-Tercüme-i Hâli* (Istanbul: Sözler Yayinevi, 1991).

Bedreddin, 'Pollagra bir Avitaminose Hastalığımıdır?', *İstanbul Seririyatı* 13 (1932), pp. 104–5.

Bigland, Douglas, 'Oedema as a Symptom', *The Lancet* (31 January 1920), pp. 314–16.

Bigland, Douglas, 'Pellagra Outbreak in Egypt', *The Lancet* (1 May 1920), pp. 947–53.

Bilge, Rüştü, '(Temaruz) ve (Sar'a)' *Askeri Sihhiye Mecmuası* 67 (1938), pp. 33–41.

Birol, Ali Esat, *Öjenik Tatbikatı: Yedinci Milli Türk Tıb Kurultayı* (Istanbul: Kader, 1938).

Burridge, W., 'Pellagra among the Prisoners in Egypt', *The Lancet* (9 October 1920), p. 764.

Çakıröz, Raci, *Çarlık ve Bolşevik Rusya'da 10 Yıl: Bnb. Raci Çakıröz'ün Hatıraları* (Istanbul: Belge Yayınları, 1990).

Çantay, Hasan Basri, *Kara Günler ve İbret Levhaları* (Istanbul: Ahmed Said Matbaası, 1964).

Çelik, Osman Şerafeddin, 'Bir Pellagra Vak'ası', *Türk Tıb Cemiyeti Mecmuası* 2 (1936), pp. 16–18.

Çelik, Osman Şerafeddin, 'Harp ve Sari Hastalıklar', *İstanbul Seririyatı* 22 (1940), pp. 8–14.

Çöl, Emin, *Çanakkale – Sina Savaşları* (Ankara: Güryılmaz Matbaası, 1977).

Doğantuğ, Mevlut, 'Ruh Hastalıklarında Anormal Reaksiyonlar', in Nazım Şakir Şakar (ed.), *Ordu Doktorunun Nöropsişiyatri Kılavuzu* (Istanbul: Askeri Basımevi, 1946), pp. 110–28.

Dwinger, Edwin Erich, *Prisoner of War: a Siberian Diary* (New York, NY: Knopf, 1930).

Enright, J. I., 'Pellagra Outbreak in Egypt: II – Pellagra amongst German Prisoners of War', *The Lancet* (8 May 1920), pp. 998–1,003.

Enright, J. I., 'War Oedema in Turkish Prisoners of War', *The Lancet* (7 February 1920), pp. 314–16.

Erbuğ, A. Hilmi, 'Kaybolan Yıllar', *Askeri Tarih Bülteni* 19 (1994), pp. 177–264.

Erev, Muhiddin, 'I. Dünya Savaşında bir Yedek Subay'ın Anıları', *Hayat Tarih Mecmuası* 3 (various issues, 1967).

Eyüb Sabri, *Esaret Hatıraları* [orig. *Bir Esirin Hatıraları*], ed. Nejat Sefercioğlu (Istanbul: Tercüman, [1922] 1978).

[Gökay], Fahreddin Kerim, *Türkiye'de Felc-i Umumi Mes'elesi* (Istanbul: Kader Matbaası, 1927).

[Gökay], Fahrettin Kerim, *Yorgun Sinirler ve Marazi Aşklar Üzerine Ruhi Tedkikler* (Istanbul: Kader Matbaası, 1928).

[Gökay], Fahrettin Kerim, *Akıl Hıfzıssıhası 'Hygiene Mentale' Noktai Nazarından Ruhi Tetkikler* (Istanbul: Kader, 1930).

[Gökay], Fahreddin Kerim, *Ruh Hastalıkları* (Istanbul: Vatandaş Matbaası, 1931).

[Gökay], Fahreddin Kerim, *Türkiye'de İntiharlar Meselesi* (Istanbul: Kader Matbaası, 1932).
[Gökay], Fahreddin Kerim, 'Milli Nüfus Siyasetinde (Eugenique) Meselesinin Mahiyeti', *Ülkü* 13: 15 (1934), pp. 206–12.
Gökay, F. Kerim, 'Raşit Tahsin Hocamız', *Tıp Dünyası* 9 (1936), pp. 3,069–76.
Gökay, Fahrettin Kerim, *Beden Yapılışı ve Karakter Münasebeti* (Istanbul: Kader Basımevi, 1936).
Gökay, Fahrettin Kerim, *Biolojinin Psişiyatride Teşhis ve Tedavi Bakımından Kıymeti* (Istanbul: Kader Basımevi, 1938).
Gökay, Fahrettin Kerim, *Kısırlaştırmanın Rolü* (Istanbul: Kader Basımevi, 1938).
Gökay, Fahreddin K, 'Türkiyenin Hijyen mental ve psişiyatri sahasındaki hizmetleri', *Tıp Dünyası* (1939), pp. 2–4.
Gökay, Fahrettin Kerim, *Türkiye'nin Hijyen Mental ve Psişiyatri Sahasındaki Hizmetleri* (reprint of an article from *Tıb Dünyası*, number 135, 1939) (Istanbul: Kader Basımevi, 1939).
Gökay, Fahrettin Kerim, 'İrade ve Sinir Sağlamlığı', in *CHP Konferanları 12* (Ankara: Ulus, 1940), pp. 3–8.
Gökay, Fahrettin Kerim, 'Irk Hıfzıshhasında İrsiyetin Rölü ve Nesli Tereddiden Korumak Çareleri', in *CHP Konferanları 12* (Ankara: Ulus, 1940), pp. 12–15.
Gökay, Fahrettin Kerim, 'Ruh Hastalıklarının Tekevvününde İrsiyet ve Bünye Noktasından Yapılan Araştırmalar', *Türk Tıb Cemiyeti Mecmuası* 6: 11 (1940), pp. 284–305.
Gökay, Fahrettin Kerim, 'Harb ve Sinir', *Tıb Dünyası* 14 (1941), pp. 4,605–12.
Gökay, Fahrettin K, 'Harpte Nöro-psişiyatri', *Tıb Dünyası* 14 (1941), pp. 4,769–71.
Gökay, Fahrettin Kerim, *Akıl Hastalıklarının Tekevvününde İrsiyet ve Alkolün Tesiri* (Istanbul: Kenan, 1942).
Gökay, Fahrettin Kerim, '21 Ocakta München Üniversitesinde Yapılan Dr. Honoris Causa Töreninde Psychiatri Kliniği Anfisinde Prof. Gökay'ın Konferansı', *Tıb Dünyası* 27 (1954), pp. 2,083–90.
Gökay, F. Kerim, 'Türk Tababeti Ruhiye Tarihi', *Tıp Dünyası* 48 (1975), pp. 368–79.
Gökçay, Hayri, *Bir Türk'ün Hatırat ve İntikamı* (Istanbul: Sıralar Matbaası, 1958).
Göze, Ahmet, *Rusya'da Üç Esaret Yılı*, 2nd edn (Istanbul: Boğaziçi, 1991).
Gündüz, Asım, *Hatıralarım* (Istanbul: Kervan, 1973).
H. Cemal, *Mehmetçiğin Esareti-yahut Esir Olma!!!* (Dersaadet/Istanbul: Matbaa-yı Nefaset, 1329/1913).
H. Cemal, *Tekrar Başımıza Gelenler* (Istanbul: Kastaş, 1991).
Harputlu, Hüseyin Tevfik, 'Birinci Dünya Savaşında Ruslar'a Esir Düşen Bir Subayın Türkistan Hatıraları', *Hayat Tarih Mecmuası* 3 and 4 (1971).
Hasan Basri Efendi, *Bir Gemi Kâtibinin Esaret Hatıraları* (Istanbul: Yapı Kredi Yayınları, 2009).
His, Wilhelm, 'Medizinisches aus der Türkei', *Deutsche Medizinische Wochenschrift* 43 (15 November 1917), p. 1,463.
Hüseyin Kenan, 'Akıl Hijyeni', *Sıhhi Sahifeler* 1: 12 (1923), pp. 168–70.
Hüseyin Kenan, 'Psikopatlar', *İstanbul Seririyatı* 3: 16 (1339/1923), pp. 385–90.
İnan, M. Rauf, *Bir Ömrün Öyküsü: Köy Enstitüleri ve Sonrası* (Ankara: Öğretmen, 1988).
İncesu, Sokrat, *Birinci Dünya Savaşında Çanakkale-Arıburnu Hatıralarım* (Çanakkale: Esen Matbaası, 1964).
İrfanoğlu, Ahmet Rıza (ed.), *Allahüekber Dağları'ndan Sibirya'ya: İrfanoğlu İsmail Efendi'nin Esaret Yılları Hatıraları (1914–1920)* (Istanbul: n.p., 2004).
İsmail Hakkı, *Şanlı Asker Ali Çavuş* (Ankara: Genelkurmay Basımevi, 1991).

İsmail Hakkı, *Yiğitlere Öğütler-Gazilere Armağan*, 2nd edn, ed. Kemaleddin Şenocak (Munich: Islamischer Verlag, 1977).

İybar, Tahsin, *Sibirya'dan Serendib'e* (Ankara: Ulus Basımevi, 1950).

İzzeddin Şadan, 'Bünyevi Psikopatilere dair Ruhi Tedkikler', *İstanbul Seririyatı* 8 (1339/1923), pp. 1,287–93.

Karaman, Sami Sabit, *İstiklâl Mücadelesi ve Enver Paşa: Trabzon ve Kars Hatıraları, 1921–1922* (Istanbul: Selüloz Basımevi, 1949).

Kenan Tevfik, 'Kadınları Kısırlaştırma Usulleri ve Bunların Akıl ve Ruh Hastalıklarındaki Tatbik Mahalleri', *Türk Ginekoloji Arşivi* 1 (1934), pp. 92–7.

Kraepelin, Emil, 'Psychiatric Observations on Contemporary Issues', *History of Psychiatry* 3 (1992), pp. 253–69.

Kuşçubaşı, Eşref, *Turkish Battle at Khaybar*, compiled by Philip H. Stoddard and H. Basri Danışman (Istanbul: Arba, 1997).

Lelean, P. S., 'Pellagra', *The Lancet* (17 July 1920), p. 157.

Mehmed Âsaf, *Volga Kıyılarında ve Muhtıra: Esâret Hâtıra ve Mâceraları*, ed., Murat Cebecioğlu (İzmir: Akademi Kitapevi, 1994).

Mehmed Emin, *Memleketimizde İntişar Etmekte Olan Mısır Hastalığı* (Istanbul: Necm-i İstiklal Matbaası, 1337/1921).

Muhtar, [Ahmed], 'Memleketimizde Trahom', *İstanbul Seririyatı* 1: 8 (1335/1919), pp. 159–61.

Muhtar, Ahmed, 'Memleketimizde Trahom', *İstanbul Seririyatı* 2: 10 (1336/1920), pp. 380–82.

Mümtaz, Hüseyin, 'Bir mülazım-ı evvelin harb ve esaret günleri: İmparatorluk'tan Cumhuriyet'e bir ömür', *Tarih ve Medeniyet* 3 (1996), pp. 28–33.

Mustafa Hayrullah, 'Harb-i Hazırın Emraz-ı 'Asabiye ve 'Akliyeye Öğretikleri', in *şişli Müessesinde Emraz-ı Akliye ve Asabiye Müsamereleri*, numara 7 (Istanbul: Hilal Matbaası, 1333/1917), pp. 8–17.

Mustafa Hayrullah, *Emraz-ı 'Asabiyye* (Istanbul: Devlet Matbaası, 1928).

Mustafa Hayrullah, *Asabiye Hastalıkları: Nuhâ, Asabimuhitiye, Sempatik Sistemi Hastalıkları, Nevrozlar* (Istanbul: Devlet Matbaası, 1929).

Nabi, Yaşar, 'Nufus Meselesi Karşısında Türkiye', *Ülkü* 13 (1939), pp. 33–9.

Niyazi İsmet, *Küçük Sıhhat Memurlarına Mahsus Trahom ve Sair Göz Sari Hastalıkları* (Ankara: T. O. Matbaası, 1934).

Noyan, Abdulkadir, 'Öjenik Münakaşası', in *Yedinci Milli Türk Tıp Kurultayı* (Istanbul: Kader, 1938), pp. 87–8.

Noyan, Abdulkadir, 'Harp Salgınları=Epidemies de guerre', *Askeri Sıhhıye Mecmuası* 69 (1940), pp. 6–7.

Noyan, Abdulkadir, *Son Harplerde Salgın Hastalıklarla Savaşlarım* (Ankara: Havadis Matbaası, 1956).

Nureddin, 'Mısır çöllerinde Türk gençleri', *Vakit* (various dates in 1920).

Ölçen, Mehmet Arif, *Vetluga Irmağı* (Ankara: Ümit Yayıncılık, 1994).

Ölçen, Mehmet Arif, *Vetluga Memoir: a Turkish Prisoner of War in Russia, 1916–1918* (Gainesville, FL: University of Florida Press, 1995).

Orfanidis, Emil, 'Irkın Tereddisine Karşı Mücadele', *Türk Tıb Cemiyeti Mecmuası* 1: 8 (August 1935), pp. 463–7.

Osman Cevdet, 'Nevrasteni – ateh', *İstanbul Dar'ül Funun Tıb Fakültesi Mecmuası* 6 (1340/1924), pp. 572–8.

Özkök, Hidayet, *Çanakkale'den-Hicaz'a Harp Hatıraları* (Kayseri: Kültür Müdürlüğü, 1992).
Price, Hereward T., *Boche and Bolshevik: Experiences of an Englishman in the German Army and in Russian Prisons* (London: John Murray, 1919).
Pye, Ernest, *Prisoner of War, 31,163 – Bedros M. Sharian* (New York, NY: Fleming H. Revell Company, 1938).
Roaf, H. E., 'A Contribution to the Pathology of Pellagra', *Journal of the Royal Army Medical Corps* 34 (1920), pp. 534–8.
S. Şükrü, 'Trahom: Trachome – Tarihçesi – Avrupa ve Asyada Saha-yı İntişarı – Türkiye'de Trahom', *İstanbul Seririyati* 8 (Kanun-i Sani, 1927), pp. 1,355–50.
Şadan, İzzettin, 'Bünyevi Psikopatlara Dair Ruhi Tedkikler', *İstanbul Seririyatı* 8: 6 (1926/1927), pp. 1,287–93.
Şadan, İzzettin, 'Schizophrenie (Erken Bunama) – E. Bleuler', *İstanbul Seririyatı* 14 (1932), pp. 189–93.
Sağlam, Tevfik, *Büyük Harpte 3. Orduda Sıhhi Hizmet* (Istanbul: Askeri Matbaa, 1941).
Said Cemil, 'Pellagra', *Ceride-i Tıbbiye-i Askeriye* 49 (1920), pp. 1,181–4.
[Şakar], Nazım Şakir, '(330-332) Üçüncü Ordu Mıntıkasında beray Müşahede ve Muayene – Mütehassına Gönderilen 412 Emraz-ı Asabiye Vakası', in *Şişli Müessesinde Emraz-ı Akliye ve Asabiye Müsamereleri*, numara 2 (Dersaadet/Istanbul: Matbaa-i Zeliç Biraderler, 1332/1916), pp. 33–4.
[Şakar], Nazım Şakir, '(330-332) Üçüncü Ordu Mıntıkasında Müşahede-i Seririyesi Tarafından İcra Kılınan 57 Emraz-ı Akliye Vakası', in *Şişli Müessesinde Emraz-ı Akliye ve Asabiye Müsamereleri*, numara 2 (Dersaadet/Istanbul: Matbaa-i Zeliç Biraderler, 1332/1916), p. 36.
[Şakar], Nazım Şakir. 'Erzurum Santral Sertababetine Vurud Eden (70,000) hastada Muayene-yi Maddiyye-i Ruhiye Yapılmış (2,000) Neferin Dejenere Derece ve Yüzdeki Nisbetleri', in *Şişli Müessesinde Emraz-ı Akliye ve Asabiye Müsamereleri*, numara 2 (Dersaadet/Istanbul: Matbaa-i Zeliç Biraderler, 1332/1916), p. 35.
[Şakar], Nazım Şakir, 'Emraz-ı Asabiye ve Akliyede Teşhis', *İstanbul Seririyatı* 2 (1337/1921), pp. 182–8.
[Şakar], Nazım Şakir, *Emraz-ı Asabiye Dersleri* (Istanbul: Kader Matbaası, 1924).
[Şakar], Nazım Şakir, *Temaruz ve Teşhisi* (Istanbul: Mekteb-i Tıbbiye-yi Askeriye Matbaası, 1340/1924).
Şakar, Nazım Şakir (ed.), *Ordu Doktorunun Nöropsişiyatri Kılavuzu* (Istanbul: Askeri Basımevi, 1946).
Şakar, Nazım Şakir, 'Orduda Temaruz (Simulation)', in Nazım Şakir Şakar (ed.), *Ordu Doktorunun Nöropsişıatri Kılavuzu* (Istanbul: Askeri Basımevi, 1946), pp. 145–62.
Sanan, Münif, 'Asabi ve Ruhi Muayene ve Teshis Usulleri', in Nazım Şakir Şakar (ed.), *Ordu Doktorunun Nöropsişiyatri Kılavuzu* (Istanbul: Askeri Basımevi, 1946), pp. 3–20.
Selçuk, Sadi, *Esaretin Acı Hatıraları* (Konya: n.p., 1955).
Serhadoğlu, M. Rıza, *Savaşçı Doktorun İzinde* (Istanbul: Remzi, 2005).
Şerif Bey, Kaymakam, *Sarıkamış İhata Manevrası ve Meydan Muharebesi* (Istanbul: Necm-i İstiklal Matbaası, 1922).
Şerif Bey, Kaymakam, *Sarıkamış İhata Manevrası*, ed. Murat Çulcu (Istanbul: Arba Yayınları, 1998).
Sorguç, Erdoğan (ed.), *Kaybolan Filistin: Yd. P. Tğm. İbrahim Sorguç'un Anıları, İstiklal Harbi Hatıratı* (Izmir: E. Sorguç, 1996).
[Şükrü], İhsan Schükry and Fahreddin Kerim [Gökay], 'Die Geschicte der Psychiatrie in

der Türkei', *Allgemeine Zeitschrift für Psychiatrie und Psychich-Gerichliche Medizin* 84 (1926), pp. 403-7.

Şükrü, Yusuf, 'Pellagra Hakkında', *Sıhhıye Mecmuası* 4 (1928), pp. 39-40.

Tanrıkurt, Asaf, *Yemen Notları* (Ankara: Güzel Sanatlar Matbaası, 1965).

Taşer, M. Fevzi, *Cepheden Cepheye - Esaretten Esarete (Ürgüplü Mustafa Fevzi Taşer'in Hatıraları)* (Ankara: Kültür Bakanlığı, 2000).

Tenner, Arthur S., 'Experiences of an Eye Surgeon in the Near East Relief in Turkey and Syria from March, 1919, to July, 1920', *The Medical Pickwick* 12 (June 1921), pp. 203-7.

Tevfik Rüşdü, 'Teksir-i Nufus', *İstanbul Seririyatı* 2 (1338/1922), pp. 101-4.

[Tiner], Şükrü Hazım, 'Nevrasteni ve 'Ateh-i Nâbehengâm', in *Emraz-ı 'Akliye ve 'Asabiye Müsamereleri*, numara 9 (Istanbul: Hilal Matbaası, 1334/1918), pp. 29-31.

[Tiner], Şükrü Hazım, 'Babinskiye nazaran isteri', *İstanbul Seririyatı* 1: 3 (1 Ağustos 1335), pp. 68-71.

[Tiner], Şükrü Hazım, 'Pellagra', *İstanbul Seririyatı* 2 (1336/1920), pp. 249-52.

Tiner, Şükrü Hazım, *Eugenik Bahsine Umumi Bir Bakış: Yedinci Milli Türk Tıb Kurultayı* (Istanbul: Kader, 1938).

Tokgöz, Server Kamil, *Öjenism, 'Irk Islahı'* (Ankara: Sümer Yayınevi, 1938).

Tonguç, Faik, *Birinci Dünya Savaşında Bir Yedek Subay'ın Anıları* (Istanbul: İş Bankası Kültür Yayınları, 1999).

Tuğaç, Hüsamettin, *Bir Neslin Dramı: Kafkas Cephesinden, Çarlık Rusyasında Tutsaklıktan Anılar* (Istanbul: Çağdaş Yayınları, 1975).

[Uzman], Mazhar Osman, 'Türkler Mütereddimi', in Mazhar Osman [Uzman], *Sıhhi Hitabeler* (Istanbul: Mahmud Bey Matbaası, 1915), pp. 80-109.

[Uzman], Mazhar Osman, 'Harb Nevrozları', in *Şehir Emaneti Şişli Müessesinde Emraz-ı akliye ve Asabiye Müsamereleri*, numara 4 (Dersaadet/Istanbul: Hilal Matbaası, 1333/1917), pp. 3-8.

[Uzman], Mazhar Osman, 'Babinki'ye Nazaran İsterya', in *Şehir Emaneti Şişli Müessesinde Emraz-ı akliye ve Asabiye Müsamereleri*, numara 6 (Dersaadet/Istanbul: Hilal Matbaası, 1333/1917), pp. 25-7.

[Uzman], Mazhar Osman, 'Nutk-u iftitahi', in *Şehir Emaneti Şişli Müessesinde Emraz-ı Akliye ve Asabiye Müsamereleri*, numara 11 (Istanbul: Sancakcıyan Matbaası, 1334), pp. 1-2.

[Uzman], Mazhar Osman, 'Harbde görülen veka'iden', in *Şehir Emaneti Şişli Müessesinde Emraz-ı akliye ve Asabiye Müsamereleri*, numara 8 (1334/1918), pp. 3-6.

[Uzman], Mazhar Osman, 'Tababet-i Akliye ve Asabiye Kongresi', *İstanbul Seririyatı* 1: 7 (1335/1919), pp. 135-8.

[Uzman], Mazhar Osman, 'Harb'den Sonra', *İstanbul Seririyatı* 2 (1336/1920), pp. 89-90.

[Uzman], Mazhar Osman, 'Sinir Hastalıkları ve Hidmeti Askeriye', *İstanbul Seririyati* 4 (1341/1921), pp. 844-9.

[Uzman], Mazhar Osman, 'Sendemi Brütüs?', *İstanbul Seririyatı* 2 (August 1337/1921), pp. 89-92.

[Uzman], Mazhar Osman, 'Üçüncü Emraz-ı Asabiye ve Akliye Kongresi', *İstanbul Seririyatı* 3 (1337/1921), pp. 112-16.

[Uzman], Mazhar Osman, 'Viladi ve Kısbi Cinnetler', *Sıhhi Sahifalar* 1: 12 (1923), pp. 170-3.

[Uzman], Mazhar Osman, *Akıl Hastalıkları* (Istanbul: Kader Matbaası, 1928).

[Uzman], Mazhar Osman, 'Nufus Bereketi Arefesindeyiz II', *Sıhhi Sahifalar* (1930), pp. 33-8.

[Uzman], Mazhar Osman, 'Mecnunlar Arasında Mücrim Tipleri, 5', *İstanbul Seririyatı* 12

(1930), pp. 2,922–4.
[Uzman], Mazhar Osman, 'Nufus Bereketi Arefesindeyiz', *Sıhhi Sahifalar* n. v. (February 1930), pp. 33–8.
[Uzman], Mazhar Osman, 'Mecnunlar Arasında Mücrim Tipleri, 3', *İstanbul Seririyatı* 12 (1931), pp. 3,776–9.
[Uzman], Mazhar Osman, 'Cumhuriyetin Sıhhat Siyaseti', in Mazhar Osman (ed.), *Sıhhat Almanakı* (Istanbul: Kader Matbaası, 1933), pp. 35–43.
[Uzman], Mazhar Osman (ed.), *Sıhhat Almanakı* (Istanbul: Kader Matbaası, 1933).
Uzman, Mazhar Osman, 'İdiş ve Kısır etme', in *Eugenic İdiş, Kısır ve Eyi Çocuk Yetişdirme Hakkında İki Konferans* (Istanbul: Kader, 1935).
Uzman, Mazhar Osman, *İdiş ve Kısır Etme* (Istanbul: Kader Matbası, 1935).
Uzman, Mazhar Osman, 'Kısır ve İdiş Etme (sterilisation et castration)', *Türk Tıb Cemiyeti Mecmuası* 1: 5 (1935), pp. 248–52.
Uzman, Mazhar Osman, *Eugenic, İdiş, Kısır ve Eyi Çocuk Yetiştirme Hakkında İki Konferans* (Istanbul: Kader, 1935).
Uzman, Mazhar Osman, 'Ruh tıbbının içtimaiyatta rolü', *İstanbul Seririyatı* 19 (1937), pp. 203–10.
Uzman, Mazhar Osman, 'Öjenik', in *CHP Konferansları 2* (Ankara: n.p., 1939), pp. 3–12.
Uzman, Mazhar Osman, 'Ord. Prof. Mazhar Osman'ın Söylevi', *Tıp Fakültesi Mecmuası* 1: 7 (1939), pp. 1,060–73.
Uzman, Mazhar Osman, 'Konferans', *İstanbul Seririyatı* 22 (June 1940), pp. 58–60.
Uzman, Mazhar Osman, *Tababeti Ruhiye*, 2 vols (Istanbul: Kader Basımevi, 1941).
Uzman, Mazhar Osman, 'Pellagra ve Sinir Sistemi Hastalıkları', *İstanbul Seririyatı* 26 (1944), pp. 3–12.
[Uzman], Mazhar Osman, *Psychiatria*, 4th edn (Istanbul: Kader Basımevi, 1947).
Vischer, Adolf L., 'Some Remarks on the Psychology of Internment: Based on Observations on Prisoners of War in Switzerland', *The Lancet* 97 (1919), pp. 696–7.
Vischer, Adolf L., *Barbed Wire Disease: a Psychological Study of the Prisoners of War* (London: Bale and Danielson, 1919).
Woodcock, H. M., 'Helminthic Infections and Pellagra', *The Lancet* (7 August 1920), p. 320.
Yoldaş, Cemil Zeki, *Kendi Kaleminden Teğmen Cemil Zeki (Yoldaş), Anılar-Mektuplar* (Istanbul: Arba, 1994).

OFFICIAL PUBLICATIONS

Başvekalet İstatistik Genel Direktörlüğü, *1935 20 İlkteşrin Genel Nufus Sayımı, Türkiye Nufusu*. (Ankara: Ulus, 1935).
Boyd, F. D., and P. S. Lelean, *Report of a Committee of Enquiry Regarding the Prevalence of Pellagra among Turkish Prisoners of War* (Alexandria: Army Printing and Stationary Department, 1919).
Carnegie Endowment for International Peace, *Report of the International Commission to Inquire into the Causes and Conduct of the Balkan Wars* (Washington, DC: Carnegie Endowment for International Peace, 1914).
Devlet İstatistik Enstitüsü, *Genel Nufus Sayımı, 1927* (Ankara: n.p., n.d.).
Genelkurmay Harp Tarihi Başkanlığı, *Türk İstiklâl Harbine Katılan Tümen ve Daha Üst Kademelerdeki Komutanların Biyografileri* (Ankara: Genelkurmay Basımevi, 1972).
Hammond-Searle, A. C., and A. G. Stevenson, *Report of Investigations on Pellagra among*

Turkish Prisoners of War in Egypt, 1920 (Alexandria: Whitehead Morris, 1921).

İstanbul Emraz-ı 'Akliye ve 'Asabiye Müessesi, *İstanbul Emraz-ı 'Akliye ve 'Asabiye Müessesi Senelik Mesa'isi: 339-340 Senelerine Mahsus* (Istanbul: Kader Matbaası, 1925).

Matbuat Umum Müdürlüğü, 'Osmanlı İmparatorluğundan Türkiye Cumhuriyetine', in *Fotoğraflarla Türkiye* (Ankara: Matbuat Umum Müdürlüğü, 1938).

Red Cross, *Reports on British Prison-Camps in India and Burma: Visited by the International Red Cross Committee in February, March and April, 1917* (London: T. Fisher Unwin, 1917).

Red Cross, *Turkish Prisoners of War in Egypt: a Report by the Delegates of the International Committee of the Red Cross* (London: HMSO, 1917).

Royal Commission, *Palestine Royal Commission Report, 1936* (London: HMSO, 1937).

Sağlık ve Sosyal Yardım Bakanlığı, *Sağlık Hizmetlerinde 50 Yıl* (Ankara: n.p., 1973).

Sıhhat ve İçtimai Muavenet Vekaleti, *Trahom Hakkında Halka Nasayih* (Dersaadet/Istanbul: Hilal Matbaası, 1340/1924).

Sıhhat ve İçtimai Muavenet Vekaleti, *Sıhhiye Mecmuası Fevkalâde Nüshası: Vekâletin 10 Yıllık Mesaisi* (n.p: n.p., 1933).

Sıhhat ve İçtimai Muavenet Vekalati, *Trahom Mücadele Talimatnamesi* (Ankara: İdeal Basımevi, 1944).

T. B. M. M. (Türkiye Büyük Millet Meclisi), *Zabıt Ceridesi*. First Term, Second Legislation Year, volume 10.

T. B. M. M. (Türkiye Büyük Millet Meclisi), *Zabıt Ceridesi*. Sixth Term, Second Legislation Year, volume 10.

Türk Dil Kurumu, *Türkçe Hekimlik Terimleri Üzerine bir Deneme* (Bursa: Yeni Basımevi, 1944).

War Office, *Statistics of the Military Effort of the British Empire During the Great War, 1914–1920* (London: HMSO, 1922).

SECONDARY SOURCES

Açıksözcü, Hüsnü, *İstiklal Harbinde Kastamonu* (Kastamonu: Kastamonu Vilayet Matbaası, 1933).

Ahıska, Meltem, 'Occidentalism: The Historical Fantasy of the Modern', *South Atlantic Quarterly* 102 (Spring/Summer 2003), pp. 351–79.

Ahmad, Feroz, *The Making of Modern Turkey* (New York, NY: Routledge, 1993).

Ahmad, Jalal Al-e, *Gharbzedegi/Weststruckness* (Costa Mesa, CA: Mazda Publishers, 1997).

Akçam, Taner, *From Empire to Republic: Turkish Nationalism and Armenian Genocide* (London: Zed Books, 2004).

Akın, Yiğit, *Gürbüz ve Yavuz Evlatlar: Erken Cumhuriyet'de Beden Terbiyesi ve Spor* (Istanbul: İletişim, 2004).

Aksakal, Mustafa, *The Ottoman Road to War in 1914* (Cambridge: Cambridge University Press, 2008).

Alemdaroğlu, Ayça, 'Politics of the Body and Eugenics Discourse in Early Republican Turkey', *Body and Society* 11 (2005), pp. 61–76.

al-Farsi, M. A., 'Nutritional and Functional Properties of Dates', *Critical Reviews in Food Science and Nutrition* 48 (November 2008), pp. 877–88.

Alkan, Mehmet Ö., 'Modernization from Empire to Republic and Education in the Process of Nationalism', in Kemal Karpat (ed.), *Ottoman Past and Today's Turkey*. (Leiden: Brill,

2000), pp. 47–132.
Altınay, Ayşe Gül, *The Myth of the Military-Nation: Militarism, Gender, and Education in Turkey* (New York, NY: Palgrave, 2005).
Altınay, Ayse Gül, and Tanıl Bora, 'Ordu, Militarizm ve Milliyetçilik', in Tanıl Bora (ed.), *Milliyetçilik* (Istanbul: İletişim Yayınları, 2002), pp. 140–54.
[Altınay], Ahmet Refik, *Tarihte Osmanlı Neferi* (Istanbul: Matbaa-yı Askeriye, 1915).
Anderson, Benedict, *Imagined Communities* (London: Verso, 1991).
Anon., *Anıtlarımız, Şehitlerimiz* (Erzurum: Atatürk Üniversitesi Yayınları, 1978).
Anon., 'Compulsory Matrimony in Turkey', *The Eugenical News* 8 (1922), pp. 22–3.
Anon., 'Marriage Day in Turkey', *Eugenical News* 5 (1920), p. 43.
Anon., 'Medical Profession and the Social Evil', *Medical News* 78 (16 March 1901), pp. 425–26.
Anon., 'Picric Acid Jaundice', *The British Medical Journal* 2 (27 July 1918), pp. 92–3.
Anon., 'The Degeneracy of the Human Species'. *The Crayon* 4 (April 1857), pp. 108–9.
Appadurai, Arjun, *Modernity at Large* (Minneapolis, MN: University of Minnesota Press, 1996).
Appadurai, Arjun, 'The Grounds of the Nation-State: Identity, Violence and Territory', in K. Goldmann and U. Hannerz, *Nationalism and Internationalism in the Post-Cold War Era* (London: Routledge: 2000), pp. 129–40
Arda, B., and C. H. Güvercin, 'Eugenics Concept: From Plato to Present', *Human Reproduction and Genetic Ethics* 14 (2008), pp. 20–6.
Aslan, Erdal, 'Devrim Tarihi Ders Kitapları', in Salih Özbaran (ed.), *Tarih Öğretimi ve Ders Kitapları* (Istanbul: Tarih Vakfı, 1995), pp. 296–8.
Atalay, Mustafa, *Cemal Gürsel ve Hayatı* (Ankara: Kültür Matbaası, 1960).
Audoin-Rouzeau, Stéphane, *Men at War: National Sentiment and Trench Journalism in France During the First World War* (Oxford: Berg, 1992).
Babington, Anthony, *Shell Shock: a History of the Changing Attitudes to War Neurosis* (London: Leo Cooper, 1997).
Barnham, Peter, *Forgotten Lunatics of the Great War* (New Haven, CT: Yale University Press, 2008).
Barrett, James W., 'Trachoma and Visual Standards during the War', *British Medical Journal* (18 August 1923), p. 303.
Batırel, Hasan F., and Mustafa Yüksel, 'Rudolf Nissen's Years in Bosphorus and the Pioneers of Thoracic Surgery', *Annals of Thoracic Surgery* 69: 2 (February 2000), pp. 651–4.
Benjamin, Walter, 'The Storyteller', in Walter Benjamin, *Illuminations: Essays and Reflections* (London: Jonathan Cape, 1970), p. 84.
Berkes, Niyazi, *Development of Secularism in Turkey* (New York, NY: Routledge, 1998).
Beşikçi, Mehmet, ''İhtiyat Zâbiti'nden 'Yedek Subay'a: Osmanlı'dan Cumhuriyet'e Bir Zorunlu Askerlik Kategorisi Olarak Yedek Subaylık ve Yedek Subaylar, 1891–1930', *Tarih ve Toplum: Yeni Yaklaşımlar* 13 (Autumn 2011), pp. 45–89.
Beşikçi, Mehmet, *The Ottoman Mobilization of Manpower in the First World War* (Leiden: Brill, 2012).
Bhabha, Homi K., 'Dissemination: Time, Narrative, and the Margins of the Modern Nation', in Homi K. Bhabha (ed.), *The Location of Culture* (London: Routledge, 1994), pp. 139–70.
Bianchi, Bruna, 'Psychiatrists, Soldiers, and Officers in Italy During the Great War', in Paul Lerner and Mark Micale (eds), *Traumatic Pasts: History, Psychiatry, and Trauma in the Modern Age, 1870–1930* (Cambridge: Cambridge University Press, 2001), pp. 222–52.

Bora, Tanıl, 'İnşa Döneminde Türk Kimliği', *Toplum ve Bilim* 71 (1996), pp. 168–94.
Bourke, Joanna, *Dismembering the Male: Men's Bodies, Britain and the Great War* (Chicago, IL: University of Chicago, 1996).
Bourke, Joanna, 'Effeminacy, Ethnicity and the End of Trauma: the Sufferings of "Shell-shocked" Men in Great Britain and Ireland, 1914–39', *Journal of Contemporary History* 35 (2000), pp. 57–69.
Brunner, Jose, 'Psychiatry, Psychoanalysis, and Politics During the First World War', *Journal of the History of Behavioral Sciences* 27 (1991), pp. 352–65.
Brunner, Jose, 'Will, Desire and Experience: Etiology and Ideology in the German and Austrian Medical Discourse on War Neuroses, 1914–1922', *Transcultural Psychiatry* 37 (September 2000), pp. 295–320.
Burke, Peter, *History and Social Theory* (Ithaca, NY: Cornell University Press, 1992).
Çağaptay, Soner, *Islam, Secularism and Nationalism in Modern Turkey: Who is a Turk?* (New York, NY: Routledge, 2006).
Çakır, Serpil, *Osmanlı Kadın Hareketi* (Istanbul: Metis Yayınları, 1993).
Çambel, Perihan, *Ögenik (Eugenics) Hakkında Düşünceler* (Istanbul: Kader Matbaası, 1946).
Carlson, Eric T., 'Medicine and Degeneration: Theory and Praxis', in Edward Chamberlin and Sander Gilman (eds), *Degeneration: the Dark Side of Progress* (New York, NY: Columbia University Press, 1985), pp. 121–44.
Chamberlin, J. Edward, and Sander L. Gilman, *Degeneration: the Dark Side of Progress* (New York, NY: Columbia University Press, 1985).
Chatterjee, Partha, *Nationalist Thought and the Colonial World: a Derivative Discourse?* (London: Zed Books, 1986).
Chatterjee, Partha, *The Nation and its Fragments: Colonial and Postcolonial Histories* (Princeton, NJ: Princeton University Press, 1993).
Chatterjee, Partha, 'Two Poets and a Death: on Civil and Political Society in the Non-Christian World', in Timothy Mitchell (ed.), *Questions of Modernity* (Minneapolis, MN: University of Minnesota Press, 2000), pp. 35–48.
Collins, Joseph, 'The Etiology, Prognosis, and Treatment of General Paresis' and 'Medical Profession and the Social Evil', *Medical Record* 69 (1906), pp. 125–31, 426.
Criss, Nur Bilge, *Istanbul Under Allied Occupation* (Leiden: Brill, 1999).
Darwin, Leonard, 'Eugenics During and After the War', *The Eugenics Review* 7 (April 1915), pp. 91–106.
Davis, Gerald, 'Prisoner of War Camps as Social Communities: Krasnoyarsk, 1914–1921', *Eastern European Quarterly* (1987), pp. 147–63.
Deak, Istvan, *Beyond Nationalism: a Social and Political History of the Habsburg Officer Corps, 1848–1918* (New York, NY: Oxford University Press, 1990).
Deweese, Devin, *Islamization and Native Religion in the Golden Horde: Baba Tükles and Conversion to Islam in Historical and Epic Tradition* (University Park, PN: Pennsylvania State University Press, 1994).
Dikötter, Frank, 'Race Culture: Recent Perspectives on the History of Eugenics', *American Historical Review* 103 (1998), pp. 467–78.
Doğantuğ, Mevlut, *Orduda Sinir ve Ruh Hastalıkları Serisinden: Erkenbunama (Şizofreni)* (Istanbul: Askeri Basımevi, 1946).
Dolev, Eran, 'The Story of the Pellagra Outbreak among the Turkish POWs at the Final Stage of the Campaign', in Yigal Sheffy and Shaul Shai (eds), *The First World War: Middle Eastern Perspective, Proceedings of the Israeli-Turkish International Colloquy, 3–6 April*

2000, Tel Aviv (Tel Aviv: Tel Aviv University, 2000), pp. 227–32.
Dolev, Eran, *Allenby's Military Medicine: Life and Death in World War I Palestine* (New York, NY: I. B. Tauris, 2007).
Dowling, John E., 'Vitamin A Deficiency and Night Blindness', *Proceedings of the National Academy of Sciences of the United States of America* 44 (1958), pp. 648–61.
Duara, Prasenjit, *Rescuing History from the Nation: Questioning Narratives of Modern China* (Chicago, IL: University of Chicago Press, 1995).
Eason, H. L., 'Ophthalmic Practice in the Mediterranean and Egyptian Expeditionary Forces, 1915–1918', *Guy's Hospital Reports* 70 (1920), pp. 63–114.
Edensor, Tim, *National Identity, Popular Culture, and Everyday Life* (Oxford: Berg, 2002).
Efendieva, Nilüfer, 'Milli Kurtuluş Mücadelesine Kadınların İştiraki (1918–1922)', in *VIII. Türk Tarih Kongresi, 11-15. X. 1976 Kongreye Sunulan Bildiriler*, 3: 1979–84 (Ankara: Türk Tarih Kurumu, 1979).
Enginün, İnci, 'Milli Mücadelede Türk Kadını', *Türk Kültürü* 20 (1982), pp. 618–24, 688–94.
Enginün, İnci, Zeynep Kerman and Selim İleri, *Kurtuluş Savaşı ve Edebiyatımız* (Istanbul: Oğlak, 1998).
Eraksoy, M., 'Mustafa Hayrullah Diker', *Journal of Neurology* 250 (2003), pp. 1,505–6.
Eren, Mehmet Ali, 'İngilizler 15 bin Türk'ü kör etti', *Aksiyon* 200 (3–9 Ekim 1998), pp. 26–30.
Erev, Muhiddin, 'I. Dünya Savaşında bir Yedek Subayın Hâtıraları: 4', *Hayat Tarih Mecmuası* 3: 8 (Ağustos 1967), pp. 58–64.
Ergin, Murat, 'Biometrics and Anthropometrics: Twins of Turkish Modernity', *Patterns of Prejudice* 42 (2008), pp. 281–304.
Ergün, Mustafa, *Atatürk Devri Türk Eğitimi* (Ankara: Ankara Üniversitesi Basımevi, 1982).
Erickson, Edward J., *Ordered to Die: a History of the Ottoman Army in the First World War* (Westport, CN: Greenwood Press, 2000).
Erickson, Edward J., *Ottoman Army Effectiveness in World War I: a Comparative Study* (London: Routledge, 2007).
Eyüboğlu, Sabahattin, *Sanat Üzerine Denemeler, Eleştiriler* (Istanbul: Cem Yayınevi, 1981).
Fanon, Frantz, 'Medicine and Colonialism', in *A Dying Colonialism* (New York, NY: Grove Press, 1965), pp. 121–46.
Ferguson, Niall, *The Pity of War: Explaining World War I* (New York, NY: Basic Books, 1999).
Fethi, Rükneddin, *Doğu Köylerinde* (Ankara: Çığır, 1938).
Findley, Carter V., 'The Advent of Ideology in the Islamic Middle East (Part II)', *Studia Islamica* 56 (1982), pp. 147–80.
Findley, Carter V., *Ottoman Civil Officialdom: a Social History* (Princeton, NJ: Princeton University Press, 1989).
Findley, Carter V., 'An Ottoman Occidentalist in Europe: Ahmet Midhat Meets Madame Gülnar, 1889', *American Historical Review* 103 (1998), pp. 15–49.
Findley, Carter V., *Turkey, Islam, Nationalism and Modernity: a History, 1789–2007* (New Haven, CT: Yale University Press, 2010).
Finlayson, Alan, 'Psychology, Psychoanalysis and Theories of Nationalism', *Nations and Nationalism* 4 (1998), pp. 154–5.
Foucault, M., *Discipline and Punish* (New York, NY: Vintage, 1980).
Foucault, M., *History of Sexuality* (New York, NY: Vintage, 1980).
Frik, Feridun, *Türkiye Cumhuriyetinde Tıb ve Hıfzısıhha Hareketleri, 1923–1938*

(Leverkusen: Universum, 1939).
Fuller, J. G., *Troop Morale and Popular Culture in the British and Dominion Armies, 1914–1918* (Oxford: Clarendon Press, 1990).
Georgeon, François, *Osmanlı-Türk Modernleşmesi (1900–1930)* (Istanbul: YKY, 2000).
Ginzburg, Carlo, *The Cheese and the Worms: the Cosmos of a Sixteenth-Century Miller.* (Baltimore, MD: Johns Hopkins University Press, 1980).
Göçek, Fatma Müge, 'Ethnic Segmentation, Western Education, and Political Outcomes: Nineteenth Century Ottoman Society', *Poetics Today* 14 (1993), pp. 507–38.
Göçek, Fatma Müge, 'Reading Genocide', in Israel Gershoni, Amy Singer and Hakan Erdem (eds), *Middle East Historiographies* (London: I. B. Tauris, 2006), pp. 101–27.
Göçek, Fatma Müge, 'Defining Parameters of a post-nationalist Turkish Historiography through the case of Anatolian Armenians', in Hans-Lukas Kieser (ed.), *Turkey Beyond Nationalism* (London: I. B. Tauris, 2006), pp. 85–103.
Göçek, Fatma Müge, *The Transformation of Turkey* (London: I. B. Tauris, 2011).
Gökalp, Ziya, *Yeni Türkiye'nin Hedefleri* (Istanbul: İstanbul Matbaası, 1977).
Gökalp, Ziya, 'Mefkurenin Harikaları', in Abdulhaluk Çay (ed.), *Makaleler VII* (Ankara: Kültür Bakanlığı Yayınları, 1982).
Gökalp, Ziya, *Turkish Nationalism and Western Civilization: Selected Essays of Ziya Gökalp*, trans. Niyazi Berkes (Westport, CT: Greenwood Press, 1959).
Göldaş, İsmail, *Milli Kurtuluş Savaşında Öğretmenler* (Istanbul: Öğretmen Dünyası Yayınları, 1981).
Gould, Stephen Jay, *The Mismeasure of Man* (New York, NY: W. W. Norton, 1996).
Günbulut, Şükrü, *Neydi Bu İşlerin Aslı? Savaş Şiirleri Antolojisi* (Istanbul: Berfin, 1999).
Gürkan, Kazım İsmail, '14 mart 1827, Türkiyede Hekimliğin (Batı)ya Dönüşü', *Tıp Araştırmaları Dergisi* 1 (1966), pp. 1–33.
Hacking, Ian, *Mad Travellers: Reflections on the Reality of Transient Mental Illness* (Cambridge, MA: Harvard University Press, 2002).
Halman, Talât Sait (trans.), *Fazıl Hüsnü Dağlarca* (Pittsburgh, PA: University of Pittsburgh Press, 1969), p. 152.
Hanioğlu, M. Şükrü, *Young Turks in Opposition* (New York, NY: Oxford University Press, 1995).
Hanioğlu, M. Şükrü, *Preparation for a Revolution: Young Turks, 1902–1908* (New York, NY: Oxford University Press, 2001).
Hansen, Randall, 'Eugenic Ideas, Political Interest, and Policy Variance: Immigration and Sterilization Policy', *World Politics* 53 (2001), pp. 237–63.
Hatemi, Hüsrev, 'Balkan Harbi Yaralıları Adlı Eser ve Dr. Yahoub', *Tıp Tarihi Araştırmaları* 4 (1990), pp. 97–9.
Hawkins, Mike, *Social Darwinism in European and American Thought, 1860–1945* (Cambridge: Cambridge University Press, 1997).
Hawkins, Mike, 'Durkheim's Sociology and theories of Degeneration', *Economy and Society* 28 (February 1999), pp. 118–37.
Heyd, Uriel, *Foundations of Turkish Nationalism: the Life and Teachings of Ziya Gökalp* (Westport, CT: Hyperion Press, 1979).
Hot, Inci, 'Ülkemizde Trahom ile Mücadele', *Tıp Etiği, Hukuku, Tarihi Dergisi* 11 (2003), pp. 22–9.
Hourani, Albert, *Arabic Thought in the Liberal Age, 1798–1939* (London: Oxford University Press, 1970).

Hüseyin Hüsnü Erkilet, *Yıldırım* (Ankara: Genelkurmay Basımevi, 2002).
Hynes, Samuel, *The Soldiers' Tale* (New York, NY: Allen Lane, 1997).
Ikuhiko Hata, 'Japanese Military and Popular Perceptions of POWs', in Bob Moore and Kent Fedorowich (eds), *Prisoners of War and Their Captors in Word War II* (Oxford: Berg, 1996), pp. 253–76.
İlhan, Suat, 'Türk Kurtuluş Hareketinin Safhaları ve Çağdaşlaşmaya Etkileri', *Atatürk Araştırma Merkezi Dergisi* 1 (1985), pp. 319–26.
[İnan], Âfet, 'Türk İstiklâli ve Lozan Muahedesi', *Belleten* 2 (1938), pp. 276–91.
Işık, Adnan, *Malatya, 1830–1919* (Istanbul: Kurtiş, 1998).
Jusdanis, Gregory, *The Necessary Nation* (Princeton, NJ: Princeton University Press, 2001).
Kadıoğlu, Ayşe, 'Milletini Arayan Devlet: Türk Milliyetçiliğinin Açmazları', in A. Ünsal (ed.), *75 Yılda Tebaa'dan Yurttaş'a Dogru* (Istanbul: Tarih Vakfı, 1998), pp. 201–11.
Kadıoğlu, Ayşe, 'Introduction: Understanding Nationalism through Family Resemblances', inAyşe Kadıoğlu and E. Fuat Keymen (eds), *Symbiotic Antagonisms* (Salt Lake City, UT: University of Utah Press, 2011), pp. xi–xxi.
Kaiser, R. J., 'Geography', in A. J. Motyl (ed.), *Encyclopedia of Nationalism*, vol. 1 (San Diego, CA: Academic Press, 2001), pp. 315–33.
Kandemir, Feridun, *Cumhuriyet Devrinde Siyasi Cinayetler* (Istanbul: Ekicigil, 1955).
Kansu, Aykut, *Revolution of 1908 in Turkey* (Leiden: Brill, 1997).
Kantorovitz, Myron, 'Alfred Grotjan as a Eugenist', *Journal of Heredity* 31 (1940), pp. 155–9.
Karahanoğulları, Onur, *Birinci Meclisin İçki Yasağı ve Men-i Müskirat Kanunu* (Ankara: Phoenix, 2008).
Karal, Enver Ziya, *Türkiye Cumhuriyeti Tarihi (1918–1960)* (Istanbul: Milli Eğitim Bakanlığı, 1960).
Karaömerlioğlu, M. Asım, 'The Village Institutes Experience in Turkey', *British Journal of Middle Eastern Studies* 25 (1998), pp. 47–73.
Karaömerlioğlu, M. Asım, 'The Peasants in Early Turkish Literature', *East European Quarterly* 36: 2 (2002), pp. 127–54.
Karaömerlioğlu, M. Asım, *Orada Bir Köy Var Uzakta, Erken Cumhuriyet Döneminde Köycü Söylem* (Istanbul: Iletisim, 2006).
[Karaosmanoğlu], Yakup Kadri, 'Hasretten Hasrete', in Yakub Kadri, Falih Rıfkı and Ruşen Eşref, *Seçme Yazılar* (Ankara: Devlet Matbaası, 1928).
Karaosmanoğlu, Yakup Kadri, *Yaban* (Istanbul: İletişim, 1998).
Karaosmanoğlu, Yakup Kadri, *Ergenkon* (Istanbul: Remzi, 1964).
Karpat, Kemal H, 'Historical Continuity and Identity Change or How to be Modern Muslim, Ottoman, and Turk', in Kemal H. Karpat (ed.), *Ottoman Past and Today's Turkey* (Leiden: Brill, 2000), pp. 1–28.
Kayalı, Hasan, *Arabs and Young Turks: Ottomanism, Arabism, and Islamism in the Ottoman Empire, 1908–1918* (Berkeley, CA: University of California Press, 1997).
Kaymaz, Nejat, 'Türk Kurtuluş Savaşının Tarihsel Konumu ve Niteliği', *Belleten* 40 (1976), pp. 599–616.
Kennedy, Foster, 'The Nature of Nervousness in Soldiers', *Journal of the American Medical Association* 71: 1 (July 1918), p. 19.
Khalidi, Rashid, 'The Arab Experience of the War', in Hugh Cecil and Peter H. Liddle (eds), *Facing Armageddon: the First World War Experienced* (London: Leo Cooper, 1996), pp. 642–55.

Killen, Andreas, *Berlin Electropolis: Shock, Nerves, and German Modernity* (Berkeley, CA: University of California Press, 2006).

Kıymaz, Ahmet, *1918–1920 Arası Romanda Milli Mücadele* (Ankara: Akçağ, 1991).

Köker, Levent, *Modernleşme, Kemalizm ve Demokrasi* (Istanbul: Iletisim, 1987).

Köknel, Özcan, *Kötü Ruhtan Ruh Sağlığına: Türkiye'de Psikiyatri Tarihi* (Istanbul: Alfa, 1998).

Koptagel-İlal, Günsel, 'Son 100 Yılda Türkiye'de Genel Çizgileriyle Psikiyatri ve Psikosomatik Hekimliğin Gelişimi', *Çerrahpaşa Tıp Fakültesi Dergisi* 12 (1981), pp. 355–72.

Köroğlu, Erol, 'Mahzendeki Geçmiş: Yakup Kadri Karaosmanoğlu'nun Romanlarında Birinci Dünya Savaşı', in Özgen Felek and Walter G. Andrews (eds), *Victoria R. Holbrook'a Armağan* (Istanbul: Kanat, 2006), pp. 39–73.

Köroğlu, Erol, *Ottoman Propoganda and Turkish Identity* (London: I. B. Tauris, 2007).

Kraut, Alan, *Goldberger's War* (New York, NY: Farrar, Straus and Giroux, 2003).

Kretschmer, Ernst, *Beden Yapısı ve Karekter* (Ankara: Maarif Vekaleti, 1942).

Kretschmer, Ernst, *(Kretschmer)' in karakter ve beden yapısı ölçüleri* (Istanbul: İstanbul Üniversitesi Yayınları, 1944).

Kutay, Cemal, *Kurtuluşun 'Kuvvacı' Din Adamları: Cumhuriyetin 75. Yılında Onlara Saygı.* (Istanbul: Aksoy, 1998).

Landau, Jacob, *Tekinalp: the Turkish Patriot, 1883–1961* (Leiden: Nederlands Historisch-Archaeologisch Instituute Istanbul, 1984).

Larcher, Maurice, *La Guerre Turque dans la Guerre Mondiale* (Paris: Berger-Levrand, 1926).

Leed, Eric J., *No Man's Land, Combat and Identity in World War I* (Cambridge: Cambridge University Press, 1979).

Lerner, David, and Richard Robinson, 'Swords and Ploughshares: the Turkish Army as a Modernizing Force', *World Politics* 13 (October 1960), pp. 19–44.

Lerner, Paul, 'Psychiatry and Casualties of War in Germany', *Journal of Contemporary History* 35 (2000), pp. 13–28.

Lerner, Paul, 'Rationalizing the Therapeutic Arsenal: German Neuropsychiatry in World War I', in Mark S. Micale and Paul Lerner (eds), *Traumatic Pasts* (Cambridge: Cambridge University Press, 2001), pp. 140–71.

Lerner, Paul, *Hysterical Men* (Ithaca, NY: Cornell University Press, 2003).

Lewis, Bernard, *The Political Language of Islam* (Chicago, IL: University of Chicago Press, 1988).

Lombroso, Caesar, *The Female Offender* (New York, NY: Appleton, 1897).

Macar, Oya Dağlar, 'Galiçya Cephesi'nde Osmanlı Birlikleri ve Sağlık Hizmetleri (1916–1917)', *Osmanlı Bilimi Araştırmaları* 10 (2009), pp. 35–58.

Mahmut Şemsi, *Harbin İstifai Tesirleri ve Zabitlerimizin, Neslimizin Islahındaki Ehemmiyetleri* (Istanbul: Askeri Matbaa, 1933).

Mahmut Şemsi, *Terbiyenin Biyolojik Temelleri* (Ankara: Çankırı Matbaası, 1934).

Maksudyan, Nazan, *Türklüğü Ölçmek: Bilimkurgusal Antropoloji ve Türk Milliyetçiliginin Irkçı Çehresi, 1925–1939* (Istanbul: Metis Yayınları, 2005).

Manson-Bahr, Philip, 'The Correlation of the Pathology and Bacteriology of Bacillary Dysentery', *Journal of the Royal Army Medical Corps* 33 (1919), pp. 117–39.

Mardin, Şerif, *Religion and Social Change in Modern Turkey* (Albany, NY: SUNY Press, 1989).

Mardin, Şerif, 'European Culture and the Development of Modern Turkey', in Ahmet Evin

and Geoffrey Dento (eds), *Turkey and the European Community* (Leske: Opladen, 1990), pp. 13–23.
Mardin, Şerif, *The Genesis of Young Ottoman Thought* (Syracuse, NY: Syracuse University Press, 2000).
Maslow, Abraham, 'A Theory of Human Motivation', *Psychological Review* 50 (1943), pp. 370–96.
McCarthy, Justin, *Muslims and Minorities: the Population of Ottoman Anatolia and the End of the Empire* (New York, NY: New York University Press, 1983).
Merridale, Catherine, 'War, Death, and Remembrance in Soviet Russia', in Jay Winter and Emmanuel Sivan (eds), *War and Remembrance in the Twentieth Century* (Cambridge: Cambridge University Press, 1999), pp. 61–83.
Merridale, Catherine, 'The Collective Mind: Trauma and Shell-shock in Twentieth-century Russia', *Journal of Contemporary History* 35 (2000), pp. 39–55.
Micale, Mark S., 'Jean-Martin Charcot and *les nèvroses traumatiques*', in Mark S. Micale and Paul Lerner (eds), *Traumatic Pasts* (Cambridge: Cambridge University Press, 2001), pp. 115–39.
Micale, Mark S., 'The Decline of Hysteria', *Harvard Mental Health Letter* 17 (2000), pp. 4–6.
Micale, Mark S., and Paul Lerner, 'Trauma, Psychiatry and History: a Conceptual and Historiographical Introduction', in Mark S. Micale and Paul Lerner (eds) *Traumatic Pasts* (Cambridge: Cambridge University Press, 2001), pp. 1–30.
Mısıroğlu, Kadir, *Kurtuluş Savaşında Sarıklı Mücahitler* (Istanbul: Sebil, 1967).
Mitchell, Timothy, 'Making the Nation: the Politics of Heritage in Egypt', in Nezar Alsayyad (ed.), *Consuming Tradition, Manufacturing Heritage* (London: Routledge, 2001), pp. 212–39.
Mitchell, Timothy, *Rule of Experts, Egypt, Techno-Politics, Modernity* (Berkeley, CA: University of California Press, 2002).
Mosse, George L., *Fallen Soldiers: Reshaping the Memory of the World Wars* (Oxford: Oxford University Press, 1990).
Mosse, George, *The Image of Man: the Creation of Modern Masculinity* (Oxford: Oxford University Press, 1996).
Mosse, George, 'Shell-shock as a Social Disease', *Journal of Contemporary History* 35 (2000), pp. 101–8.
Natter, Wolfgang, *Literature at War, 1914–1940* (New Haven, CT: Yale University Press, 1999).
Nemal, Arın, 'Jin. Ord. Prof. Dr. Wilhelm Gustav Liepmann'ın (1878–1939) İstanbul Üniversitesi'ndeki hizmet süreci ve Sosyal Jinekoloji Üzerine Düşünceleri', *Türk Aile Hekimliği Dergisi* 12 (2008), pp. 153–62.
Nesin, Aziz, *Bu Yurdu Bize Verenler*, 5th edn (Istanbul: Adam, 1988).
Neumann, Christoph K., 'Tarihin Yararı ve Zararı Olarak Türk Kimliği: Bir Akademik Deneme', in Salih Özbaran (ed.), *Tarih Öğretimi ve Ders Kitapları* (Istanbul: Tarih Vakfı, 1995), pp. 98–106.
Noyan, Abdülkadir, 'Vitaminsizlik Hastalıkları: Ordu ve Memleketimizde Durumu', *Anadolu Kliniği* 11 (1944), pp. 43–52.
O'Hanlon, Rosalind, 'Recovering the Subject: Subaltern Studies and Histories of Resistance in Colonial South Asia', *Modern Asian Studies* 22 (1988), pp. 189–224.
Oktay, Ahmet, *Cumhuriyet Dönemi Edebiyatı, 1923–1950* (Ankara: Kültür Bakanlığı, 1993).
Örs, Yaman, 'Regional Report: Psychiatry and Philosophy in Turkey – Godotian

Expectations?', *Philosophy Psychiatry and Psychology* 5 (1998), pp. 267–71.
Öz, Baki, *Kurtuluş Savaşında Alevi-Bektaşiler* (Istanbul: Can, 1995).
Özaydın, Zuhal, 'Osmanlı Hilal-i Ahmer Cemiyeti Salnamesine göre Osmanlı Hilal-i Ahmer Cemiyetinin Kuruluşu', *Tıp Tarihi Araştırmaları* 4 (1990), pp. 70–89.
Özdemir, Hikmet, *The Ottoman Army, 1914–1918* (Salt Lake City, UT: University of Utah Press, 2008).
Özel, Ahmet,*Türkiye Diyanet Vakfı İslam Ansiklopedisi* (Istanbul: Türkiye Diyanet Vakfı, 1995), s.v. 'Esir'.
Özel, Mehmet, *Cephelerden Kurtuluş Savaşı'na: İmparatorluktan Cumhuriyet'e* (Ankara: Kültür Bakanlığı, 1992).
Özer, Ahmet, *İki Kumandan: Yüzbaşı Re'fet, Binbaşı Asım* (Izmir: Işık Yayınları, 1997).
Özgiray, Ahmet, '1918–1920 Senelerinde İstanbul'un Sosyo-Ekonomik Problemleri ve Beyaz Rus Göcü', *Birinci Milli Türkoloji Kongresi, Istanbul, 6–9 February 1978* (Istanbul: Kervan, 1980), pp. 319–22.
Özgüç, Ağah, *Başlangıcından Bu Güne Türk Sinemasında İlkler* (Istanbul: Yılmaz, 1990).
Özgüç, Ağah (ed.), *80. Yılında Türk Sineması* (Ankara: T. C. Kültür Bakanlığı, 1995).
Özkırımlı, Umut, *Theories of Nationalism: a Critical Introduction* (New York, NY: St. Martin's Press, 2000).
Özkırımlı, Umut, *Contemporary Debates on Nationalism* (Basingstoke: Palgrave, 2005).
Özpekcan, Meliha, 'Büyük Millet Meclisi Tutanaklarına Göre Türkiye Cumhuriyeti'nde Sağlık Politikası', *Yeni Tıp Tarihi Araştırmaları* 7 (2001), pp. 105–61.
Öztan, G. Gürkan, 'Türkiye'de Öjeni Düşüncesi ve Kadın', *Toplum ve Bilim* 105 (2006), pp. 265–82.
Pehlivanlı, Hamit, *Kurtuluş Savaşı İstihbaratında Askeri Polis Teşkilatı* (Ankara: Genelkurmay Basımevi, 1992).
Pick, Daniel, *Faces of Degeneration: a European Disorder, c. 1848–1918* (Cambridge: Cambridge University Press, 1993).
Pick, Daniel, *War Machine: Rationalization of Slaughter in the Modern Age* (New Haven, CT: Yale University Press, 1996).
Prakash, Gyan, 'Writing Post-Orientalist Histories of the Third World: Perspectives from Indian Historiography,' *Comparative Studies in Society and History* 32 (1990), pp. 383–404.
Prakash, Gyan, 'Subaltern Studies as Postcolonial Criticism', *American Historical Review* 99 (1994), pp. 1,475–90.
Prost, Antoine, 'The Algerian War in French Collective Memory', in Jay Winter and Emmanuel Sivan (eds), *War and Remembrance in the Twentieth Century* (Cambridge: Cambridge University Press, 1999), pp. 161–76.
Quataert, Donald, *The Ottoman Empire, 1700–1922* (Cambridge: Cambridge University Press, 2000).
Rabson, S. Milton, 'Alfred Grotjahn, Founder of Social Hygiene', *Bulletin of the New York Academy of Medicine* 12 (February 1936), pp. 43–58.
Rachomimov, Alon, 'The Disruptive Comforts of Drag: (Trans) Gender Performances among Prisoners of War in Russia, 1914–1920', *American Historical Review* 111 (April 2006), pp. 362–82.
[Ran], Nazım Hikmet, *Kuvâyı Milliye: Destan* (Istanbul: Bilgi Yayinevi, 1986).
Reid, James J., *Crisis of the Ottoman Empire* (Stuttgart: Franz Steiner Verlag, 2000).
Rodriguez, Julia, *Civilizing Argentina: Science, Medicine, and the Modern State* (Chapel Hill,

NC: University of North Carolina Press, 2006).
Roudebush, Marc, 'A Battle of Nerves', in Paul Lerner and Marc Micale (eds), *Traumatic Pasts: History, Psychiatry, and Trauma in the Modern Age, 1870–1930* (Cambridge: Cambridge University Press, 2001), pp. 253–79.
Şahiner, Necmettin, *Son Şahitler Bediüzzaman Said Nursi'yi Anlatıyor* (Istanbul: Yeni Asya Yayınları, 1978).
Şapolyo, Enver B., *Türkiye Cumhuriyeti Tarihi* (Istanbul: Yeni Matbaa, 1958).
Schilcher, Linda Schatkowski, 'The Famine of 1915–1918 in Greater Syria', in John Spagnolo (ed.), *Problems of the Modern Middle East in Historical Perspective: Essays in Honour of Albert Hourani* (Oxford: Ithaca Press, 1992), pp. 229–58.
Scott, James C., *Domination and the Arts of Resistance: Hidden Transcripts* (New Haven, CT: Yale University Press, 1992).
Şener, Erman, *Kurtuluş Savaşı ve Sinemamız* (n.p.: Dizi Yayınları, 1970).
Sert, Gürkan, 'İkinci Milli Tıp Kongresinde Dr. Vefik Hüsnü (Bulat)'ın Sunduğu 'Türkiye Trahom Coğrafyası' adlı eserin Türk Tıp Tarihi Açısından Değerlendirilmesi', in *38. Uluslararası Tıp Tarihi Kongresi Bildiri Kitabi* (Ankara: Türk Tarih Kurumu, 2002), pp. 1,517–19.
Shephard, Ben, *A War of Nerves: Soldiers and Psychiatrists in the Twentieth Century* (Cambridge, MA: Harvard University Press, 2003).
Shorter, Frederic, 'Turkish Population in the Great Depression', *New Perspectives on Turkey*, 23 (2004), pp. 103–24.
Showalter, Elaine, 'Hysteria, Feminism, and Gender', in Sander Gilman (ed.), *Hysteria Beyond Freud* (Berkeley, CA: University of California Press, 1993), pp. 286–344.
Sivan, Emmanuel, 'Private Pain and Public Remembrance in Israel', in Jay Winter and Emmanuel Sivan (eds), *War and Remembrance in the Twentieth Century* (Cambridge: Cambridge University Press, 1999), pp. 177–204.
Smith, W., 'National Symbols', in A. J. Motyl (ed.), *Encyclopedia of Nationalism*, vol. 1 (San Diego: Academic Press, 2001), p. 521–30.
Somersan, Naci, 'Prenuptial Medical Examination in Turkey', *The Eugenics Review* 29 (1937–38), pp. 261–3.
Spivak, Gayatri Chakravorty, 'Can the Subaltern Speak?', in Cary Nelson and Lawrence Grossberg (eds), *Marxism and Interpretation of Culture* (London: Macmillan, 1988), pp. 271–313.
Spivak, Gayatri, 'Practical Politics of the Open End', in Martin McQuillan (ed.), *Deconstruction: a Reader* (New York: Routledge, 2000), pp. 397–404.
Stites, Richard, 'Days and Nights in Wartime Russia: Cultural Life, 1914–17', in Aviel Roshwald and Richard Stites (eds), *European Culture in the Great War* (Cambridge: Cambridge University Press, 1999), pp. 8–31.
Stone, Martin, 'Shellshock and the Psychologists', in W. F. Bynum, Roy Porter and Michael Shepherd (eds), *The Anatomy of Madness: Essays in History of Psychiatry* (London: Tavistock, 1985), pp. 242–71.
Sungur, Mehmet, *et al.*, 'Common Features of PTSD Cases Amongst a Group of Military Staff Referred From the Southeast Region of Turkey', *Journal of Cognitive Psychotherapy* 9 (1995), pp. 279–84.
Suny, Ronald G., 'Constructing Primordialism: Old Histories for New Nations', *Journal of Modern History* 73 (2001), pp. 8,562–96.
Tamari, Salim, 'With God's Camel in Siberia: the Russian Exile of an Ottoman Officer from

Jerusalem', *Jerusalem Quarterly* 35 (2008), pp. 31-50.
Tamir, Yael, *Liberal Nationalism* (Princeton, NJ: Princeton University Press, 1993).
Tansel, Fevziye, 'İstiklal Harbinin Anadolulu Mücahit Kadınları', *Türk Kültürü* 30 (1992), pp. 81-90.
Taşkıran, Cemalettin, *Ana Ben Ölmedim* (Istanbul: Türkiye İş Bankası Yayınları, 2001).
Temel, Mehmet, *İşgal Yıllarında İstanbulun Sosyal Durum* (Ankara: T. C. Kültür Bakanlığı, 1998).
Thom, Burton, 'Strain in Spirochetes', *American Journal of Syphilis* 5 (1921), pp. 9-19.
Thompson, Elizabeth, *Colonial Citizens: Republican Rights, Paternal Privileges, and Gender in French Syria and Lebanon* (New York, NY: Columbia University Press, 1999).
Toprak, Zafer, *Türkiye'de 'Milli İktisat', 1908-1918* (Ankara: Yurt Yayınları, 1982).
Toprak, Zafer, 'İstanbul'da Fuhuş ve Zührevi Hastalıklar, 1914-1933', *Tarih ve Toplum* 39 (March 1987), pp. 31-40.
Trouillot, Michel-Rolph, *Silencing the Past: Power and Production of History* (Boston: Beacon, 1995).
Turda, Marius, *Modernism and Eugenics* (New York, NY: Palgrave, 2010).
Türk Ansiklopedisi (Ankara: Maarif Matbası, 1943-84), s.v. 'Dünya Harbi, I', 'İstiklal Harbi', 'Gümüşpala, Ragıp', 'Gürsel, Cemal', 'Sunay, Cevdet'.
Uğurel-Şemin, Refia, *Ordu Alfa Testleri 'Army Alpha Tests': Alfa Testlerinin Türkçeye Adaptasyonu, Çevrilmesi ve Üniversite, Yüksek Mühendis Okulu ve Bazı Liselere Tatbiki* (Istanbul: Rıza Çoşkun Matbaası, 1943).
Uğurel-Şemin, Refia, *Stanford-Binet Ölçeğinin İstanbul Çocuklarına Uygulanması* (Istanbul: İstanbul Üniversitesi, 1987).
Ünal, Muhittin, *Kurtuluş Savaşında Çerkeslerin Rolü* (Istanbul: Cem Yayınevi, 1996).
Ünsal, Artun, 'Kayıp Kimliğin Pesinde Türkiye', in Artun Ünsal (ed.), *75 Yılda Tebaa'dan Yurttaş'a Doğru* (Istanbul: Tarih Vakfi, 1998), pp. 181-200.
Urla, Jacqueline, and Jennifer Terry, 'Introduction: Mapping Embodied Deviance', in Jacqueline Urla and Jennifer Terry (eds), *Deviant Bodies* (Bloomington, IN: Indiana University Press, 1995), pp. 1-18.
Uyar, Mesut, and Edward J. Erickson, *A Military History of the Ottomans: From Osman to Ataturk* (Santa Barbara, CA: ABC-CLIO, 2009).
Uzer, Umut, 'The Geneology of Turkish Nationalism', in Ayşe Kadıoğlu and E. Fuat Keymen (eds), *Symbiotic Antogonisms* (Salt Lake City, UT: University of Utah Press, 2011), pp. 103-32.
Varlık, Bülent M., 'Esaret Gazeteleri', *Tarih ve Toplum* 34 (July 2000), pp. 26-9, appendix.
Volkan, Vamık, *Blood Lines: From Ethnic Pride to Ethnic Terrorism* (New York, NY: Farrar, Straus and Giroux, 1997).
Walker, Alan S., *Australia in the War of 1939-1945. Series 5 – Medical: Volume 1: Clinical Problems of War* (Canberra: Australian War Memorial, 1962).
Webster Brown, Mabel, and Frankwood Williams (eds), *Neuropsychiatry and the War* (New York, NY: National Committee for Mental Hygiene, 1918).
Webster Brown, Mabel, and Frankwood Williams (eds), *Neuropsychiatry and the War – Supplement I (October 1918)* (New York, NY: National Committee for Mental Hygiene, 1918).
Weiland, Hans, and Leopold Kern, *In Feindeshand: Die Gefangenschaft im Weltkriege in*

Einzeldarstellungen (Vienna: n.p., 1931).
Weindling, Paul, 'Social Hygiene and the Birth Rate in Wartime Germany', in Richard Wall and Jay Winter (eds), *The Upheaval of War: Family, Work and Welfare in Europe, 1914–1918* (Cambridge: Cambridge University Press, 1988), pp. 417–38.
Werman, David S., 'Freud's "Narcissism of Minor Differences": a Review and Reassessment', *Journal of the American Academy of Psychoanalysis* 16 (1988), pp. 451–9.
Winter, Jay, 'Shell-shock and the Cultural History of the Great War', *Journal of Contemporary History* 35 (2000), pp. 7–11.
Winter, Jay, and Emmanuel Sivan. 'Setting the Framework', in Jay Winter and Emmanuel Sivan (eds), *War and Remembrance in the Twentieth Century* (Cambridge: Cambridge University Press, 1999), pp. 6–39.
Yalman, Mehmed Emin, *Turkey in the World War* (New Haven, CT: Yale University Press, 1931).
Yanıkdağ, Yücel, 'Ottoman Prisoners of War in Russia, 1914–22', *Journal of Contemporary History* 34 (1999), pp. 69–86.
Yanıkdağ, Yücel, 'World War I: Ottoman Empire', in Jonathan F. Vance (ed.), *Prisoners of War and Internment: a Dictionary* (Santa Barbara, CA: ABC-CLIO, 2001).
Yanıkdağ, Yücel, 'Educating the Peasants: the Ottoman Army and Enlisted Men in Uniform', *Middle Eastern Studies* (November 2004), pp. 91–107.
Yanıkdağ, Yücel, 'Mısır'daki Osmanlı Esirlerinde Görülen Pelagra Hastalığı: I. Dünya Savaşında Tibbi Oryantalizm ve İngiliz Doktorlar', *Toplumsal Tarih* 153 (September 2006), pp. 26–33.
Yanıkdağ, Yücel, 'From Cowardice to Illness: Diagnosing Malingering in the Ottoman Great War', *Middle Eastern Studies* 48 (March 2012), pp. 205–25.
Yeni Türk Ansiklopedisi (Istanbul: Ötüken Yayınevi, 1985), s.v. 'Birinci Dünya Savaşı', 'Milli Mücadele'.
Yerkes, Robert M., 'Psychological Examining in the United States Army', *Memoirs of the National Academy of Sciences* 15 (1921), pp. 1–890.
Yergök, Ziya, *Tuğgeneral Ziya Yergök'ün Anıları: Sarıkamış'tan Esarete (1915–1920)*, trans. Sami Önal (Istanbul: Remzi, 2005).
Yıldız, Ahmet, *Ne Mutlu Türküm Diyebilene* (Istanbul: İletişim, 2001).
Yılmaz, Faruk, *Kurtuluş Savaşı ve Sonrasında Niğde* (Niğde: n.p., 1998).
Young, Allan, 'W. H. R. Rivers and the War Neurosis', *Journal of the History of Behavioral Sciences* 35 (1999), pp. 359–78.
Yurtsever, Cezmi, *Gözlerim Eyvah. Mısır'daki Esir Kamplarında Gözleri Kör edilen 15 Bin Türk Askerinin Belgesel Hikayesi* (Istanbul: Yeni Zamanlar Dagitim, 2009).
Žižek, Slavoj, 'Eastern Europe's Republics of Gilead', *New Left Review* (September–October 1990), pp. 50–62.
Žižek, Slavoj, *Tarrying with the Negative* (Durham, NC: Duke University Press, 1993).
Zürcher, Erik J., *The Unionist Factor: the Role of the Committee of Union and Progress in the Turkish National Movement, 1905–1926* (Leiden: Brill, 1984).
Zürcher, Erik Jan, *Turkey: a Modern History* (New York, NY: I. B. Tauris, 1994).
Zürcher, Erik Jan, 'Between and Death and Desertion: the Experience of the Ottoman Soldier in World War I', *Turcica* 28 (1996), pp. 235–58.
Zürcher, Erik Jan, 'Little Mehmed in the Desert: the Ottoman Soldier's Experience', in Hugh Cecil and Peter Liddle (eds), *Facing Armageddon: the First World War Experienced*

(London: Leo Cooper, 1996), pp. 230–41.
Zürcher, Erik Jan, 'The Ottoman Conscription System, 1844–1914', *International Review of Social History* 43 (1998), pp. 437–49.
Zürcher, Erik Jan, 'Young Turks, Ottoman Muslims and Turkish Nationalists: Identity Politics, 1908-1938', in Kemal H. Karpat (ed.), *Ottoman Past and Today's Turkey* (Leiden: Brill, 2000), pp. 150–79.
Zürcher, Erik Jan, 'Birinci Dünya Savaşında Amele Taburları', in Erik Jan Zürcher (ed.), *Savaş, Devrim ve Uluslaşma* (Istanbul: Bilgi, 2009), pp. 201–14.

UNPUBLISHED SECONDARY SOURCES

Arıkan, Mustafa, 'Asker Mektupları', MA thesis, Selçuk Üniversitesi, 1986.
Aybers, Orhan, 'What did the Governmental Apparatus Comprehend from a Healthy Society during the 1930s in Turkey', PhD dissertation, Middle East Technical University, 2003.
Eskicumalı, Ahmet, 'Ideology and Education: Reconstructing the Turkish Curriculum for Social and Cultural Change, 1923–1946', PhD dissertation, University of Wisconsin, 1994.
Güven, Esin, 'I. Dünya Savaşı'dan Rusya'daki Türk Esirleri ve Rusya Türkleri', MA thesis, Marmara University, 1996.
Güvenç-Salgırlı, Sanem, 'Eugenics as Science of the Social: a Case from 1930s Istanbul', PhD dissertation, Binghamton University, 2009.
Karaömerlioğlu, Asım M., 'The Cult of the Peasant: Ideology and Practice, Turkey, 1930–1946', PhD dissertation, Ohio State University, 1999.
Koçak, Filiz, 'Türkiye'de Sağlık Politikası'nın Gelişimi, 1850–1950', PhD dissertation, Yıldız Teknik University, 1995.
Köroğlu, Erol, 'Tarih, İdeoloji ve Popüler Roman: Burhan Cahit Morkaya ve Yüzbaşı Celâl', Boğaziçi University Institute of Modern Turkish History, 5 November 1999.
Köroğlu, Erol, 'Retorik Bir Araç Olarak Tarih: Birinci Dünya Savaşının Modern Türk Edebiyatında Ele Alınışı', Orient-Institut Der Deutschen Morgenlandischen Gesellschaft Abteilung Istanbul, 17 May 2000.
Kutlu, Cemil, 'I. Dünya Savaşında Rusyadaki Türk Savaş Esirleri ve Bunların Yurda Döndürülmeleri Faaliyetleri', PhD dissertation, Atatürk University, 1997.
Lerner, Paul, 'Hysterical Men: War, Neurosis and German Mental Medicine, 1914–1921'. PhD dissertation, Columbia University, 1996.
Mehmed Feyyaz Efendi, '*Hatırat*' (1919), unpublished manuscript.
Oğuz, N. Yasemin, 'Cumhuriyet dönemi Türk Psikiyatrisine evrimsel bir bakış', paper presented at the Fourth Turkish Congress of the History of Medicine, Istanbul, 18–20 September 1996.
Yanıkdağ, Yücel, '"Ill-Fated Sons" of the Nation: Ottoman Prisoners of War in Russia and Egypt, 1914–1922', PhD dissertation, Ohio State University, 2002.
Yanıkdağ, Yücel, 'When Cowardice Became Sickness: the Changing Medical Discourse of Malingering in the Ottoman Great War and Beyond', paper delivered at Princeton University, Near Eastern Studies, Brown Bag Talk, 6 April 2009.

INDEX

A. Rıza
  on pellagra, 122, 155, 164n15, 165n25
Adana, and trachoma, 148, 150
Adıyaman, and trachoma, 147, 150
Akçura, Yusuf, 20, 45n98, 112n11
Aksakal, Mustafa, 15
Aksiyon, 161–2
alcohol
  and degeneracy, 213, 221, 228, 235
  prohibition of, 237
Alevi, 81
Allenby, Edmund, General, 121, 164n8
Anatolia
  diseases in, 3, 10, 119, 147, 155, 230
  effect of wars, 214, 224, 260
  efforts to uplift, 91, 95
  invasion of, 107, 225
  poverty of, 59, 89
  trachoma in, 147–9, 153, 155, 159
  as war zone, 2, 9, 16, 21
Anderson, Benedict, 7, 8
Antalya, and trachoma, 148, 150
Appadurai, Arjun, 150
Arab rebellion *see* Arab revolt
Arab
  Ottomans in military, 17, 151, 199, 200, 207n139, 224
  and Turkish conflicts, 53–60
Arab revolt, 53, 58–9, 74n41

al-Aref, Aref, 31
Armenian
  deportations of, 224, 255
  doctors in military, 178
  doctors in prison camps, 57, 142, 161–3
  recruits, 17, 74n29, 196
  refugees in Egypt, 197, 207n122, 207n124
Asia
  peoples and religions of, 86–7, 107–9
  Turkey as leader of, 108–9
Atatürk, Mustafa Kemal
  and blind prisoner of war, 142
  death and illness of, 11n5, 39n3, 248n136
  and Gallipoli campaign, 257, 259
  and military service, 142, 262
  and sports, 265
  and War of Independence, 271n62
auto-suggestion (imitation), 175
Ayberk, Nuri Fehmi, and trachoma, 151, 152, 160
Aydemir, Şevket Süreyya, 81, 112n11, 113n47, 183, 206n119

Babinski, Joseph, 172, 175, 181, 186
Bakırköy mental institution, 2, 194, 195–6, 206n116, 237

295

Balkan Wars, 14–15, 79, 214
  prisoners of war in, 15, 269n14, 252
  and 'Ten-Year War', 254
barbed wire disease, 192, 195
Binet-Simon testing, 236, 247n132
Birol, Ali Esat
  and eugenics, 238
  military service, 265–6
  operations on soldiers, 265–6
birth control, 230, 234, 248n143; *see also* fertility
birth rate, 224, 225; *see also* fertility
Bolshevik Revolution *see* Russian Revolutions
British, image of, 51–3
[Bulat], Vefik Hüsnü, 149
Bulgaria
  advancement of, 93–4, 225
  and Balkan Wars, 14–15, 252
  in Egypt, Bulgarian nationals, 132, 134, 140
  and Great War, 16
bureaucrats *see* civil servants
buried alive neurosis, 185–6, 204n68–9
Burma, prisoners in, 18, 40n28, 112n11, 119, 137, 166n57

camptocormie, 178; *see also* Grabetyan, Yahoub
captivity *see* prison camps and prisoners of war
casualties, Great War *see* Great War
casualties, War of Independence *see* War of Independence
Çelik, Osman Şerafeddin, 155, 231
census, of 1927, 224–5, 262
Central Asia
  peoples of, 38, 45n93, 104, 105–6
  and Turks, 117n106, 213
Charcot, Jean-Martin, 172–4, 175, 198
Charles Beard, 173
Chatterjee, Partha, 7–8, 79, 159
CHP *see* Republican People's Party
Christian minorities *see* non-Muslims and *reaya*
cinema
  in prison camps, 31

  in Turkey, 271n62
civil servants, 82, 100, 110, 116n91
  and positive eugenics, 234
civilisation
  absence of, among peasants, 80, 90, 95, 98
  and degeneracy, 211, 241
  and disease, 120, 150, 151, 153, 157, 159, 241
  doctors as propagandist of, 222–3
Committee of Union and Progress (CUP)
  and concept of the people, 79, 98, 115n78
  and ideology, 78–9, 98, 101, 111n8
  and Islam, 79
creosol
  and blindness of prisoners, 161–3
  as delousing agent, 141–4

Dağlarca, Fazıl Hüsnü, 147
degeneracy
  and alcohol, 235
  and atavism, 217
  of Turks, 208–9, 213–14, 223–4, 262–3
degenerates
  extinction and sterility of, 210, 211, 218
  infection, source of, 218
  institutionalisation of, considered, 219
  procreation of, 218, 219, 226, 230
  surviving the war, 171, 189–90, 217, 219, 222, 227
  in Turkey, estimated number of, 219, 246n108, 262
degeneration
  definition, evolving, 210–11
  dementia praecox, 210, 213
  individual, 209–10, 211
  and law of progressivity, 209, 212–13
  levels of, 190, 215
  and modernity, 211, 241
  physical, 214
  threat of, 210, 218
delousing, 142–4; *see also* creosol
dementia praecox, 3, 182, 184–5, 213; *see also* schizophrenia
diathèse, constitutional disposition, 174, 202n13

disease carries *see* prisoners of war
doctors, generalists, 158, 159, 184
 criticism of, 188, 220
Durkheim, Émile, 99, 211
Düşünsel, Feridun Fikri, 96, 115n76
dysentery, 3, 17, 119, 123, 130, 131, 155, 165n39, 166n60
dysgenic, 226, 227, 228, 233, 235, 241, 242, 245n82, 262
 in Turkey, estimated number of, 231
 see also eugenics

Eason, H. L., 140–1, 144–5
education
 importance of, 89–96, 102
 early Turkish republic, 257, 259
electrotherapy, 176, 187
epilepsy, 183, 189, 209, 211
Ergenekon (place), 104–5, 117n104
Erickson, Edward, 16, 18, 19
Erkilet, Hüseyin Hüsnü, 17
eugenics
 defined, 227, 245n80
 and dysgenics, 226, 227, 228, 233, 235, 241, 242, 245n82, 262
 Germany, 227–8, 229, 231, 247n123
 and hereditary diseases, 5, 230, 231, 232, 238, 239
 and hereditary disposition, 176, 186, 228
 and internment (institutionalisation), 219, 231
 and marriage, 227–8
 negative, 227, 237–41
 positive, 227, 232
 and reproduction control, 228–9
 scholarship on, 246n110
 and Second World War, 237, 247n135
 and sterilisation, 230, 248n143
 United States *see* United States
 and war, 223, 227, 237, 272n82
 and women, 228, 229, 248n146
European prisoners of war, 65–6, 68, 123, 136–7, 140
Eyüb Sabri Bey, 142, 145, 162–3

Faik [Kaltakkıran], 141, 154

fertility, 224, 225, 230, 233–4, 247n145
films *see* cinema
First World War *see* Great War
Foucault, Michel, 248n150
 and bio-politics, 12n16, 266, 268
funeral, 50–1, 69

Galicia front, 18, 40n20
Gallipoli, 18, 60, 167n91, 173, 178, 179, 180, 182–3, 186, 253
 in nationalist historiography, 257, 259
Garabetyan, Yahcub, 178, 203n31
Gaupp, Robert, 176, 201n3, 215, 229
gaye (aim), 96, 98–100, 109, 110, 267
general paresis, 156–58
Germany
 émigré scientists from, 239
 alliance with Ottomans *see* Ottoman Empire
 psychiatry, 172, 174–7
Göçek, Fatma Müge, 254
Gökalp, Ziya
 on degeneration, 211–12
 and development of society, historical, 113n30
 in Malta, 115n84
 mefkure, 99, 211–12
 on national culture, 96, 111n10, 113n35, 115n78, 211–12
 and populism, 115n78
Gökay, Fahrettin Kerim
 on (constitutional) body types in Turkey, 216–17
 on eugenics, 228–9, 239, 246n110
 on hysteria, 186
 and Kretschmer, 216
 on marriage, 233
 on mental testing of students, 236
 as public figure, 235–6, 240, 248n149
 on recruitment, 221
 on schizophrenia, 243n18
 on sterilisation, 228, 229, 239, 248n143
 on Turkish soldiers, 263
 on women, 233
government (state)
 Ottoman, as enemy of Turkish people
 under Ottomans, 89, 100, 110

Grand National Assembly
  and prisoners of war, 41–2, 144, 154, 237, 251
  and Village Institutes, 96, 115n76
Great War
  casualties, 19–20
  demographic impact, 218, 224, 260
  economic effects, 260
  and nationalist historiography, 254–9, 261
  Ottoman entry into, 15–16
  psychiatric problem estimates, 178–9
  responsibility for entering, 255–6
Greece
  invasion of western Anatolia, 2, 84, 85, 91, 107, 224, 256
Greeks, Anatolian, 58, 158, 213
Grotjahn, Alfred, 188, 219, 235
Gülhane, 238
Gümüşpala, Ragıp, 249–50
Gürsel, Cemal, 250

Hanioğlu, Şükrü, 111n6, 111n8
Harb Mecmuası, 185
Haydarpaşa Hospital, 185
heredity, 212–13
hierarchical order, social
  class system, as imagined, 94
  educational difference, 82, 226
Hikmet, Nazım *see* Ran, Nazım Hikmet
Hüseyin Kenan
  on degeneracy, 212–13, 247n148
  on eugenics, 231
  on hysteria, 204n72
  on psychopaths, 180–1
hygiene, 25, 90, 120, 149, 151, 153, 218, 235, 236, 249
hysteria
  defined, 173, 175
  as fear reaction, 174, 181, 186
  male, 173–4
  among Ottoman troops, 178, 180, 181–2, 183–4
  symptoms, 173
  see also malingering

identity
  banal aspects, 4, 47, 70
  construction, 110, 258
  cultural, 8, 78
  and identification, 12n17, 46, 54, 55,72
imperialism
  European, as threat to Islam, 107–8
  European, as threat to Ottoman Empire, 85
İnan, Afet, 262
India, 102, 119, 137, 155, 166n57, 194, 195
industrialisation, 15, 16, 85, 98, 116n91, 157
industrialised war, 178, 180, 181, 263
İnönü, İsmet, 237
Islam, 54–5, 59, 65, 68–70, 78–9, 80, 103–5
  and Arabs, 54–5, 59
  and folk beliefs, 113n38
  misinterpreted, 86–8, 113n38
  and modernisation, 85
  and progress, 87–8
  reform of, proposed, 86–8
  and Turks, as defenders of, 54–5, 59
Islamic modernism, 78, 111n2, 113n43, 116n92
Istanbul
  Allied occupation, 1, 115n84, 140, 141,158, 193, 224, 260
  buildings and locations, Bakırköy, 2, 194, 195–6, 206n116, 237
  buildings and locations, Toptaşı, 195–6, 237
  repatriation to, 1–2
  residents of, as exempt from military service, 223
  war and post-war conditions, 2, 260
Italy, war neurotics, 179
Izmir
  Greek invasion of, 2, 84, 91
  prisoners' concern for, 91
  repatriation to, 140

Jerusalem, 31, 140, 144, 196
jihad, 104
  against ignorance, 98, 109

Karaosmanoğlu, Yakub Kadri, 258–9, 261
Kaufmann machine, 176, 187–8; *see also* electrotherapy
Kayalı, Hasan, 111n8
Kemal, Mustafa *see* Atatürk, Mustafa Kemal
Köroğlu, Erol, 258, 269n30, 271n56
Kraepelin, Emil, 172
   on degeneration, 156, 198–9
   on dementia praecox, 210
   eugenics, 245n93
   on war neurosis, 217
Krafft-Ebing, Richard von, 156
Kretschmer, Ernest, 195, 215–16
   and constitution and body types, 215–16, 243n35
Kurds, 17, 111n8, 207n139, 224

LaPaix (Şişli) Hospital, 176, 185, 202n21, 214
Law on Hygiene, 153, 232–3, 246n114
Lawrence, T. E., 59
Le Bon, Gustave, 78, 211
literacy
   expansion of, 90–1, 93, 94–5
   and illiteracy, 93, 193, 271n62
   soldiers, among, 11n11, 104, 253–4
Lombroso, Caesar, 229, 235, 243n37

madrasa, 88, 207n139; *see also* village school
Mahmut Şemsi
   on deaths of educated classes (*münevver*), 226
   and eugenics, 234
malaria, 119, 131, 144, 147, 153, 160
malingering, 181, 188–90, 197, 199–200
   and hysteria, 174, 175, 176, 181–2, 186–7, 188
Malta, 115n84, 154, 206n108
Manuelyan, Bağdasar, 231, 245n75
marriage
   arranged, 228, 234
   as compulsory, 232, 246n113
   as fruitful with children, 233–4
   neuro-psychiatrists' views on, 227, 232, 246n112
   as stately matter, 227–8, 232, 234
'Marriage Day', 224–5

Marriage Hygiene Law, 232–3, 246n114
Maudsley, Henry, 211, 217, 218
Mazhar Osman
   on castration, 230
   on degeneracy, 177–8, 213–14, 218, 220–2
   on eugenics, 228–9
   on hysteria, 188
   on malingering, 188, 254, 263
   marriage hygiene law, 232–3
   military nation, 222, 264
   on military service, 244n51, 264
   on procreation, 247n121
   on psychopathy, 217–18, 219–21
   as public figure, 236, 240, 247n127
   on sports, 264–5
   on sterilisation, 238
   on war neurosis, absence of, 180
   on wars' effects, 223, 225, 264
   on willpower, 218
   on women, 229, 245n94
medical examination of recruits, 197, 219–21, 265
medical Orientalism *see* Orientalism, medical
mefkure, 98–9, 211–12
Mehmet Şeref Bey, 141, 154
Mental Hygiene Society, 235–6
military
   casualties, 18–19
   conscription, 16–18, 262, 266
   conscription 'exemptions', 207n139, 223, 226
   conscription, reforms suggested for, 220–1
   desertion, 82, 190, 200, 269n18
   ethnic make-up of, 17
   food shortages, 16, 21, 124, 132–3, 135
   labour battalions, 17
   losses to disease, 17
   mobilisation, 15–16
   nation, as reflection of, 208–9, 210
   and non-Muslims, 17, 18, 19, 117n102, 199, 207n139, 223
   officers and officer candidates, 16
   service and insanity, 197
   strength, 18
   see also military service

military coup, 1960, 249–50
'military nation', 222, 254, 262–3, 264
'military selection', 223–4, 226, 245n75
military service
    degenerative and demographic effect of, 223–4, 264
    eugenic qualities of, 264–5
    and mental health, 197, 220–1
    Turks, as falling on, 207n139, 223–4
Millet-i Müsellaha see 'military nation'
Morel, Benedict-Augustin
    and degeneracy, 177, 209, 217, 243n37
münevver class, 226, 230, 234
Munich Conference, 1916, 174–7
music, 102–4
Mustafa Hayrullah, 175
    on disposition to mental illness, 212
    on hysteria, 186
    on neurasthenia, 212

national extinction, 84–5
national health, 208–9
National Struggle, 224; *see also* War of Independence
nationalism, 70
    'anti-colonial', 7, 79–80, 159, 256
    Arab, 55–6, 57–9
    belatedness of, among Ottomans, 85–6
    scholarship on, 7–8, 12n17
Nazım Hikmet *see* Ran, Nazım Hikmet
Nazım Şakir
    on degeneracy, 214–15, 216
    and electrotherapy, 187–8
    and hysterics and war neurotics, 182, 183, 184, 214
    lethargic encephalitis, 119, 163n2
    on malingering, 188–9, 199–200, 263
    on mistreatment of hysterics, 181, 187–8
neurasthenia
    causes of, 173
    and class, 173, 184
    defined, 173
    and degeneracy, 212
    and modernity, 173
    and Ottoman soldiers, 180, 181, 183–4, 185, 208
    and schizophrenia connection, 184
    symptoms, 173
    and will power, 211–12
night blindness, 139–40
non-Muslims *see* military, non-Muslims and *reaya*
Noyan, Abdülkadir 122, 155, 158, 237–8

ophthalmia, 140–5
Oppenheim, Hermann, 172, 174, 175–6
Orfanidis, Emil, 231
Orientalism, medical, 154, 156–7, 159, 161
Ottoman Empire
    alliance with Germany, 15
    declaration of war, 15
    and the Great War, 14–20
    as multi-ethic empire, 6, 17, 116n95, 199

Palestine front, 18, 21, 39, 74n29, 123, 124, 132, 133, 135, 196
    and trachoma, 140, 144, 148, 155
peasants
    and agriculture, 90, 95, 96
    education of, in camps, 89–93
    and identity, 80–1
    and ignorance, 80–4, 86, 88–9, 95
    malingering as trait among, 189
    as outside of the nation, 83–4
    'pathological' behaviour of, 82–3
    and religion, 80–1, 113n38
    as soldiers, 17, 80–3
    uplifting of, after the war, 89, 95–6
pellagra
    casualties, 121–3, 124, 125–6
    causation (aetiology), 120–1
    commissions establishment of, 121
    defined, 120
    and diet factor, 132–9, 155, 161
    endemicity, 124–5
    and Germans, 136–7, 140
    and inter-current diseases, 123, 130–1
    symptoms, 120, 127–8
    as wasting disease, 128–9, 135
pension neurosis (Germany), 174, 177, 178
pithiatism, 175; *see also* Babinski, Joseph
population, effects of Great War *see* Great War
population fears, 225, 233

population of Turkish Republic *see* census
prison camp
  conditions, Egypt, 26, 28–9, 30–1, 33
  conditions, Russia, 23–25, 29, 30–1, 33–2
  food, Egypt, 29, 34, 42n55, 43n65, 132–5, 137, 166n60, 167n75–6
  food, Russia, 26–9, 33, 35, 56–7
  housing, 23, 25, 26, 33
  labour, 128, 132, 137–8; *see also* prisoners of war, labour for Russian families
  mental problems manifested in, 191–4
  schools, 89–93, 95
prisoners of war
  activities, 30–4
  as disease carriers, 3, 119, 148, 159, 261
  diseases among, 130–1
  escapes, 2, 37–9, 44n89, 44n92, 45n93, 45n94, 45n97, 75n48, 76n72, 112n11, 196, 207n122, 269n18
  ethnic make-up of, 17
  ethnic relations among, 53–60
  European, 4, 25, 26, 30, 31, 34, 65, 66–7, 70, 71, 133, 136
  funeral of, 69
  homoeroticism, among, 65–6, 67
  international aid for, 34, 39, 45n98, 61, 75n52
  inter-rank relations among, 60–2
  labour for Russian families, 30, 50, 68, 73n15
  numbers of, 19–20
  policing of each other's behaviour, 63–72
  repatriation of, 2, 226, 260–1
  shame, 251–2, 254
  transportation of, 21–3; *see also teplushki*
procreation
  incentives for, 233–4
  as patriotic duty, 234–5; *see also* marriage
prostitution, 158, 210, 229; *see also* syphilis
psychiatry
  heredity, views on, 177, 200, 212, 235
  influence of, 237
  and military doctors, 219
  and modernity and civilisation, 153, 222–3, 241

  and neurology, 201n1
  and state, 222–3
psycho-neurosis, 131, 184
psychopathy, 188, 198–9, 209, 217, 219, 233, 241, 246n108, 267
  and hysteria, 217

race as ethnicity, 105, 213–14
RAMC, 122, 126–7
Ran, Nazım Hikmet, 255–6, 260
reaya, 89, 110, 114n48
religion
  and Europeans, 86
  and Germans, 68
  practice of, in captivity, 68, 193–4
  and Russians, 50, 68
Republican People's Party, 35, 240, 250
Russia
  Ottoman image of, 47–51, 52–3
  peasants, 29, 48, 49, 83
  women, 22, 41n31, 49–51, 68–9, 76n72
Russian revolutions, 27, 33, 61, 65

Şadan, İzzeddin
  on atavism, 217–18
  on degeneracy, 217
  on psychopathy, 217
Said Nursi, 250
Saydam, Refik, 149–50, 236–7
schizophrenia
  and degeneracy, 184–6, 198, 199, 206n117, 208–10, 213, 228, 233
  and dementia praecox, 184
  development of, 197–8
  and marriage, 233
  and prisoners of war, 3, 194, 195, 226, 241
  and sex, 198
  and sterilisation, 238
  symptoms, 182
schools, religious *see* village schools
Second National Medical Congress, 149
Second World War, 11n5, 180, 189, 237, 248n135, 252
self-criticism
  as Muslims, 85–8
  as Ottomans, 82–5

Seventh Turkish National Congress of Medicine, 11n5, 237, 238, 248n136, 265–6
Sevres Treaty, 85, 112n23
shell shock, 172–3, 201n8; *see also* war neurosis and hysteria
Shorter, Frederic, 247–8n135, 248n143
Sinai front, 124, 132, 135
Şişli Hospital *see* La Paix (Şişli) Hospital
social Darwinism, 78, 201
social-demographic engineering, 209, 232–41, 268
social hygiene, 219
Spain, 41n36, 159
sports
  Mazhar Osman on, 264–5
  militarisation of, 264–5
  Mustafa Kemal Atatürk on, 265
  prison camps, 31, 33
sterilisation *see* women
suicide
  and degeneration, 235
  rates, 260
Şükrü Hazım *see* Tiner, Şükrü Hazım
Sunay, Cevdet, 250
syphilis
  in Anatolia, 147
  and civilisation, 156–8
  and degeneration, 213, 229
  and eugenics, 229–30, 232, 246n114
  and Marriage Hygiene Law, 246n114
  and prisoners of war, 130
  and war, 230

TBMM *see* Grand National Assembly
'talking cure', 176, 188
Tanzimat, 78
tavuk karası see night blindness
teplushki, 22–3, 25, 41n34, 191–2
Tevfik Rüşdü
  on devastation of Anatolia, 225
Tiner, Şükrü Hazım
  and Alpha testing, 266
  and degenerates, 226
  and degeneration, 219, 246n108
  and dementia praecox, 185–6
  and eugenics, 171

hysteria, 181–2, 186–8
pellagra and trachoma, 120
theatre
  in Egyptian camps, 30–1, 91
  in Russian camps, 30–1, 60, 66–7
Toptaşı *Bimarhanesi*, 195, 196, 237
trachoma
  causation, 141
  diffusion worldwide, 152–3, 159–60
  and ethnic groups, 151
  infection rates, 146–7, 150
  in Ottoman Anatolia, 146–7, 152
  and Ottoman troops, 140–1, 144, 148
  and poverty, 149, 151
  and prisoners of war, 145–6, 148
  and republican Anatolia, 147, 149
  Struggle Against, 149–53
  and village dispensaries, 150, 151, 152
Traitement brusque, 175; *see also* electrotherapy and Nazım Şakir
tuberculosis, 3, 14, 123, 130, 131, 147, 233, 153
Turan, 105–6
Turkish History Thesis, 262
Turkish language, 95–6, 106
typhus, 17, 24, 42n43, 163n4, 260

ümera
  in Egypt, 61–2
  in Russia, 60–1, 62
United States
  diplomats in Egypt, 39
  diplomats in Russia, 22, 24, 42n56, 193
  eugenics in, 227, 231, 239
  medical mission in Turkey, 148
  missionaries, 214
  soldiers, 221, 266
Uyar, Mesut, 116

Village Institutes, 96–8, 115n73–4, n76
village schools, 88, 91, 93

war neurosis
  causes, 174–6
  and European soldiers, 178–9
  and Ottoman troops, 178, 179, 181
  and prisoners of war, 175–6, 181

symptoms, 172
and trench warfare as causative factor, 178
War of Independence, 218, 222, 224, 254–9, 261, 272n64
  casualties, 257, 270n42
  in film, 271n62
  foundation of nation-state, 257–8
  myth of, 256, 257, 259, 261
  and repatriated prisoners, 250–1, 253
  women, 258
War of Liberation *see* War of Independence
war profiteering, 56–7, 97, 260
war rich *see* war profiteering
war volunteers, 197

will power, 176, 181, 187–8, 189–90, 211–12, 218
women
  and 1927 census, 224
  and crime, 229
  and marriage, 228, 230
  Ottoman Empire, 98, 115n77
  Russia *see* Russia, women
  and sex, 229, 245n94
  sterilisation, 230, 238–9, 248n146

Young Ottomans, 78

Žižek, Slavoj, 8, 12n17, 110
Zürcher, Erik Jan, 111n8

EU representative:
Easy Access System Europe
Mustamäe tee 50, 10621 Tallinn, Estonia
Gpsr.requests@easproject.com

www.ingramcontent.com/pod-product-compliance
Lightning Source LLC
Chambersburg PA
CBHW052149300426
44115CB00011B/1590